Stroke Management in Vietnam

Anthony Rudd • Thanh Ngoc Le
Ngoc Huy Nguyen
Editors

Stroke Management in Vietnam

Key Considerations for the Implementation of Healthcare Services

Springer

Editors
Anthony Rudd
King's College London
London, UK

Thanh Ngoc Le
VNU University of Medicine and Pharmacy
Cau Giay District, Hanoi, Vietnam

Ngoc Huy Nguyen
Phu Tho Department of Health
Viet Tri City, Phutho province, Vietnam

ISBN 978-981-96-0220-9 ISBN 978-981-96-0221-6 (eBook)
https://doi.org/10.1007/978-981-96-0221-6

This Springer imprint is published by the registered company Springer Nature Singapore Pte Ltd.
The registered company address is: 152 Beach Road, #21-01/04 Gateway East, Singapore 189721, Singapore

Preface

I am delighted to have edited this book, which is the first to be published on stroke in Vietnam. Stroke is the top cause of death in Vietnam and the most important cause of acquired disability, while published data of stroke has been limited. While it is a disease that often affects older people not infrequently, it affects younger people and children. Vietnam has a rapidly developing economy, and while that brings improving living standards for the population, unfortunately it also brings with it an increasing susceptibility to disease of high-economy countries such as hypertension and diabetes mellitus, the presence of which greatly increases the risk of someone developing a stroke. It is vital that Vietnam develops its health service to both improve stroke prevention and to deliver high-quality acute stroke care and rehabilitation. This book has been a collaboration between many colleagues in Vietnam as well as friends and colleagues from the UK. We hope that we can continue to work together to both improve stroke care in both of our countries and to foster good research that crosses international frontiers.

This is an important book, being the first to specifically address the huge problem of stroke in Vietnam and providing information for health care planners, physicians, nurses and therapists. Stroke is already one of the most important health care issues for the country, and with changing demographics is likely to become even more of a problem. Our population is ageing and this will increase the prevalence of the disease, and we are increasingly adopting 'Western' lifestyle habits which may also increase the incidence. But, as the book points out, the majority of stroke is preventable through changes in diet, exercise and management of problems such as hypertension. And stroke once it happens is also treatable, providing we manage patients quickly and effectively. I hope this book stimulates interest in the disease and that we can attract the brightest clinicians to specialise in the disease, and especially to conduct research so that future generations of Vietnamese people do not have to suffer from what can be a terrible disease for both the patient and their family.

Worldwide, stroke is one of the leading causes of death and disability causing huge suffering to patients and families as well as being a major economic burden in all countries. It is estimated that over three quarters of all strokes are preventable through effective primary prevention of hypertension, type 2 diabetes mellitus, obesity and other risk factors. And while until recently it was often seen as an untreatable condition, developments over the past 30 years have meant that many people who have stroke can now be treated acutely to completely reverse the effects of the stroke. And even for those people who do suffer disability, well-organised nursing and rehabilitation can enable them to return to a good quality of life. But for these treatments to be effective, there needs to be a well-organised and well-funded health service delivering prevention, acute treatment and rehabilitation.

This book summarises the key research and developments in stroke care. Much of the evidence comes from Europe and the United States, but the fact is that in most respects a stroke patient in Europe has much the same needs as a stroke patient in Vietnam or anywhere else. This book can be the first book of stroke written in English in medical universities in Vietnam for medical students, master students and PhD students.

We hope that the contents of this book stimulates students and qualified health professionals to see how important stroke is as a disease and how exciting and satisfying working with stroke patients can be. We also hope that health managers and political leaders also see that investing in effective stroke care is an important investment that pays enormous rewards for patients, families and society as a whole.

Ngoc Huy Nguyen
Phutho Department of Health
Phutho, Vietnam

VNU University of Medicine and Pharmacy
Hanoi, Vietnam

Thanh Ngoc Le
VNU University of Medicine and Pharmacy
Hanoi, Vietnam

Anthony Rudd
King'College London, London, UK

Contents

Chapter 1
Epidemiology of Stroke in Vietnam

Ngoc Huy Nguyen, Anthony Rudd, and Thong Van Nguyen

1.1 Introduction

Stroke is a significant public health concern in Vietnam due to a high incidence and prevalence of death and disability in the population. Since early 2008 in Vietnam, cerebrovascular diseases have been a major concern by both the Vietnam Association of Cardiology and the Vietnam Association of Neurology. The Vietnam Association of Stroke was established in 2008 in collaboration with the Vietnam Association of Neurology and support from World Stroke Organization (WSO). Since then, stroke has been a priority area for many hospitals and clinicians. The first stroke education program in Vietnam ran from 2008 to 2011, when 8596 doctors were trained and received the certificate signed by the WSO and the Vietnam Ministry of Health. Scientific Conferences on stroke in Vietnam are organized annually for stroke scientists and doctors and abstracts are published in the Vietnamese edition of the International Journal of Stroke. Studies on stroke epidemiology in Vietnam have been limited. This chapter reviews these studies identifying the most important issues relevant to clinicians, health administrators, and politicians.

N. H. Nguyen (✉)
Phutho Department of Health, Phutho, Vietnam

VNU University of Medicine and Pharmacy, Hanoi, Vietnam
e-mail: ngochuynguyen8888@gmail.com

A. Rudd
King's College, London, UK

T. Van Nguyen
Vietnam Stroke Association, Hanoi, Vietnam

Stroke Center, Phutho General Hospital, Phutho, Vietnam

A. Rudd et al. (eds.), *Stroke Management in Vietnam*,
https://doi.org/10.1007/978-981-96-0221-6_1

1.2 Stroke Incidence and Prevalence

Data of stroke incidence and prevalence in Vietnam is limited. There are no studies that focus on the incidence and prevalence of stroke in whole country's population. Cong NH firstly published in 1995 that the incidence and prevalence in Southern Vietnam was 161 and 415 per 100,000 people, respectively [1]. Another study by Le VT, Le TL, Nguyen TH et al., in 1999 on stroke in South Vietnam showed that stroke prevalence was 6.08 per 1000 inhabitants in three different regions of southern Vietnam (one site in a Hô Chi Minh City and two rural areas in the Tiên Giang and Kiên Giang provinces) and prevalence increased with age. Mortality and incidence, after age adjustment, were 1.31 and 2.5 per 1000 inhabitants, respectively [2]. However, the data in that study based on collected epidemiology data on strokes using a door-to-door survey, therefore those authors has presented that the data on prevalence and mortality must be considered carefully [2].

In a recent study on population-based incidence rates of first-ever stroke (FES) in central Vietnam done by Yamanashi H, Ngoc MQ, Huy TV et al., they have shown that stroke incidence data in Southeast Asia countries is limited but that the crude annual incidence rate of FES was 90.2 per 100,000 population. The age-adjusted incidence of FES was 115.7 (95% CI 95.9–139.1) when adjusted to the WHO world populations. The study highlights a considerable proportion of FES cases in Vietnam attributed to intracerebral hemorrhage, with an age-adjusted incidence rate of 36.9 per 100,000, the highest reported since 2000 in other LMICs [3]. Interestingly, a study on prevalence of atrial fibrillation in older hospitalized patients in Vietnam showed prevalence of AF in older hospitalized patients in Vietnam of 3.9%, Anticoagulation for stroke prevention is underused in these patients.

1.3 Epidemiology of Risk Factors for Stroke

There are many risk factors for stroke which are divided into two types: non-modifiable factors (e.g., age, gender, race, and genetic predisposition) and modifiable or potentially modifiable lifestyle-related factors such as tobacco smoking, alcohol consumption, poor diet, physical inactivity, overweight, and obesity. These factors strongly relate to the prevalence of stroke. The prevalence of common risk factors of stroke such as smoking, hypertension, high body mass index is increasing in Vietnam [4]. A study in 2012 in Danang, Vietnam focused on symptoms and risk factors in 1.621 adults. This showed that the prevalence of hypertension was 27.3%, tobacco use was 26.2%, and 16.1% of individuals were overweight.

Notably, more than two-thirds of those with hypertension were unaware of their condition. The study found that rural residence, education, hypertension, high cholesterol, severe chest pain, former smoking, and being overweight were associated with a higher prevalence of stroke symptoms. Dietary salt intake is closely linked to the development of cardiovascular disease and stroke [5]. This study suggested that achieving salt reduction could reduce the prevalence of hypertension by 1.2–3.5%, leading to a reduction in the number of incident strokes each year by 80,000 to 257,000 strokes.

The paper by Duy Ton Mai, Ngoc Khue Luong, Trong Khoa Nguyen et al., reports that the risk factors for stroke in Vietnam, as in studies from other parts of the world, include age over 50 years, previous history of stroke, large artery atherosclerosis, and cardioembolism [6]. A paper from Phu Tho in Vietnam by Ngoc et al. [7] reports high levels of alcohol and smoking among the 192 patients reported.

An analysis of stroke prevalence in Vietnam reveals disparities based on age, gender, and socioeconomic status. Younger age groups are increasingly affected by stroke, highlighting the need for targeted prevention strategies for this demographic. Additionally, gender disparities in stroke prevalence indicate the importance of understanding specific risk factors and treatment approaches for both men and women. Socioeconomic status also plays a significant role, with disparities in access to healthcare and resources affecting stroke incidence and outcomes.

1.4 Stroke Trends and Statistics in Vietnam

In Vietnam, according to the Ministry of Health, there are about 200,000 incident strokes each year, with 50% of patients being left with long-term disability. Currently, stroke in adults aged 18–50 years old accounts for 15% of all cases of stroke. The number of stroke cases in young people is increasing by 2% per year especially in people under 45 years old. Potential reasons may include behavioral factors such as lack of exercise, alcohol abuse, and fatty food consumption. Hospital recorded cases in young adults suggest the number of male patients is higher four times than female patients. The patients are often in good health, but suddenly get symptoms of stroke. A patient shared that she never thought she would have a stroke and that she thought her symptom of headache was due to her increased workload. Another example was a man who had two strokes and on both occasions failed to go to the hospital and therefore did not receive appropriate acute treatment. However, most stroke cases in young people have mild symptoms and they do come to the hospital within the first 6 h, golden hours, in terms of the availability of reperfusion therapy. The latest data from Vietnam Association of Stroke reported that the number of recorded stroke cases has increased between 20% and 25% in the last three recent years with 70% of stroke patients admitted hospitals within the first 6 h of onset of stroke and so potentially eligible for reperfusion treatment.

1.5 Public Health Implications of Stroke in Vietnam

Stroke has significant public health implications in Vietnam. The impact of stroke on the Vietnamese population includes long-term disability, decreased quality of life, and increased healthcare costs. Furthermore, stroke can lead to a loss of productivity and income for both the individual and their family, contributing to the economic burden of the disease. Implementing effective prevention strategies, improving access to quality healthcare services, and raising public awareness about the risk factors and symptoms of stroke are essential for reducing the burden of this condition in Vietnam.

In Vietnam, hospitals are classified into public and private hospitals, general and specific hospitals with four classes: special class, class I, class II, class III. Vietnam had fewer than 10 stroke units in early 2017, but by 2021, the country had 81 stroke units in 2021 [6, 8]. In 2017, the ANGELS program was initiated in Vietnam. Quality criteria were implemented to meet the standards and criteria of stroke treatment across the world.

According to healthcare providers with extensive experience, patients prefer to see public physicians they know well in their own private clinics. Furthermore, addressing the social determinants of health, such as education, income, and access to healthcare, is crucial in reducing the disparities in stroke incidence and outcomes among different socioeconomic groups in Vietnam. Public health interventions targeted at these determinants could help mitigate the impact of stroke on the population and promote health equity.

For World stroke day in October, Vietnam organizes many annual conferences, meetings to share knowledge and scientific research. The Memorandum of Understanding with the Department of Medical Service Administration has been signed aiming to raise the awareness of stroke in Vietnam.

Stroke can happen to anyone and at every age including children. Addressing risk factors is crucial to reduce the risk of the disease. According to Vietnam Association of Cardiovascular disease, 50% of people with hypertension are unaware of their condition.

1.6 The Future of Stroke Management in Vietnam

The future of stroke management in Vietnam involves several key initiatives to improve stroke care and reduce the burden of stroke on individuals and the healthcare system. These initiatives include the development of national guidelines for stroke diagnosis and treatment, with Vietnamese translation [1]. The World Stroke Organization (WSO) is committed to building partnerships at the global, regional, and national levels to scale up and deliver improvements in the prevention, treatment, and longer term management of the disease to reduce the burden of stroke [2]. In 2016, the Ministry of Health in Vietnam issued Circular 47 which mandates the building of stroke units in Vietnam. The ANGELS program, which supported by the World Stroke Organization has already worked with 18 stroke-ready hospitals in Vietnam to help address quality of stroke patient care [2]. The program has achieved significant results, and the plan is to continue to improve policies, strive to reach stroke benchmark goals, and to implement solutions in the future to build a better stroke system of care infrastructure in Vietnam [2]. The number of stroke units in

Vietnam is currently 110 operating across the country but mostly located in Ho Chi Minh City and Hanoi. Each stroke unit in Vietnam cares for over 2000 patients per annum, compared to 300 patients per unit in the USA. It is suggested that the ideal figure should be about 500 per unit [4]. To address this issue, Thang estimates that Vietnam needs 400 stroke units, or at least 200 units more to have 1000 patients a year per stroke unit [4].

Prevention is also a critical aspect of stroke management in Vietnam. The Ministry of Health (MOH) has identified non-infectious diseases as a significant health risk, with the fatality rate caused by non-infectious diseases accounting for 74% of deaths [4]. To prevent stroke recurrence, patients need to increase physical exercise, lose weight to fight obesity, eat less fat, sweets, and sugar, and eat more vegetables and fruits [4].

In conclusion, the future of stroke management in Vietnam involves several key initiatives to improve stroke care and reduce the burden of stroke on individuals and the healthcare system. These initiatives include the development of national guidelines for stroke diagnosis and treatment, improving policies and stroke benchmark goals, increasing the number of stroke units, and implementing prevention strategies to reduce the risk of stroke recurrence.

Stroke presents significant public health implications for Vietnam, affecting individuals, families, and the healthcare system. Addressing these implications requires a multi-faceted approach that encompasses prevention, management, and addressing social determinants of health.

References

1. Cong NH. Stroke care in Vietnam. Int J Stroke. 2007;2(4):279–80.
2. Le VT, Le TL, Nguyen TH, Nguyen HH, Dao TX, Nguyen VT, et al. Strokes in South Vietnam: an epidemiologic study. Rev Neurol. 1999;155(2):137–40.
3. Yamanashi H, Ngoc MQ, Huy TV, Suzuki M, Tsujino A, Toizumi M, et al. Population-based incidence rates of first-ever stroke in Central Vietnam. PLoS One. 2016;11(8):e0160665.
4. Fitzpatrick AL, Ngo QV, Ly KA, Ton TG, Longstreth WT Jr, Vo TT, et al. Symptoms and risk factors for stroke in a community-based observational sample in Viet Nam. J Epidemiol Glob Health. 2012;2(3):155–63.
5. Aminde LN, Phung HN, Phung D, Cobiac LJ, Veerman JL. Dietary salt reduction, prevalence of hypertension and avoidable burden of stroke in Vietnam: modelling the health and economic impacts. Front Public Health. 2021;9:682975.
6. Ton MD, Phuong DV, Dung NT, Thang NH, Cuong TC, Hai DQ, et al. Sex disparity in stroke outcomes in a multicenter prospective stroke registry in Viet Nam. Int J Stroke. 2023;18(9):1102–11.
7. Ngoc NH, An NQ. Risk factors of ischemic cerebral vascular accident. Genet. Mol. Res. 2021;20(1). gmr 18742.
8. Ton MD, Co DX, Khue LN, Khoa NT, Thang NH, Thanh NN. Current state of stroke care in Vietnam. Vasc Intervent Neurol. 2022;2(2):331.

Chapter 2
Diagnosis of Stroke in Vietnam

Anthony Rudd, Ngoc Huy Nguyen, and Ton Duy Mai

2.1 The Definition of Stroke

Until the beginning of the twentieth century, the term apoplexy was used for what we now know as stroke. One of the first references that we know of is from the ancient Greek philosopher Hippocrates who wrote ""Persons are most subject to apoplexy between the ages of forty and sixty" and "it is impossible to remove a strong attack of apoplexy, and not easy to remove a weak attack" That stroke was an untreatable condition remained the common belief until the end of the twentieth century when the meta-analysis of stroke unit care was published, showing that specialist medical and nursing care saved lives and reduced long- term disability and the NINDS trial showing that intravenous tissue plasminogen activator was an effective treatment for some patients with ischaemic stroke.

In 1970, the World Health Organisation defined stroke as "*rapidly developed clinical signs of focal (or global) disturbance of cerebral function, lasting more than 24 h or leading to death, with no apparent cause other than of vascular origin*" [1]. Although still widely used, the World Health Organisation definition relies heavily on clinical symptoms and is now considered outdated due to significant

A. Rudd (✉)
King's College, London, UK
e-mail: anthony.rudd@kcl.ac.uk

N. H. Nguyen
Phutho Department of Health, Phutho, Vietnam

VNU University of Medicine and Pharmacy, Hanoi, Vietnam

T. D. Mai
VNU University of Medicine and Pharmacy, Hanoi, Vietnam

Stroke Center, Bach Mai Hospital, Hanoi, Vietnam

Hanoi Medical University, Hanoi, Vietnam

A. Rudd et al. (eds.), *Stroke Management in Vietnam*,
https://doi.org/10.1007/978-981-96-0221-6_2

advances in our ability to image the brain acutely after stroke. This is particularly the case for our understanding of Transient Ischaemic Attack (TIA). The diagnosis of TIA is discussed in more detail in Chap. 8 but the previous definition as "*a sudden, focal neurologic deficit that lasts for less than 24 h, is presumed to be of vascular origin, and is confined to an area of the brain or eye perfused by a specific artery*" is no longer fit for purpose. 24 h is an entirely arbitrary time point, bearing little relation to the type or extent of pathology within the brain. At least half of patients with clinically defined TIA have evidence of irreversible ischaemic damage on MRI. The American Heart Association/American Stroke Association removed time as a defining factor and produced their current definition of transient ischaemic attack as "*a transient episode of neurological dysfunction caused by focal brain, spinal cord or retinal ischaemia, without acute infarction*" [1]. However, even this is not perfect as increasingly sensitive imaging methods are able to now show acute infarction in patients that previous scanners would have missed. One of the main implications for changing definitions of both stroke and TIA is that it makes it difficult to use epidemiological data comparing incidence and prevalence data over times when definitions have changed.

Another controversy about the definition of stroke is whether silent stroke, ischaemic damage seen on brain imaging that does not correlate with any symptoms, should be included in the definition. The American Stroke Association includes silent stroke in their definition while the Europeans and the World Health Organisation currently do not. This is not just an academic argument of little consequence. Is a patient with a small silent infarct seen on a brain scan done for some other reason now labelled as having stroke? If so, what implications does that have for their treatment, their psychological well-being and their ability to get insurance and borrow money to buy a house? Or if it is not labelled a stroke is there a risk that it won't be taken seriously and potentially treatable risk factors for cerebrovascular disease will be ignored? And as with research into TIA how will it be feasible to undertake longitudinal epidemiological studies in stroke with definitions that change regularly?

The definitions of both stroke and TIA are therefore currently contentious. It is important that clinicians are aware of the debate and are clear when reading research papers what definitions are being used.

2.2 Stroke Subtypes

Making a diagnosis of stroke is insufficient at a clinical level. Stroke is a syndrome with many subtypes each having their own clinical presentation, epidemiology, prognosis and in some cases treatment.

The first and most important diagnostic stage is to differentiate between ischaemic stroke (Fig. 2.1) and haemorrhagic stroke and for haemorrhagic stroke between primary intracerebral haemorrhage and subarachnoid haemorrhage.

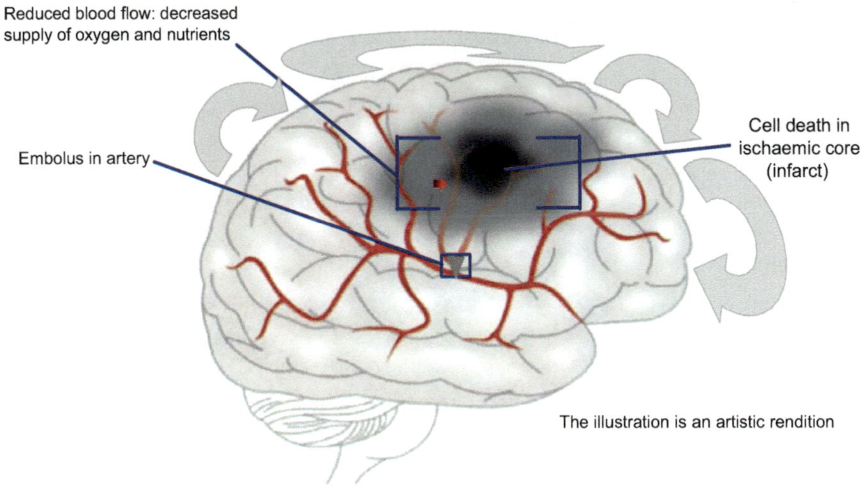

Fig. 2.1 How ischaemic stroke affects the brain

2.3 Understanding Stroke Subtypes and the Clinical Features of Stroke

In order to understand stroke, it is essential that the clinician has a good understanding of brain anatomy, both in terms of the topographical distribution of neurological function and the blood supply to the brain (Figs. 2.2, 2.3, 2.4, 2.5, 2.6, 2.7, and 2.8). Using a good history and clinical examination it should be possible to localise with some precision where in the brain the stroke has happened and therefore which cerebral artery territory is likely to have been responsible. This book is not attempting to provide a detailed description of neuroanatomy, rather it is highlighting the importance of understanding it and encouraging all clinicians treating stroke patients to ensure that this key level of knowledge is adequate. There is a temptation to rely totally on brain imaging establish a diagnosis. Our view is that this is not the correct approach. Use your clinical skills to make the diagnosis which can then be confirmed using investigations.

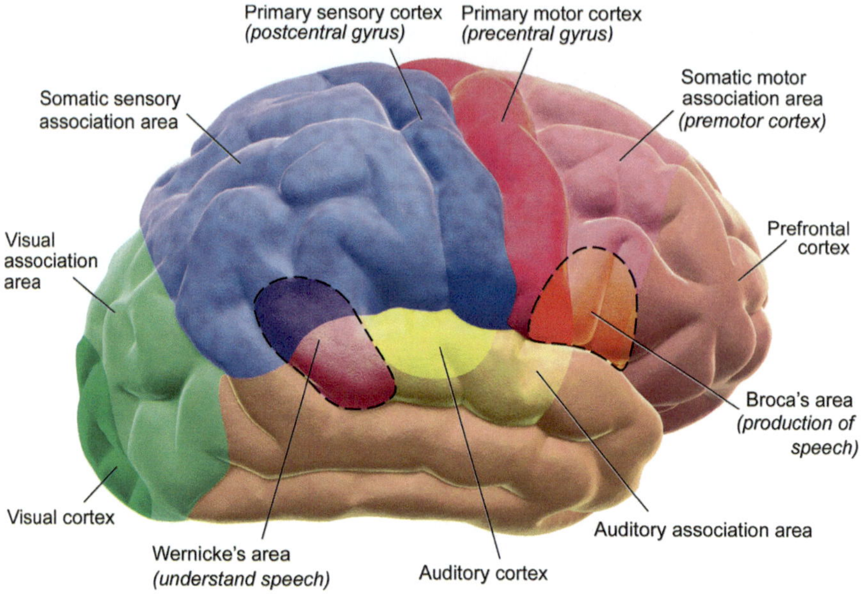

Fig. 2.2 Overview of topographical layout of the brain. By BruceBlaus. When using this image in external sources it can be cited as: Blausen.com staff (2014). "Medical gallery of Blausen Medical 2014". WikiJournal of Medicine 1(2). https://doi.org/10.15347/wjm/2014.010. ISSN 2002-4436. - Own work, CC BY 3.0, https://commons.wikimedia.org/w/index.php?curid=60100749

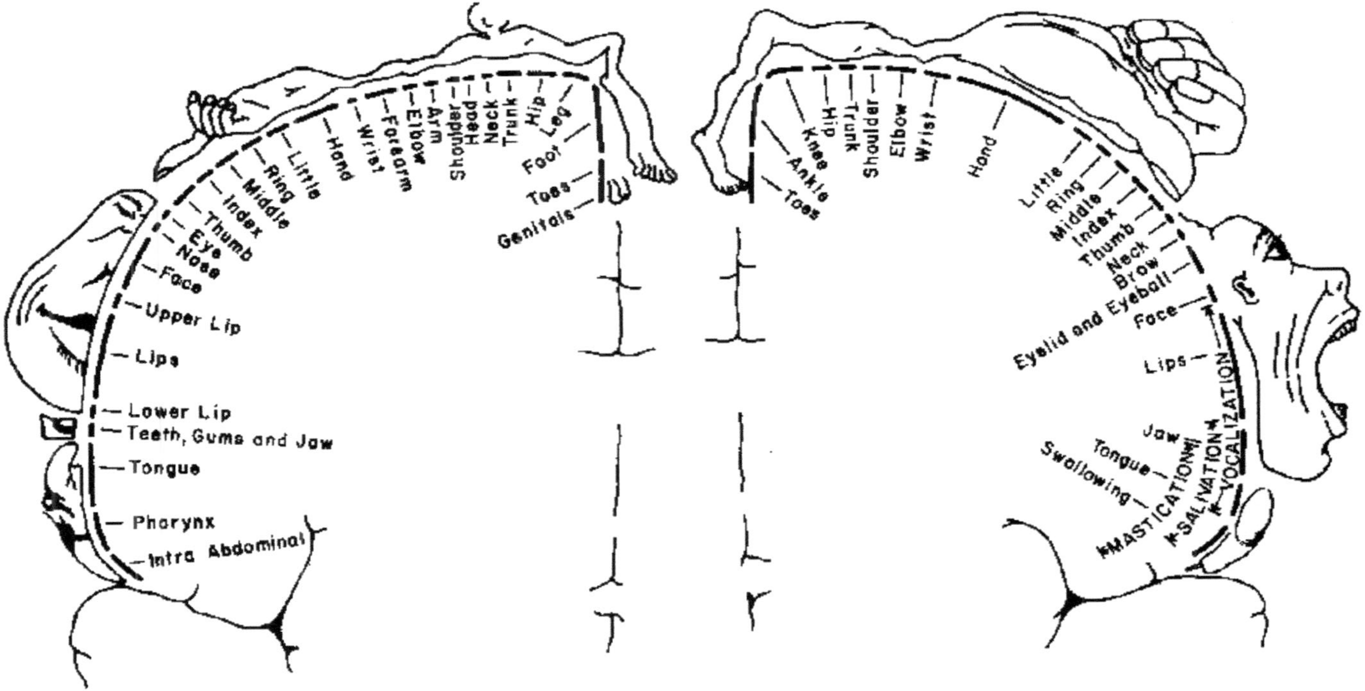

Fig. 2.3 Representation of the homunculus over the cerebral cortex. Image on the left is the motor strip and on the right the sensory strip

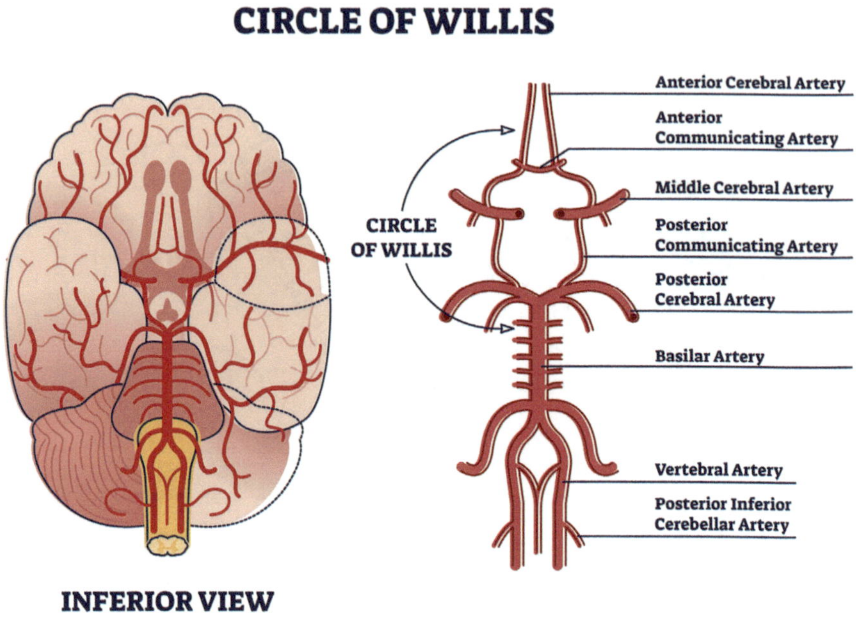

Fig. 2.4 Diagrammatic representation of the Circle of Willis

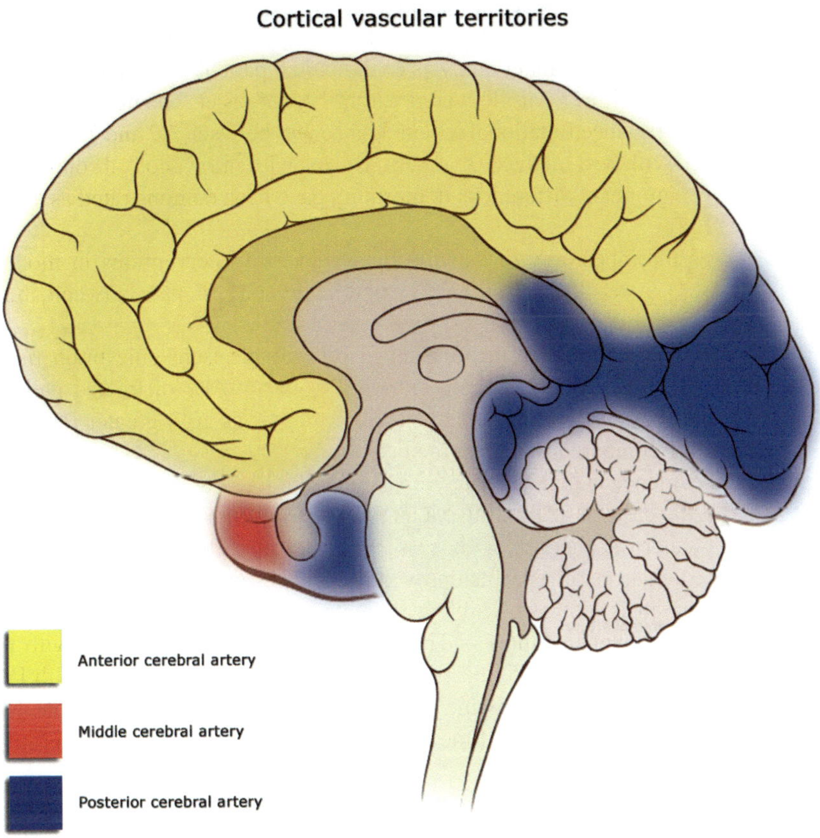

Fig. 2.5 Anterior, middle and posterior cerebral artery territories. https://www.istockphoto.com/fr/vectoriel/cercle-danastomose-circulatoire-willis-avec-du-sang-dans-le-sch%C3%A9ma-de-contour-gm1339953297-420152177. Case courtesy of Frank Gaillard, Radiopaedia.org, rID: 36100 (top). By derivative work: Frank Gaillard (talk)Brain_human_sagittal_section.svg: Patrick J. Lynch, medical illustrator - Brain_human_sagittal_section.svg, CC BY 2.5, https://commons.wikimedia.org/w/index.php?curid=4874896

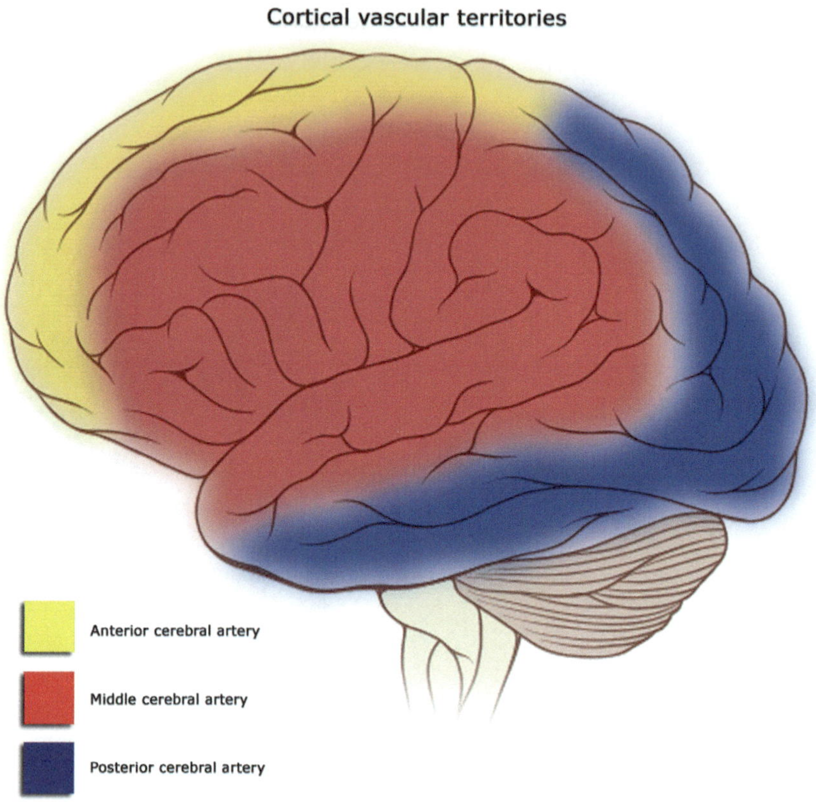

Fig. 2.5 (continued)

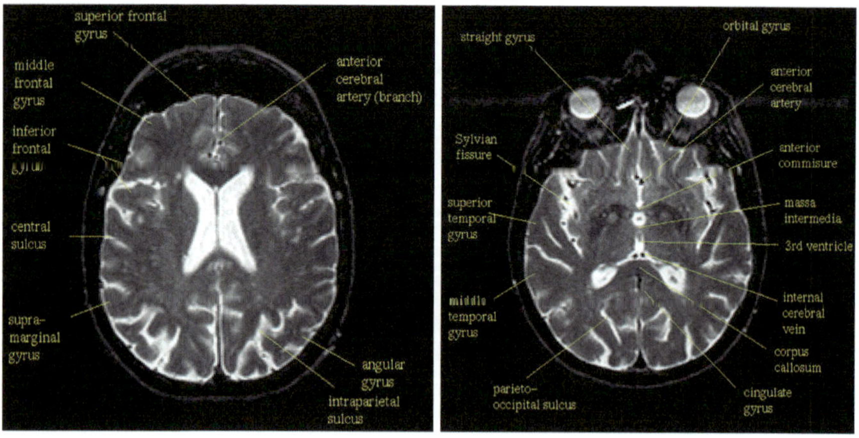

Figs. 2.6 and 2.7 Anatomical markers as seen on CT imaging

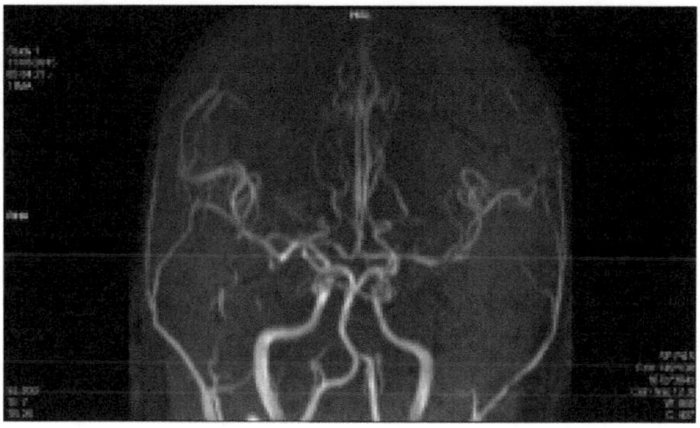

Fig. 2.8 Arteriogram showing normal cerebral circulation

2.4 Clinical Features of Stroke Subtypes

The article by Parmar [1] provides a useful summary of how stroke should be classified. The first and most important diagnostic stage is to differentiate between haemorrhagic and ischaemic stroke. In Europe and the USA, haemorrhagic stroke accounts for about 15% of stroke with ischaemic stroke being 85%. In Vietnam, the rate of haemorrhagic stroke is higher at about 20% of all stroke [3].

2.5 Classification of Ischaemic stroke

Two commonly used classifications are used.

The Oxfordshire Community Stroke Project (OCSP) categorises stroke by the territory and is based purely on the clinical presentation (Table 2.1). It is the most widely used clinical classification and is one that all clinicians involved in stroke should be familiar with [4].

Table 2.1 The Oxfordshire Community Stroke Project (OCSP) classification

Total anterior circulation infarct (TACI) includes all of
• Unilateral motor, sensory deficit, or both affecting at least two of face, arm, and leg
• Higher cerebral dysfunction (e.g., dysphagia (swallowing disorder), dyspraxia (coordination disorder), neglect, dyscalculia (difficulty in understanding numbers))
• Homonymous hemianopia
If consciousness is impaired, higher cerebral dysfunction and visual fields are assumed
Partial anterior circulation infarction (PACI)
Two of the three components of TACS or pure higher cortical dysfunction, or pure motor or sensory deficit, but not as extensive as for lacunar syndromes (see below)
Lacunar infarction (LACI)
• Pure motor or pure sensory deficit affecting at least two of face, arm or leg
• Sensorimotor deficit
• Ataxic hemiparesis
• Dysarthria (slurred speech), clumsy hand syndrome
• Acute onset movement disorder
Posterior circulation syndrome (POCS)
• Isolated hemianopia
• Brain stem signs
• Cerebellar ataxia (inability to coordinate balance, gait, extremity, and eye movements)

2.6 The TOAST Classification

A more comprehensive classification which combines the anatomical distribution of the stroke with the underlying aetiology is the Trial of Org 10,172 in Acute Stroke Treatment (TOAST) [5] system. It is now the most widely used classification system both clinically and in stroke research.

1. Large-vessel atherothrombosis;
2. Cardioembolism;
3. Small-vessel disease;
4. Other determined causes;
5. Undetermined causes.

The undetermined causes also include cases involving more than one primary mechanism

Large-vessel atherothrombosis is where atherosclerotic plaques develop in the carotid vertebral, basilar or anterior, middle or posterior cerebral arteries either causing occlusion of that vessel locally or as a result of the plaque embolising to a more distal vessel. The most common sites for the formation of atherosclerotic plaques are the bifurcation of the carotid artery into the internal and external carotid artery, the start of the vertebral artery, and the M1 and M2 sections of the middle cerebral artery.

Cardioembolism occurs as a result of thrombi formed within the heart, embolising to the brain. The most common causes are atrial fibrillation leading to thrombus formation in the left atrial appendage and prosthetic valves but also includes atrial myxoma and mural thrombus developing after myocardial infarction.

Small-vessel disease refers to occlusive disease involving the microcirculation of the brain. Common locations for small-vessel disease include deep areas of the hemispheric white matter, the internal capsule, the pons and the thalamus, reliant primarily on branches of the posterior cerebral arteries. Infracts are smaller than 1.5 cm and depending on the location within the brain, produce one of the classic lacunar syndromes:

1. Pure motor symptoms (usually face and arm, or arm and leg, comprising 33–50% of all small-vessel strokes);
2. Pure sensory;
3. Mixed sensorimotor;
4. Ataxic hemiparesis (weakness of one side with disproportionate clumsiness (ataxia) of the same side);
5. Clumsy hand dysarthria, clumsiness of either hand, which is out of proportion to any weakness of the limb, combined with slurred speech.

Other determined causes include strokes caused by extracranial arterial dissections, non-atheroscleotic vasculopathies, hypercoagulable states or haematologic disorders.

Undetermined causes include patients where full investigations have not shown a cause. About 40% of ischaemic strokes in most case series are of undetermined cause.

2.7 Differentiating Haemorrhagic Stroke from Ischaemic Stroke

Differentiating between ischaemic and haemorrhagic stroke is such a critical stage in delivering effective treatment and secondary prevention that it needs to done accurately in 100% of cases. While some clinical features such as sudden onset headache, neck stiffness and sudden decreased conscious level are much more common in haemorrhagic stroke than ischaemic stroke no clinical scale has yet been reported that can provide the 100% confidence that is required. This is the main reason why brain imaging is required for all suspected stroke patients and why such imaging should be performed as soon as possible after the onset of symptoms. Early brain scanning with either CT or MR will identify nearly all haemorrhages immediately. CT scanning early after an ischaemic stroke may appear normal but combined with the history and examination this is sufficient to establish the diagnosis.

2.8 Key Investigations in Suspected Acute Stroke

2.8.1 Imaging

The most important investigation is brain imaging. For most patients, CT is the investigation of choice. It is easily available in most hospitals, quick to perform, tolerated by most patients and relatively cheap. It will differentiate accurately between haemorrhage and infarction and may provide useful information as to the ischaemic stroke subtype. Figures 2.10, 2.11, 2.12, 2.13, 2.14, 2.15, 2.16, 2.17, 2.18, and 2.19 illustrate typical examples of how CT and MRI can provide high-quality diagnostic information about the type and location of stroke. Where endovascular thrombectomy is being considered then combining a plain CT with a CT angiogram is the most widely used investigation to identify large-vessel occlusion.

MRI is the investigation of choice for children with suspected stroke and in adults with suspected posterior circulation stroke where CT tends to be insensitive because of surrounding thick bone. MR will also show clear evidence of infarction earlier after a stroke than CT, particularly using diffusion weighted imaging sequences. Where imaging has been delayed for more than 7–10 days after the stroke a small haemorrhage may already have been cleared by phagocytes and on CT may have the appearance of an infarct. For this reason, MR is preferred for late imaging [6] (Fig. 2.9).

2.8.2 *Blood Tests*

The most urgent blood test that should be done immediately in all cases of suspected stroke is a blood glucose as hypoglycaemia can mimic stroke. Failure to identify it can result in unnecessary death or long term disability.

All patients known or suspected to be on oral anticoagulants should have clotting studies performed as soon as possible after the onset of symptoms. For patients with haemorrhage reversal of the anticoagulant may be important and for patients with infarction being considered for intravenous thrombolysis it is important to ensure that the INR is below 1.6.

Other blood tests are less urgent but all patients will need urea and electrolytes, liver function tests, thyroid function, C reactive protein and full blood count. Selected patients will need arrange of other tests depending on the suspected stroke aetiology.

2.8.3 *Other Imaging Studies*

Where cardio-embolic stroke is suspected, then the patient should have a transthoracic echocardiogram (TTE). If Patent Foramen Ovale is being considered, then a TTE bubble study and or a transoesophageal echocardiogram (TOE) is needed.

Internal carotid stenosis should be excluded using carotid Doppler studies for any patient where carotid endarterectomy or carotid stenting would be considered but do not do the test if the patient would be inappropriate for an intervention or the patient would refuse treatment. Carotid Doppler can also be used to identify large-vessel dissection if this has not already been identified on CT or MRI.

Patients with primary intracerebral haemorrhage may need arteriography to exclude an underlying cause such as an arteriovenous malformation or cavernoma

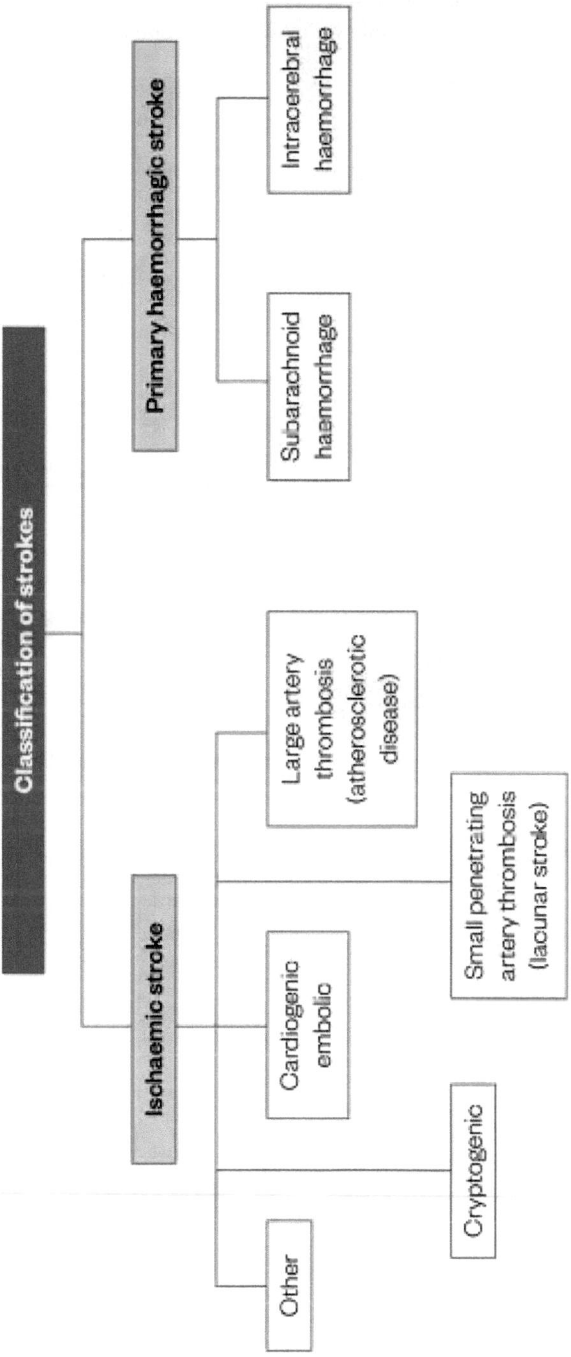

Fig. 2.9 Classification of strokes [2]

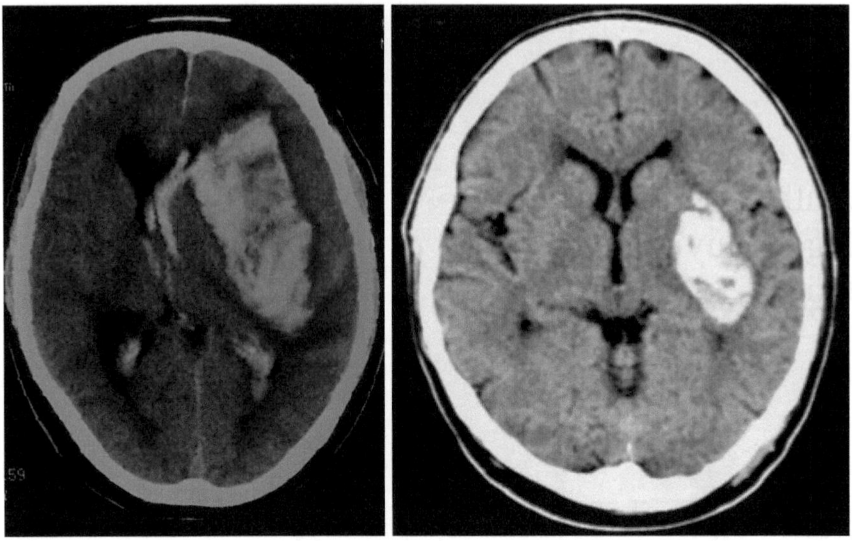

Fig. 2.10 CT of a large left hemisphere intracerebral haemorrhage with intraventricular extension and mass effect and on the right a left basal ganglia haemorrhage

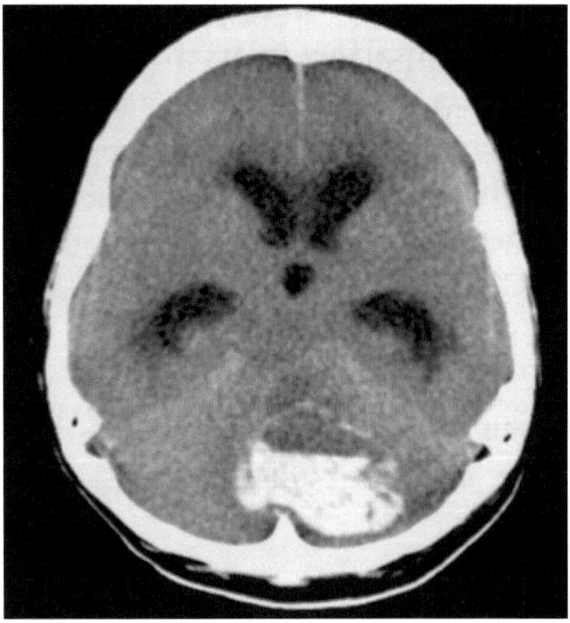

Fig. 2.11 CT showing an cerebellar haemorrhage with associated hydrocephalus

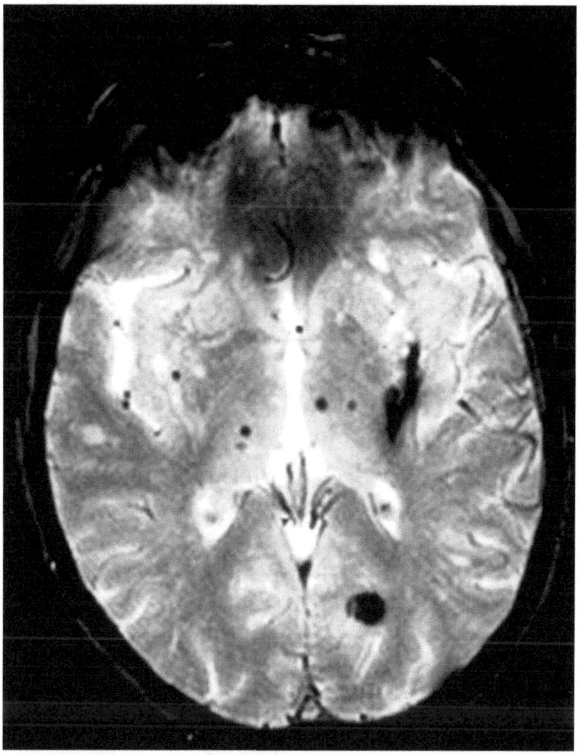

Fig. 2.12 MRI showing multiple micro-haemorrhages

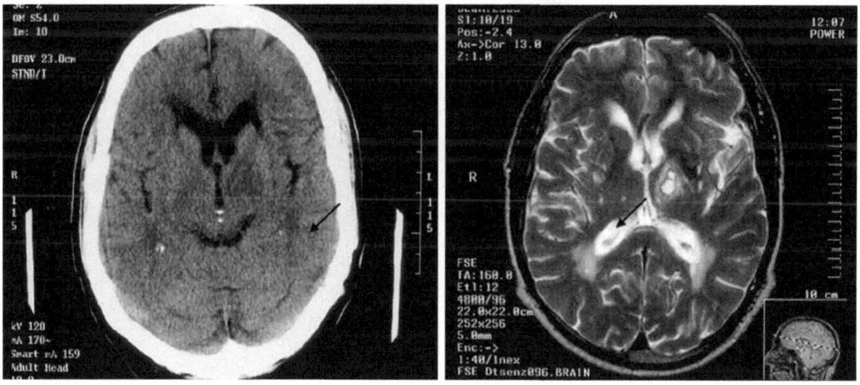

Fig. 2.13 CT scan done 10 days after the onset of symptoms showing appearances consistent with a left sided capsular infarct. The MRI on the right done immediately after the CT shows the lesion was small primary intracerebral haemorrhage

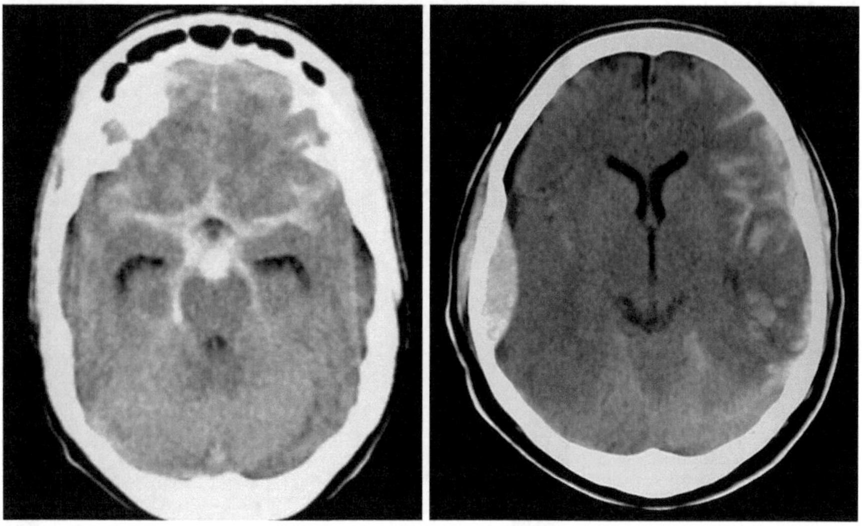

Fig. 2.14 Two CT scans of patients with subarachnoid haemorrhage. The patient on the right also has a right sided subdural haematoma

Fig. 2.15 An established left anterior cerebral artery territory infarct

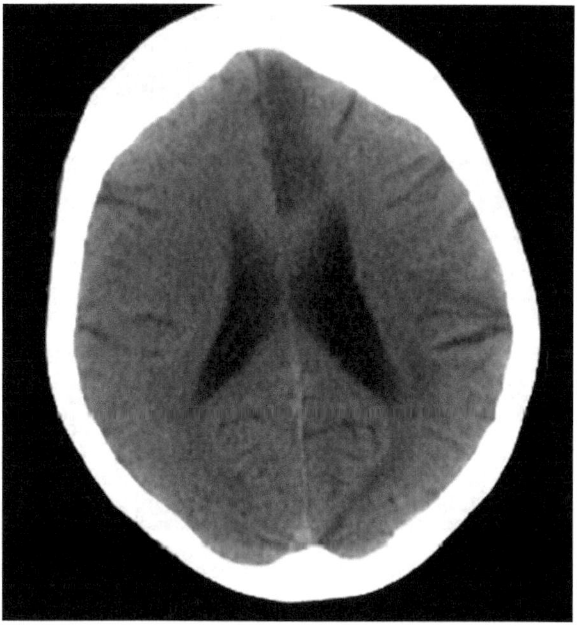

and for most patients with subarachnoid haemorrhage this is needed urgently to identify an aneurysm that may rebleed.

There is a tendency, especially among doctors with less experience and confidence to over investigate their patients. My general rule is that if an investigation is

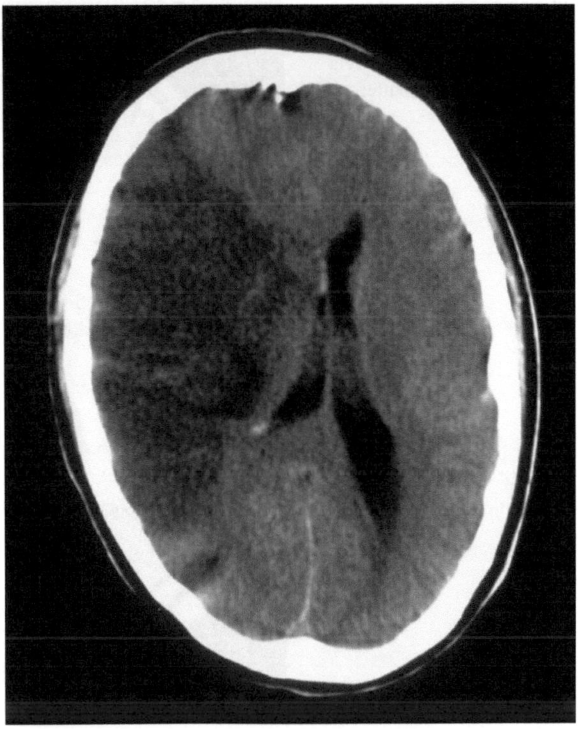

Fig. 2.16 A large right middle cerebral artery infarction with mass effect

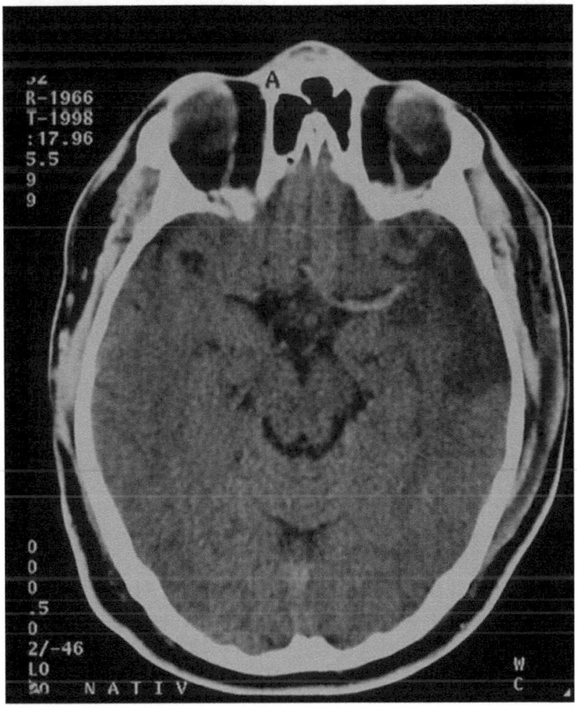

Fig. 2.17 Left hemisphere infarction with a hyperdense left middle cerebral artery

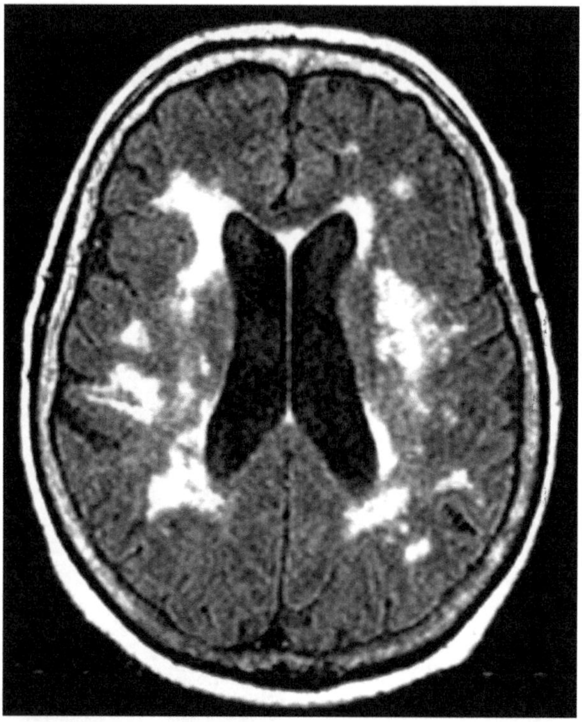

Fig. 2.18 MRI showing extensive small-vessel disease and lacunar infarcts in the deep white matter bilaterally

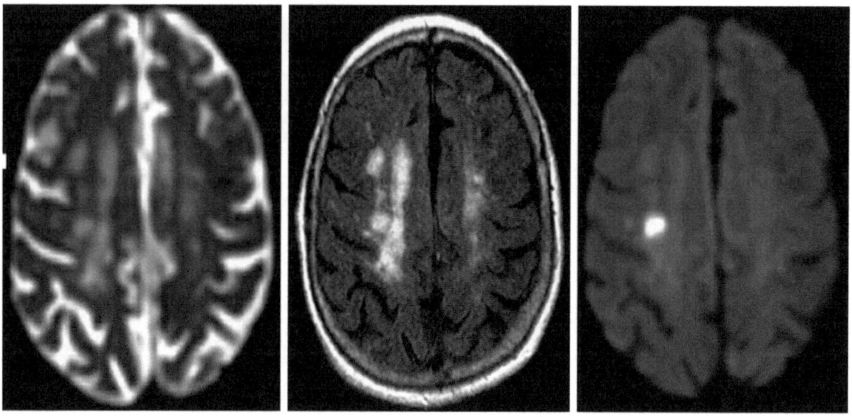

Fig. 2.19 MRI showing extensive small-vessel disease on T2 weighted image (left) and flair imaging (middle). DWI on the right shows the acute ischaemic lesion in the deep white matter on the right

not going to change management (and that includes being able to explain to a patient important information about their stroke), then don't do the test. Never do a test because it is there or you think it is "routine". Always know why you are doing a test and how it might help you or the patient. This is particularly important for patients who are approaching the end of their lives. Know when to stop.

References

1. Sacco RL, Kasner SE, Broderick JP, et al. An updated definition of stroke for the 21st century: a statement for healthcare professionals from the American Heart Association/American Stroke Association. Stroke. 2013;44(7):2064–89.
2. Parmar P. 2018. https://pharmaceutical-journal.com/article/ld/stroke-classification-and-diagnosis.
3. Mai DT, Dao XC, Luong NK, Nguyen TK, Nguyen HT, Nguyen TN. Current state of stroke care in Vietnam. Stroke. 2022;2:331. https://doi.org/10.1161/SVIN.121.000331.
4. Bamford J, Sandercock P, Dennis M, Burn J, Warlow C. Classification and natural history of clinically identifiable subtypes of cerebral infarction. Lancet. 1991;337(8756):1521–6. https://doi.org/10.1016/0140-6736(91)93206-o.
5. Adams HP, Bendixen BH, Kappelle LJ, Biller J, Love BB, Gordon DL, Marsh EE. Classification of subtype of acute ischemic stroke. Definitions for use in a multicenter clinical trial. TOAST. Trial of Org 10172 in acute stroke treatment. Stroke. 1993;24(1):35–41. https://doi.org/10.1161/01.str.24.1.35.
6. Latchaw RE, Alberts MJ, Lev MH, et al. Recommendations for imaging of acute ischemic stroke: a scientific statement from the American Heart Association. Stroke. 2009;40(11):3646–78. https://doi.org/10.1161/STROKEAHA.108.192616. Epub 2009 Sep 24.

Chapter 3
Management of Acute Ischaemic Stroke in Vietnam

Ngoc Huy Nguyen, Anthony Rudd, Thong Van Nguyen, and An Quang Nguyen

3.1 Organisation of Acute Care Services

1. **Prehospital care**: Critical for effective acute stroke management is early recognition of the possibility of the diagnosis by the patient or other people with the patient and then responding appropriately. The patient needs to be taken as quickly as possible to a stroke centre. All these aspects of prehospital care are covered in detail in Chap. 6.
2. **Emergency department**: It has been shown that having systems in place where the prehospital clinicians pre-alert the emergency department staff results in more effective and efficient care when the patient arrives. If possible, the necessary booking in of the patient to the hospital can be done while the patient is on route. One model that we think works best is where the stroke team is present in the emergency department when the patient arrives. A stroke specialist nurse can perform a quick triage to establish that stroke is a likely diagnosis and then ensure that the stroke pathway is followed as efficiently as possible. The nurse or doctor seeing the patient should be trained to be able to make decisions about

N. H. Nguyen (✉)
Phutho Department of Health, Phutho, Vietnam

VNU University of Medicine and Pharmacy, Hanoi, Vietnam
e-mail: ngochuynguyen8888@gmail.com

A. Rudd
King's College, London, UK

T. Van Nguyen
Vietnam Stroke Association, Hanoi, Vietnam

Stroke Center, Phutho General Hospital, Phutho, Vietnam

A. Q. Nguyen
Phutho Medical College, Phutho, Vietnam

A. Rudd et al. (eds.), *Stroke Management in Vietnam*,
https://doi.org/10.1007/978-981-96-0221-6_3

which patients are suitable for intravenous thrombolysis and endovascular thrombectomy. Any system that requires initial triage by a non-specialist team before handing over to the stroke/neurology team is going to be less efficient than having the specialists as the one and only assessment team in the emergency department. The key elements that need to be performed are as follows:

(a) A history from the patient or if necessary, a witness getting as accurately as possible the time of onset or the time the patient was last seen well. A brief description of the symptoms and their course should be obtained. A drug history including specifically whether the patient was taking anticoagulants.
(b) A quick physical examination including the National Institute of Health Stroke Score (NIHSS) and blood pressure.
(c) Blood taken for blood glucose (should have been done in the ambulance if the patient was brought in by paramedics) and a test for coagulation (ideally point of care INR). The other blood tests are less urgent, but it makes sense to send them on arrival. There is no need to wait for anything apart from the blood glucose and clotting before treating an appropriate patient with intravenous thrombolysis.
(d) Brain imaging. For most patients, an unenhanced CT is adequate for making initial decisions about treatment. If the patient may be suitable for endovascular thrombectomy, they should also have CT angiography (CTA). More information about imaging is given in the chapter on diagnosis (Chap. 2). Not all patients presenting with a prehospital diagnosis of stroke will require brain imaging and for this reason we are not keen on systems that take a patient directly to the scanning department. Up to 40% of patients presenting to the department with possible stroke will not have stroke. A competent assessment should be able to manage patients with diagnoses such as Bell's palsy, non-organic stroke, peripheral nerve injuries, Guillain Barre syndrome, and the many other possible diagnoses without subjecting the patient to an unnecessary scan.
(e) The emergency department should be organised in a way that intravenous thrombolysis can be initiated in the department. Well organised services have reported routine door to needle times of 20–30 min.
(f) Once the patient has been diagnosed and where appropriate revascularisation treatment initiated the patient should be transferred directly to a stroke unit (see Chap. 15). One of the most important interventions after acute stroke is offering specialist stroke unit care. It is appropriate for nearly all stroke patients including both ischaemic and haemorrhagic stroke. Stroke unit care compared to general medical or neurological care saves lives and reduces long-term disability. The key elements that make stroke unit care so effective are probably skilled nursing care and effective multidisciplinary care involving doctors, nurses, and therapists.

3.2 What Are the Most Important Interventions for Acute Stroke Patients?

- Revascularisation using intravenous thrombolytics and endovascular thrombectomy are the interventions that have been subjected to the most research and get the most publicity. But at a population level, some of the other aspects such as maintenance of homeostasis and high quality basic care in a specialist stroke unit will save more lives and reduce disability to a greater extent. For every 100 patients, up to 20% may be suitable for intravenous thrombolysis. The number needed to treat (NNT) for one good outcome based on systematic reviews is on about 7 (for patients treated between 0 and 4.5 h. So, out of the 100 patients, 20 should be treated of whom 3 will respond leaving hospital free of disability rather than leaving with long-term severe deficits. 10% of the remaining patients (although likely less than this as there is considerable overlap with the patients suitable for IVT) will be appropriate for ET. The NNT is between 2 and 7. So of the 100 patients 10 will be treated of whom about 4 will have their lives transformed from disabled to independence. About 30% will spontaneously recover with good basic medical care. Ten of the 100 patients will die as a result of the severity of their stroke regardless of the quality of treatment they receive. Therefore, over half of the patients will survive but not benefit from acute interventions. They may, however, benefit from the specialist high quality, but basic care and rehabilitation provided on a stroke unit. The population benefit for the population of Vietnam at about 96 million each year is estimated in Table 3.1. The message is that while revascularisation is important, we should not be ignoring the many patients who will not benefit and ensure that the rest have access to specialist stroke units.

Table 3.1 Impact of stroke treatments on outcome for the population of Vietnam (approx. 96 million with 120,000 strokes a year)

Intervention	Maximum impact Extra independent survivors if all patients were eligible	Proportion eligible for treatment (%)	Actual impact Extra independent survivors per year
Stroke unit	6000	80	4800
Aspirin	1200	80	960
rtPA within 0–4.5 h	19,200	20	3840
Mechanical thrombectomy	13,200	10	1320

3.3 Maintenance of Homeostasis

3.3.1 Hydration

Acute stroke is commonly followed by dehydration, partly because the patient may have been unwell for some time before being taken to hospital and partly because once in hospital hydration may not be the first thing that gets dealt with. There may also be dysphagia and cannot swallow or they have reduced thirst sensation or reduced conscious levels. A paper by Bhalla et al. [1] showed quite a strong association between higher plasma osmolality (>296 mmol/l) measured in the week after stroke and 3 month mortality with an odds ratio of death of 2.4 (95% CI 1–5.9). Similar data from an Israeli patient registry [2] showed significant associations between hydration and modified Rankin scores and mortality after stroke at one year accounting for stroke severity. Lin et al. [3] reported an intervention study where patients were actively hydrated and showed that the percentage of patients with an mRS score of 2 or lower was significantly higher in the hydration group than that in the control group. Further evidence for the importance of maintaining hydration comes from the Sentinel Stroke National Audit Programme from the UK. With a database of over 32,000 patients, Bray et al. [4] showed that giving antiplatelet treatment and adequate fluid and nutrition for the first 2 h was associated with a 45% (95% CI 0.49–0.61) reduction in 3-month mortality compared to those patients who did not have those care processes documented or given. While all of these studies had methodological flaws it does appear that allowing a patient to become dehydrated is a risk factor for poorer outcomes.

3.3.2 Oxygenation

Correcting hypoxia is important. While there is little evidence to prove that statement, it seems self-evident that at a time when hypoxia secondary to poor blood supply to the brain is causing ischaemic damage allowing low oxygen saturations to occur cannot but increase the risk of cerebral infarction. However, the question arises as to whether giving oxygen to nonhypoxic patients is helpful is different. The Stroke Oxygen Study published by Roffe [5] showed no benefit for oxygen supplementation. A systematic review and meta-analysis of normobaric oxygenation trials after stroke by Mahmood et al. [6] showed no significant effect on early recovery, functional outcome, or mortality in acute stroke. A Cochrane review of hyperbaric oxygen after acute ischaemic stroke by Bennett et al. [7] including 11 RCTs involving 705 participants showed no significant differences in the case fatality rate at 6 months in those receiving HBOT compared with the control group (risk ratio (RR) 0.97, 95% confidence interval (CI) 0.34–2.75, *P* value 0.96). There were major methodological flaws in many of the studies and the conclusions were that further research was needed before dismissing it as a potentially useful treatment.

3.3.3 Blood Pressure

Theoretically, it could be argued that blood pressure should be allowed to be high or raised to improve cerebral circulation after an acute ischaemic stroke. Alternatively, it could be argued that blood pressure should be kept low to reduce the risk of cerebral oedema and haemorrhagic transformation. 75% of patients have high blood pressure in the first week after a stroke and at least 50% of patients presenting with stroke have prior hypertension. Bath et al. [8] in Cochrane review of 26 trials involving 17,011 participants concluded that there is insufficient evidence that lowering blood pressure during the acute phase of stroke improves functional outcome. That it is reasonable to withhold blood pressure-lowering drugs until patients are medically and neurologically stable, and have suitable oral or enteral access, after which drugs can then be reintroduced and that further trials are needed to identify which people are most likely to benefit from early treatment, in particular whether treatment started very early is beneficial.

Guidelines state that blood pressure should be controlled to below 185/110 mmHg before giving intravenous thrombolytic agents <180/105 mmHg for the following 24 h. But this is not based on RCT evidence being largely based on trials of thrombolytics given for myocardial infarction. Observational data from the Safe Implementation of Thrombolysis in Stroke (SITS) register [9] showed that a higher SBP post-thrombolysis is associated with symptomatic ICH and poor outcome. A U-shaped relationship was seen between SBP 2–24 h after thrombolysis and major disability and death, with the most favourable outcomes occurring in those with SBP 141–150 mmHg [10].

3.3.4 Temperature

Raised temperature above 37.5° occurs in up to 50% ischaemic stroke patients. It is often multifactorial related to presence of infection and the size of infarct and is known to be associated with worse outcomes. Therapeutically induced hypothermia has shown some promise in animal models and some patients with hypoxic encephalopathy but the evidence in stroke patients is inconclusive for the following three questions:

- In hyperthermic patient with acute ischemic stroke, does treatment of hyperthermia compared with no treatment of hyperthermia improve functional outcome and/or survival?
- In normothermic patients with acute ischemic stroke, does prevention of hyperthermia with antipyretics compared with no prevention of hyperthermia improve functional outcome and/or survival?
- In patients with acute ischemic stroke, does induction of hypothermia compared with no induction of hypothermia improve functional outcome and/or survival?

A meta-analysis of five studies [10] with a total of 789 patients giving paracetamol to acute ischaemic stroke patients prophylactically to prevent fever did result in a modest reduction in temperature but had no impact on functional outcomes. Again, this is an area where we need some well conducted trials.

Work on induced hypothermia is ongoing. It is a complex intervention usually requiring sedation and ventilation. It is not yet a treatment that can be recommended for routine use.

3.3.5 *Blood Glucose*

In contrast to acute myocardial infarction, tight glycaemic control has not been shown to improve outcome in stroke [11] and studies have warned against aggressive lowering with insulin infusions due to the risk of hypoglycaemia. This has led the UK National Clinical Guidelines [12] to recommend a broadening of the target range for blood glucose in acute stroke to be changed for the previously recommended level from 4 to 11 mmol/L to 5–15 mmol/L with close monitoring to avoid hypoglycaemia.

3.4 Swallowing Assessment and Nutrition

Dysphagia (swallowing difficulty associated with foods, fluids, and saliva) is common after acute stroke with an incidence between 40 and 78%. There is an association between dysphagia and poor outcomes including a higher risk of longer hospital stay, chest infection, disability, and death [13]. Evidence from the UK national audit shows that delays in the screening and assessment of dysphagia are associated with an increased risk of stroke-associated pneumonia [14]. Prompt detection of dysphagia in patients with acute stroke is therefore essential. In patients with dysphagia on initial screening, a specialist swallowing assessment is indicated that includes consideration of function and cognition and a broader range of food and fluids of varying texture. The UK National Clinical Guidelines [12] have a long list of recommendations including:

- Patients with acute stroke should have their swallowing screened, using a validated screening tool, by a trained healthcare professional within 4 h of arrival at hospital and before being given any oral food, fluid, or medication.
- Until a safe swallowing method is established, patients with swallowing difficulty after acute stroke should be considered for alternative fluids and have a

comprehensive specialist assessment of their swallowing completed by a specialist in dysphagia management within 24 h of admission.

- They should be considered for a nasogastric tube for fluids and nutrition within 24 h.
- Patients with swallowing difficulty in the acute phase of stroke should only be given food, fluids, and medications in a form that minimises the risk of aspiration.
- Patients with acute stroke should be screened for the risk of malnutrition on admission and at least weekly thereafter. Screening should be conducted by trained staff using a structured, standardised, validated tool.
- Patients with acute stroke who are at low risk of malnutrition on admission, and are able to meet their nutritional needs orally, should not routinely receive oral nutritional supplements.
- Patients with acute stroke who are at risk of malnutrition or who require tube feeding or dietary modification should be referred to a dietitian for specialist nutritional assessment, advice and monitoring.
- Patients with stroke who are at risk of malnutrition should be offered nutritional support. This may include oral nutritional supplements, specialist dietary advice, and/or tube feeding in accordance with their expressed wishes or, if the patient lacks mental capacity, in their best interests.
- Patients with stroke who are unable to maintain adequate nutrition and hydration orally should be:
  - Referred to a dietitian for specialist nutritional assessment and advice.
  - Be assessed for nasogastric tube feeding within 24 h of admission.

3.5 Head Positioning

The issue is whether head position can influence cerebral blood flow and cerebral perfusion. One systematic review [15] has examined four small non-randomised trials of head position in acute patients with ischaemic stroke. The trials studied cerebral blood flow using transcranial Doppler but did not report on functional outcome. In the international multicentre cluster randomised trial HeadPoST [16] of 11,093 patients hospitalised with acute stroke, there was no significant difference between the lying-flat head position and the sitting-up position for the first 24 h with respect to the primary outcome of disability at 90 days. There were also no significant differences in mortality or in the rates of serious adverse events, including pneumonia. The UK Stroke Guidelines [12] therefore recommend that patients admitted to hospital with acute stroke should be allowed to adopt either a sitting-up or lying-flat head position in the first 24 h, according to comfort. Stroke units should not have a policy or practice that favours either head position.

3.6 Mouth Care

Mouth care (also referred to as oral care) refers to the promotion and maintenance of a clean oral cavity including the teeth, gums, cheeks, tongue, and palate. A clean mouth requires the removal of traces of food and debris and dental plaque. A clean mouth is pleasant for the person with stroke and maintains the health of the mouth, teeth, and gums. Poor oral hygiene can lead to dental caries, periodontal gum disease, the development of ulceration, soreness, cracked lips, and fungal infections and is associated with increased bacteria in the mouth and in saliva. In people with dysphagia, this may increase the risk of aspiration pneumonia. People with problems chewing and swallowing and soreness of the mouth report a decrease in the range of food they are able to eat. A clean and healthy mouth can prevent discomfort and help to achieve good nutrition. Maintaining good oral hygiene can be difficult following a stroke because of cognitive impairment, dysphagia or arm weakness and can be made worse by inadequate control of saliva and medication side effects such as xerostomia (dry mouth). Members of the multidisciplinary team should be trained to ensure provision of adequate mouth care. The UK guidelines therefore make the following recommendations

- People with stroke, especially those who have difficulty swallowing or who are tube fed, should have mouth care at least three times a day (particularly after mealtimes), which includes removal of food debris and excess secretions, and application of lip balm.
- People with stroke, including those who have full or partial dentition and/or wear dentures and especially those who have difficulty swallowing or who are tube fed, should have mechanical removal of plaque at least twice a day by the brushing of teeth and cleaning of gums and tongue with a low foaming, fluoride-containing toothpaste. Chlorhexidine dental gel may be prescribed short term and requires regular review.

3.7 Revascularisation

3.7.1 Intravenous Thrombolysis

3.7.1.1 Intravenous Thrombolysis Within 4.5 h of Onset Need Case Example

Treatment with thrombolysis should only be given in units where staff are trained and experienced in the provision of stroke thrombolysis and have a thorough knowledge of the contraindications to treatment and the management of complications such as neurological deterioration. The inclusion and exclusion criteria are summarized in Table 3.2.

Table 3.2 Indications and exclusion criteria for intravenous thrombolysis [17]

Indications for intravenous thrombolysis after acute ischaemic stroke
1. Acute ischaemic stroke within 4.5 h after the onset of symptoms
2. Age over 18 (but only because there have been no trials of thrombolysis in children)
3. Measurable neurological deficits. Some recommendations set a specific NIHSS score above which it is indicated but our opinion is that this is too rigid and does not take into account individual impact of deficits. For example, isolated hemianopia may not be important for some but would be for a patient whose livelihood depended on their ability to drive
Contraindications for intravenous thrombolysis after acute ischaemic stroke
• Any suggestion of haemorrhage on brain imaging
• Ischemic stroke or severe head trauma in the previous 3 months
• Previous intracranial haemorrhage
• Intra-axial intracranial neoplasm
• Gastrointestinal malignancy
• Gastrointestinal haemorrhage in the previous 21 days
• Intracranial or intraspinal surgery within the prior 3 months
• Symptoms suggestive of subarachnoid haemorrhage
• Persistent blood pressure elevation (systolic ≥185 mmHg or diastolic ≥110 mmHg)
• Active internal bleeding
• Presentation consistent with infective endocarditis
• Stroke known or suspected to be associated with aortic arch dissection
• Acute bleeding diathesis including platelet count <100,000/mm
• Current anticoagulant use with an INR >1.7 or PT >15 s or aPTT >40 s
• Therapeutic doses of low molecular weight heparin received within 24 h (e.g., to treat VTE and ACS); this exclusion does not apply to prophylactic doses (e.g., to prevent VTE)
• Current use (i.e., last dose within 48 h in a patient with normal renal function) of a direct thrombin inhibitor or direct factor Xa inhibitor with evidence of anticoagulant effect by laboratory tests such as aPTT, INR, ECT, TT, or appropriate factor Xa activity assays

The evidence supporting treatment are summarised in the European Stroke Organisation Guidelines on intravenous thrombolysis for acute ischaemic stroke [17]. Two reviews provide evidence the treatment: a systematic review and meta-analysis of study level data from ten randomised controlled trials (RCTs) by Wardlaw et al. [18] (6887 patients) and an individual patient data meta-analysis from 9 RCTs by Emberson et al. [19] (6756 patients). These reviews included patients with a wide range of ages and stroke severities.

The study level meta-analysis demonstrated that alteplase within 6h of stroke onset reduced the risk of death or disability defined as a mRS score of 3–6 (odds ratio (OR) 0.84, 95% CI: 0.77–0.93, $P=0.0006$, $I^2=63\%$), and that the effect was greatest within 3h (OR 0.68, 95% CI: 0.53–0.87, $P=0.002$, $I^2=0.0\%$). The individual participant data meta-analysis was consistent with these results. It showed that alteplase significantly increased the odds of excellent outcome (no or non-disabling symptoms, mRS score 0–1) at 3months and at 6months in the third International Stroke Study (IST-3), with earlier treatment resulting in greater proportional benefit (p for interaction=0.016). Alteplase significantly increased the odds of an excellent outcome when given within 3 h (OR 1.75, 95% CI: 1.35–2.27, $p<0.0001$) from 3 to 4.5 h (OR 1.26, 95% CI: 1.05–1.51, $P=0.0132$ but not after 4.5 h (OR 1.15, 95% CI: 0.95–1.40, $P=0.15$).

3.7.1.2 Intravenous Thrombolysis Between 4.5 and 24 h

Unless there is advanced imaging showing a mismatch between perfusion and diffusion indicating potentially salvageable tissue treatment should not be given.

The UK National Clinical Guidelines for Stroke published in 2023 [12] summarises the evidence-based criteria for extending the time window for intravenous thrombolysis in Table 3.3. The recommendation in these guidelines is

Patients with acute ischaemic stroke, regardless of age or stroke severity, who were last known to be well more than 4.5 h earlier, should be considered for thrombolysis with alteplase if:

treatment can be started between 4.5 and 9 h of known onset, or within 9 h of the midpoint of sleep when they have woken with symptoms.

and

they have evidence from CT/MR perfusion (core-perfusion mismatch) or MRI (DWI-FLAIR mismatch) of the potential to salvage brain tissue. This should be irrespective of whether they have a large artery occlusion and require mechanical thrombectomy.

Table 3.3 Evidence-based criteria for using intravenous thrombolysis between 4.5 h and 9 h after onset of symptoms and for wake-up stroke [12]

	Imaging		Imaging criteria
Wake-up stroke	>4.5 h from last seen well, no upper limit	MRI DWI-FLAIR mismatch	DWI lesion and no FLAIR lesion
Wake-up stroke or unknown onset time	>4.5 h from last seen well, and within 9 h of the midpoint of sleep. The midpoint of sleep is the time halfway between going to bed and waking up	CT or MRI core-perfusion mismatch	Suggested: mismatch ratio greater than 1.2, a mismatch volume greater than 10 mL, and an ischaemic core volume <70 mL
Known onset time	4.5–9 h	CT or MRI core-perfusion mismatch	Suggested: mismatch ratio greater than 1.2, a mismatch volume greater than 10 mL, and an ischaemic core volume <70 mL

3.7.1.3 Which Thrombolytic Agent Should Be Used and What Dose?

The very early trials of intravenous thrombolysis over 50 years ago used streptokinase and resulted in an excess of deaths in the treatment group. Whether this is a problem with the drug or whether the dose was too high remains unanswered. This is unfortunate because if it is a dose problem then a cheap thrombolytic drug is being denied to patients in countries where the high cost of the alternative agents is a barrier to their use.

Alteplase (tissue plasminogen activator) was the first drug to be shown to be effective in acute ischaemic stroke in the ground breaking NINDS trial [20] and has been the only drug available until recently. The dose used in this trial was 0.9 mg/kg and this has remained the dose in all Western countries. However, the ENCHANTED trial [21] evaluating the lower dose of 0.6 mg/kg has shown that in a predominantly Asian population the lower dose was equally effective with a lower rate of intracerebral haemorrhage. Major symptomatic intracerebral haemorrhage occurred in 1.0% of the participants in the low-dose group and in 2.1% of the standard dose group ($P = 0.01$); fatal events occurred within 7 days in 0.5% and 1.5%, respectively ($P = 0.01$) although mortality at 90 days did not differ significantly between the two groups (8.5% and 10.3%, respectively; $P = 0.07$).

A number of trials have now been reported comparing alteplase with tenecteplase show equivalence in effect and with no additional side effects. It has the advantage of being given as a single bolus rather than with alteplase which is given with 10% of the dose as a bolus and the remaining 90% as an infusion over an hour.

The ACT trial [22] recruited 1600 patients from 22 stroke centres in Canada within 4.5 h of symptom onset and were given either intravenous tenecteplase 0.25 mg/kg or alteplase 0.9 mg/kg. 1577 patients completed study with an mRS score of 0–1 achieved in 32.7% in the tenecteplase group vs. 29.6% in the alteplase group. Symptomatic intracerebral haemorrhage 6.1% vs. 1.3%, and mortality 19.9% vs. 18.1%. There were no significant differences. The ATTEST2 [23] trial was similar in design and recruited 1858 patients eligible for thrombolysis within 4½ h to standard dose of alteplase, 0.9 mg/kg or a bolus dose of tenecteplase (0.25 mg/kg). Tenecteplase was again non-inferior to alteplase (rtPA). The TASTE A trial [24] had 104 patients randomised to alteplase or tenecteplase given in a mobile stroke unit and resulted. in a superior rate of early reperfusion in the tenecteplase group compared with alteplase. The remain a number of unanswered questions which include what the ideal dose of tenecteplase is (0.25 mg/k or 0.4 mg/kg?), whether it is equally effective in the extended time window setting and in wake-up strokes and whether it is also equivalent to alteplase when used as bridging therapy before thrombectomy. Trials are underway but at the time of writing not reported into these questions.

3.8 Endovascular Thrombectomy

The evidence from RCTs for the effectiveness of mechanical thrombectomy (MT) after proximal middle and anterior cerebral artery occlusion is now very strong. Early trials failed to demonstrate efficacy possibly due to the use of older devices and patient selection. More recent trials using modern devices such as stent retrievers and aspiration devices have transformed the way thrombectomy is now perceived. The HERMES [25] meta-analysis of individual patient data from five RCTs demonstrated benefit if MT was delivered within 12 h of onset. The number needed to treat (NNT) to produce functional independence was between 3.2 and 7.4 patients when compared with best medical treatment. But, as with intravenous thrombolysis no statistically significant differences in mortality have been demonstrated as a consequence of MT.

This makes thrombectomy one of the most powerful interventions in modern medicine. There were similar rates of symptomatic ICH (4.4%) between those treated with MT or not.

Trials using advanced imaging to identify salvageable ischaemic brain tissue demonstrated good functional outcome ranging from 44–70% of treated patients with MT. Overall good functional outcome at 90 days was 20% greater (absolute benefit) with MT compared with best medical therapy.

While the evidence is that MT can be beneficial up to 24 h after onset of symptoms it is still the case, as with intravenous thrombolysis, that the earlier treatment is given the greater the chances of success. For every hour delay in MT, there is a reduction in the chances of reperfusion by 20%. The UK stroke guidelines support the use of MT given as soon as possible in patients with clinically significant neurological deficit (National Institutes of Health Stroke Scale (NIHSS) ≥6), with the procedure commencing within 5 hours of symptom onset in combination with IVT in confirmed occlusion of the proximal anterior circulation. In addition to this, MT can be used using the same time frame and criteria when IVT is also contraindicated.

For those who present within 24 h, including those with wake-up stroke, there is increasing evidence for offering MT if perfusion based imaging techniques show potentially salvageable brain tissue. The DAWN trial [26] randomised patients presenting between 6–24 h and the DEFUSE 3 trial [27] presenting within 6–16 h. Absolute benefits (good functional outcome) for patients in the DAWN trial compared with standard medical care equated to 36% and with DEFUSE 3 showing 28%.

Using this evidence, the UK National Clinical Guidelines for Stroke [12] make the following recommendations:

- Patients with acute anterior circulation ischaemic stroke and a proximal intracranial large artery occlusion (ICA and/or M1) causing a disabling neurological deficit (NIHSS score of 6 or more) of onset between 6 and 24 h ago, including wake-up stroke, and with no previous disability (mRS 0 or 1) should be considered for intra-arterial clot extraction (using a stent retriever and/or aspiration techniques, combined with thrombolysis if eligible) providing the following imaging criteria are met:

- between 6 and 12 h: an ASPECTS score of 3 or more, irrespective of the core infarct size;
- between 12 and 24 h: an ASPECTS score of 3 or more and CT or MRI perfusion mismatch of greater than 15 mL, irrespective of the core infarct size.

The evidence base for thrombectomy for patients with posterior circulation ischaemic stroke is less strong but recent trials do suggest that it may be beneficial. Langezaal et al. [28] reported a trial of 300 patients with basilar artery occlusion within 6 h of onset of symptoms and failed to find a significant difference between those treated with MT and those managed medically. But there were very wide confidence intervals and the authors conclude that there could still be a substantial benefit despite the lack of a positive outcome from this trial. Jovin et al. [29] published a trial of MT for basilar artery occlusion 6–24 h after onset of symptoms and showed a higher percentage with good functional status at 90 days than medical therapy but was associated with procedural complications and more cerebral haemorrhages. A further trial from China by Tao et al. [30] randomised 340 patients in a 2:1 ratio to either thrombectomy and best medical therapy or best medical therapy alone, with additional eligibility criteria of an NIHSS of 10 or more, PC-ASPECTS of 6 or more and in a time window of up to 12 h after stroke onset. Patients over 80 years of age additionally had to have PC-ASPECTS of 8 or more and a pre-stroke mRS of 0–1. The trial demonstrated superiority of thrombectomy with an absolute difference in mRS 0–3 of 23.2%. The recommendation regarding the use of ET for posterior circulation stroke in the UK National Clinical Guidelines [12] based on some of these data is:

- Patients with acute ischaemic stroke in the posterior circulation within 12 h of onset should be considered for mechanical thrombectomy (combined with thrombolysis if eligible) if they have a confirmed intracranial vertebral or basilar artery occlusion and their NIHSS score is 10 or more, combined with a favourable PC-ASPECTS score and Pons-Midbrain Index. Caution should be exercised when considering mechanical thrombectomy for patients presenting between 12 and 24 h of onset and/or over the age of 80 owing to the paucity of data in these groups.

A recent systematic review and meta-analysis of studies looking at whether giving intra-arterial thrombolytics during MT is beneficial failed to demonstrate any statistical advantage although there was a trend towards better outcomes [31].

3.9 Should Patients Receive Intravenous Thrombolysis Prior to Thrombectomy?

Two recent meta-analyses [32] of six RCTs support the administration of thrombolysis within 4.5 h of onset in eligible patients prior to thrombectomy. None of the individual studies had shown benefit that reached statistical significance. The meta-analysis indicated superior reperfusion rates, trends to improved clinical outcome and no statistical increase in adverse safety outcomes with bridging thrombolysis. All the randomised trials recruited patients presenting directly to thrombectomy centres. No randomised trial has yet addressed the question of whether patients presenting initially to an acute stroke centre should proceed directly to mechanical thrombectomy without bridging thrombolysis given that there are likely to be some additional delays in delivering the ET.

3.10 Organisation of Intravenous Thrombolysis and Endovascular Thrombectomy Services

Delivering acute stroke care effectively requires well-organised services that can provide the specialist input quickly and efficiently. Few if any countries have enough stroke specialist physicians and nurses to be able to provide 24 h cover, 7 days a week in all hospitals that might receive acutely ill patients. It is estimated that theoretically up to 20% of acute ischaemic stroke patients might benefit from intravenous thrombolysis and with some overlap about 10–15% in most populations would be eligible for ET. No services have so far reported achieving this sort of level of intervention for either intravenous or intra-arterial treatments. In the UK, for example, at a national level only about 12% of patients are thrombolysed nationally and between 2% and 3% of patients are treated with ET [33]. In Vietnam, these figures are about…. The main reasons behind the low rates of treatment are the lack of personnel with sufficient experience to do INT and ET, the lack of hospitals with the equipment necessary to do complex procedures, the late presentation of many patients and patients being taken to hospitals that are not equipped to deliver them.

Reorganisation of services to concentrate specialist stroke care in a small number of specialist centres, especially for ET has been shown to significantly improve performance at regional and national levels. The experience in London where the 32 hospitals that previously delivered acute care was reduced to just eight centres over night produced dramatic improvements in the process of care and outcomes at lower cost [34]. Similar results have been obtained reorganising care in other parts of the UK and in other countries. Centralising care in specialist centres is particularly important for ET where the skilled personnel and equipment is a major issue. The positive outcomes of the trials, all performed in specialist centres by some of the world's most expert clinicians are unlikely to be replicated if the procedures are performed by staff who have little experience and with access to less than ideal equipment. It is essential that all hospitals providing acute stroke care continuously monitor the quality of their processes and outcomes, preferably through a national audit with a near 100% participation rate. A report by Ngoc NH et al. of the delivery of intravenous thrombolysis (1145 patients) and endovascular thrombectomy (269 patients) from 29 clinics in Vietnam shows outcomes that are in line with outcomes from the research trials.

3.11 Neuroprotection

Research into drugs that are neuroprotective or perhaps better termed 'cytoprotective', given that it is important to maintain viability of several different types of cells in the brain and not just neurons, has been very disappointing. Despite huge sums of money developing and testing possible agents, pharmaceutical companies have yet to identify a single agent that works on human stroke patients. All of those that have been tested in RCTs have shown benefit in animal models, but these have never transferred to the clinical setting. There have been problems with design and conduct of both preclinical and clinical trials. In the preclinical setting using animal models of stroke that are not the same as stroke in the typical patient, e.g., young animals without comorbidities and using infarct size rather than functional measures are part of the problem. Many of the studies have had small sample sizes, were not blinded and had inadequate dose ranging. The issues with the clinical trials were that most trials tested the drug too late after the onset of symptoms, did not use advanced imaging, used just a single dose and again with small sample sizes. Because of these problems, it is entirely possible that some of the agents tested could have had useful effects if they had been trialled adequately.

There is one agent that has shown some promise. Hill et al. [35] showed in a multicentre, double-blind RCT that the drug given either prior to IVT bridging or at the ET centre had no significant benefit overall but did seem to help patients who did not receive tPA where there was a 9.5% absolute benefit for the Nerinetide patients. Plasma levels of the drug were much lower in the tPA patients as the drug may have been inactivated by the tPA and plasminogen. A further trial is ongoing in patients who do not receive tPA.

For future trials of cytoprotective agents, consideration should be given to giving the drug as early as possible, preferably in the ambulance or in a mobile stroke unit if prior brain imaging is necessary, giving the drug at the time of ET and infusing it after successful reperfusion of the ischaemic brain.

3.12 Antiplatelets After Acute Ischaemic Stroke

Recent evidence supports the early use of dual antiplatelet therapy in patients with TIA or minor ischaemic stroke. The CHANCE trial [36] showed in a Chinese population of patients with TIA or minor ischaemic stroke (NIHSS 0–3) that dual antiplatelet therapy started within 24 h of onset for 21 days resulted in a significant reduction in ischaemic stroke from 11.7% (aspirin group) to 8.2% (aspirin-clopidogrel group) with no significant difference in haemorrhagic stroke. A 300-mg loading dose of clopidogrel was used in this trial. The POINT trial [37] in patients with TIA or minor ischaemic stroke (NIHSS 0–3) demonstrated that dual antiplatelet therapy started within 12 h of onset and continued for 90 days resulted in a significant reduction of ischaemic stroke from 6.5% (aspirin group) to 5.0% (aspirin-clopidogrel group). Pooled analysis of these trials demonstrated the benefit of dual antiplatelet therapy up to at least 21 days. The THALES trial [38], showed in patients with a high-risk TIA or minor ischaemic stroke (NIHSS 0–5) that dual antiplatelet therapy with aspirin and ticagrelor started within 24 h of onset resulted in a significant reduction in composite outcome of stroke or death from 6.6% (aspirin group) to 5.5% (aspirin-ticagrelor group) within 30 days. Severe bleeding was more frequent with ticagrelor with an absolute risk increase of 0.4% in these three trials.

3.13 Clopidogrel Resistance

A substantial proportion of patients with TIA and stroke in some populations may be resistant to clopidogrel. Clopidogrel resistance and non-responsiveness is linked to a genetic polymorphism in the cytochrome *CYP2C19* loss-of-function allele. Ticagrelor is not affected. The CHANCE 2 trial [39] in a cohort of Chinese patients with this genetic profile showed that the risk of ischaemic stroke was significantly reduced from 7.6% in patients treated with clopidogrel for 90 days) plus aspirin for 21 days to 6.0% in those randomised to ticagrelor for 90 days plus aspirin for 21 days. On the basis of this evidence, the UK National Clinical Stroke Guidelines [12] make the following recommendations:

- For patients within 24 h of onset of TIA or minor ischaemic stroke and with a low risk of bleeding, the following dual antiplatelet therapy should be given: Clopidogrel (initial dose 300 mg followed by 75 mg/day) plus aspirin (initial dose 300 mg followed by 75 mg/day for 21 days) followed by monotherapy with clopidogrel 75 mg once daily OR Ticagrelor (initial dose 180 mg followed by 90 mg twice daily) plus aspirin (300 mg followed by 75 mg daily for 30 days) followed by antiplatelet monotherapy with ticagrelor 90 mg twice daily or clopidogrel 75 mg once daily at the discretion of the prescriber;
- For patients with TIA or minor ischaemic stroke who are not appropriate for dual antiplatelet therapy, clopidogrel 300 mg loading dose followed by 75 mg daily should be given;
- A proton pump inhibitor should be considered for concurrent use with dual antiplatelet therapy to reduce the risk of gastrointestinal haemorrhage;
- For patients with recurrent TIA or stroke while taking clopidogrel, consideration should be given to the possibility of clopidogrel resistance.

3.14 Management of Cerebral Oedema and Malignant Middle Cerebral Artery (MCA) Syndrome

Extensive cerebral ischaemia, particularly in the middle cerebral artery territory is sometimes associated with the development of severe cerebral oedema resulting in raised intracranial pressure and the risk of causing further neurological damage or death through coning of the brain through the foramen magnum. Cerebral oedema is one of two sorts; cytotoxic oedema which is what is seen after cerebral ischaemia and vasogenic which is typically seen associated with cerebral tumours. Vasogenic oedema often responds dramatically to steroids but this is not the case with cytotoxic oedema. Many centres use mannitol and or steroids to reduce the risk of developing oedema or to try and mitigate its effects when it occurs. Unfortunately, neither of these drugs has been shown to be effective and steroids could increase cerebral damage through its effect on glucose metabolism. A Cochrane review [40] of the mannitol trials concludes that the studies have all had methodological flaws and there is a case for better conducted and powered research but in the meantime it is not recommended that it is used outside of a trial setting.

Malignant MCA syndrome if left untreated is usually fatal or results in very profound long-term disability. The Cochrane review of trials of hemicraniectomy which were all done on patients under the age of 60 years [41] showed significant benefits although many patients still had severe residual disability. The DESTINY II trial Jüttler et al. [42] of decompressive hemicraniectomy for older patients with severe space-occupying MCA territory infarction showed a substantial survival benefit for patients over the age of 60 years similar to that seen in the young patients. Decisions to undertake major life-saving surgery need to be carefully considered on an individual basis, but patients should not be excluded from treatment by age alone. The guidelines recommendations are:

- Patients with middle cerebral artery (MCA) infarction who meet the criteria below should be considered for decompressive hemicraniectomy. Patients should be referred to neurosurgery within 24 h of stroke onset and treated within 48 h of stroke onset:
  - pre-stroke mRS score of 0 or 1;
  - clinical deficits indicating infarction of the MCA
  - an NIHSS score of more than 15
  - a decrease in the level of consciousness to a score of 1 or more on item 1a of the NIHSS;
  - signs on brain imaging of an infarct of at least 50% of the MCA territory with or without additional infarction in the territory of the anterior or posterior cerebral artery on the same side, or infarct volume greater than 145 mL.

3.15 Case 1

A 35-year-old Polish man was admitted to hospital having been previously fit and independent. He had collapsed with right sided weakness. Admission CT showed early signs of left MCA territory infarction with a hyperdense artery. The admission occurred before the evidence for ET had been published and facilities for thrombectomy were not available at the admitting hospital. Over the first 12 h in hospital, he deteriorated with reduced conscious level and the development of epileptic seizures.

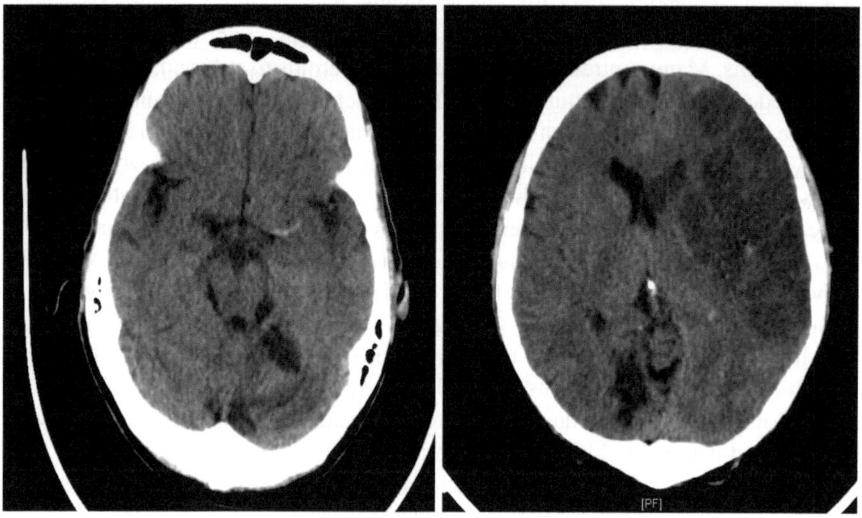

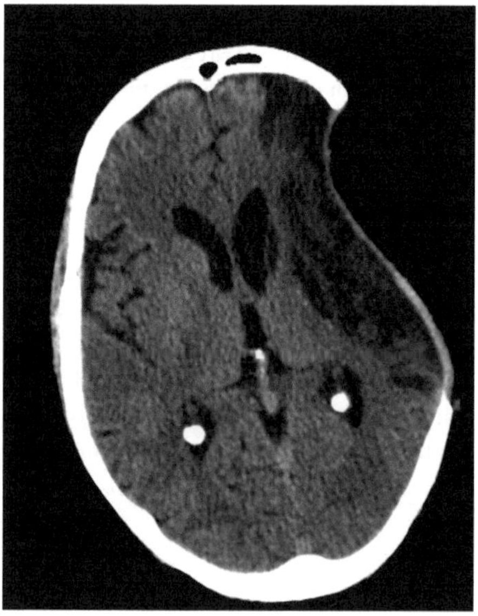

Scans showing the initial hyperdense left MCA and the signs of extensive MCA territory infarction. The final scan was done after removal of a bone flat.

In the weeks after surgery, the patient improved and was discharged from hospital after 3 months able to walk short distances but with a paretic arm and moderate motor and sensory aphasia.

3.16 Venous Stroke or Cerebral Venous Thrombosis

Cerebral venous thrombosis (CVT) is the cause of between 0.5 and 0.7% of strokes but is more common among young people, especially women. Classic presenting features include headache, seizures, and focal neurological deficits. Risk factors include a prothrombotic tendency such as haematological disorders, pregnancy, dehydration and malignancy. It is often diagnosed late because of a lack of clinical suspicion and that it can often be missed on brain imaging unless specific venous phase images are requested. Case series suggest that anticoagulation is the treatment of choice for CVT, even when haemorrhage is seen on brain imaging, with a reduction in death and dependency [43]. A Cochrane review by Coutinho et al. [44] identified two small trials of anticoagulation after CVT. Although not reaching statistical significance, there was a trend towards a positive benefit from anticoagulation for at least three months.

The UK National Clinical Guidelines make the following recommendations:

- Any patient suspected of cerebral venous thrombosis should be investigated with CT or MRI including venography.
- Patients with cerebral venous thrombosis (including those with secondary cerebral haemorrhage) should receive full-dose anticoagulation (initially full-dose heparin and then warfarin with a target INR of 2–3) for at least three months unless there are comorbidities that preclude their use.

3.17 End-of-Life Care for Devastating Stroke

Between 5 and 10% of patients admitted to hospital with stroke will have such severe haemorrhage or infarction that death is inevitable regardless of what treatment is given. In the UK about 14% of patients will die in hospital. High quality stroke care includes recognising when death is inevitable and then providing high quality palliative care aiming to treat symptoms effectively even if this means shortening life expectancy. There are major cultural differences in the way that dying patients are managed between countries but the basic principles should be the same. No patients should suffer unnecessarily when they are dying. Everything should be done to ensure that their last days are spent as comfortably both physically and mentally as possible. To deliver good care requires a multidisciplinary team including specialist palliative care physicians and nurses, stroke physicians and nurses and therapists. The views of the patient and their family must guide care. Many patients express the preference to die at home rather than in hospital and this should be accommodated wherever possible. The range of symptoms that need to be addressed include pain, depression, anxiety, nausea, and confusion. Hunger is rarely an issue and so long as mouth care is good thirst is also usually not a problem even when the decision has been made to withdraw food and liquids. Even when there is a risk of aspiration from dysphagia patients should be offered oral nutrition and hydration. Once it is decided that death is inevitable, it is rarely appropriate to continue with intravenous, nasogastric or gastrostomy feeding and hydration. Three good articles are recommended reading for this topic [45–47].

The UK National guidelines make the following recommendations:

- Services providing acute and long-term care for people with stroke should provide high quality end-of-life care for those who need it.
- Staff caring for people dying of stroke should be trained in the principles and practice of end-of-life care, including the recognition of people who are approaching the end of life.
- Decisions to withhold or withdraw life-prolonging treatments after stroke including artificial nutrition, and hydration should whenever possible take the persons prior expressed wishes and preferences into account and should be taken in the best interests of that person.
- People with stroke with limited life expectancy, and their family where appropriate, should be offered advance care planning, with access to specialist inpatient and community palliative care services when needed.

References

1. Bhalla A, Rudd AG, Wolfe CDA. The influence of raised plasma osmolality on clinical outcome after acute stroke. Stroke. 2000;31:2043–8.
2. Eizenberg Y, et al. Admission hydration status and ischemic strokeoutcome—experience from a national registry of hospitalized stroke patients. J Clin Med. 2021;10:3292.
3. Lin CJ, et al. Favorable outcome of blood urea nitrogen/creatinine-based hydration therapy 3 months after acute ischemic stroke. Am J Emerg Med. 2016;34(12):2414–8.
4. Bray BD, Ayis S, Campbell J, Hoffman A, Roughton M, Tyrrell PJ, Wolfe CD, Rudd AG. Associations between the organisation of stroke services, process of care, and mortality in England: prospective cohort study. BMJ. 2013;346:f2827.
5. Roffe C, Ali K, Warusevitane A, Sills S, et al. The SOS pilot study: a RCT of routine oxygen supplementation early after acute stroke–effect on recovery of neurological function at one week. PLoS One. 2011;6(5):e19113. https://doi.org/10.1371/journal.pone.0019113.
6. Mahmood A, Neilson S, Biswas V, et al. Normobaric oxygen therapy in acute stroke: a systematic review and meta-analysis. Cerebrovasc Dis. 2022;51(4):427–37. https://doi.org/10.1159/000521027.
7. Bennett MH, Weibel S, Wasiak J, et al. Hyperbaric oxygen therapy for acute ischaemic stroke. Cochrane Database Syst Rev. 2014;11:CD004954.

8. Bath PM, Krishnan K. Interventions for deliberately altering blood pressure in acute stroke. Cochrane Database Syst Rev. 2014;3:CD000039.
9. Appleton P, et al. Blood pressure management in acute stroke. Stroke Vasc Neurol. 2016;1:e000020.
10. Fang J, Chen C, Cheng H, et al. Effect of paracetamol (acetaminophen) on body temperature in acute stroke: a meta-analysis. Am J Emerg Med. 2017;35(10):1530–5.
11. Gray CS, Hildreth AJ, Sandercock PA, et al. Glucose-potassium-insulin infusions in the management of post-stroke hyperglycaemia: the UK Glucose Insulin in Stroke Trial (GIST-UK). Lancet Neurol. 2007;6(5):397–406.
12. National Clinical Guidelines for Stroke for the United Kingdom and Ireland. 2023. https://www.strokeguideline.org.
13. Martino R, Foley N, Bhogal S, Diamant N, Speechley M, Teasell R. Dysphagia after stroke: incidence, diagnosis, and pulmonary complications. Stroke. 2005;36(12):2756–63.
14. Bray BD, Smith CJ, Cloud GC, Enderby P, James M, Paley L, et al. The association between delays in screening for and assessing dysphagia after acute stroke, and the risk of stroke-associated pneumonia. J Neurol Neurosurg Psychiatry. 2017;88(1):25–30.
15. Olavarria VV, Arima H, Anderson CS, et al. Head position and cerebral blood flow velocity in acute ischemic stroke: a systematic review and meta-analysis. Cerebrovasc Dis. 2014;37(6):401–8.
16. Anderson CS, Arima H, Lavados P, Billot L, Hackett ML, Olavarría VV, et al. Cluster-randomized, crossover trial of head positioning in acute stroke. N Engl J Med. 2017;376(25):2437–47.
17. Berge E, Whiteley W, Audebert H, et al. European Stroke Organisation (ESO) guidelines on intravenous thrombolysis for acute ischaemic stroke. Eur Stroke J. 2021;6(1):I-LXII.
18. Wardlaw JM, Murray V, Berge E, del Zoppo G, Sandercock P, Lindley RL, et al. Recombinant tissue plasminogen activator for acute ischaemic stroke: an updated systematic review and meta-analysis. Lancet. 2012;379(9834):2364–72.
19. Emberson J, Lees KR, Lyden P, Blackwell L, Albers G, Bluhmki E, et al. Effect of treatment delay, age, and stroke severity on the effects of intravenous thrombolysis with alteplase for acute ischaemic stroke: a meta-analysis of individual patient data from randomised trials. Lancet. 2014;384(9958):1929–35.
20. National Institute of Neurological Disorders and Stroke rt-PA Stroke Study Group. Tissue plasminogen activator for acute ischemic stroke. N Engl J Med. 1995;333(24):1581–7.
21. Anderson CS, Robinson T, Lindley RI, et al. Low-dose versus standard-dose intravenous alteplase in acute ischemic stroke. N Engl J Med. 2016;374(24):2313–23.
22. Bala F, et al. Safety and efficacy of tenecteplase compared with alteplase in patients with large vessel occlusion stroke: a prespecified secondary analysis of the ACT randomized clinical trial. JAMA Neurol. 2023;80(8):824–32.
23. Huang X, Cheripelli BK, Lloyd SM, Kalladka D, Moreton FC, Siddiqui A, et al. Alteplase versus tenecteplase for thrombolysis after ischaemic stroke (ATTEST): a phase 2, randomised, open-label, blinded endpoint study. Lancet Neurol. 2015;14(4):368–76.
24. Bivard A, Zhao H, Churilov L, et al. Comparison of tenecteplase with alteplase for the early treatment of ischaemic stroke in the Melbourne Mobile Stroke Unit (TASTE-A): a phase 2, randomised, open-label trial. Lancet Neurol. 2022;21(6):520–7.
25. Goyal M, Menon BK, van Zwam WH, et al. Endovascular thrombectomy after large vessel ischaemic stroke: a meta-analysis of individual patient data from five randomised trials. Lancet. 2016;387:1723–31.
26. Nogueira RG, Jadhav AP, Haussen DC, et al. Thrombectomy 6 to 24 hours after stroke with a mismatch between deficit and infarct. N Engl J Med. 2018;378(1):11–21.
27. Albers GW, Marks MP, Kemp S, et al. Thrombectomy for stroke at 6 to 16 hours with selection by perfusion imaging. N Engl J Med. 2018;378(8):708–18.
28. Langezaal LCM, van der Hoeven EJRJ, Mont'Alverne FJ, et al. Endovascular therapy for stroke due to basilar-artery occlusion. N Engl J Med. 2021;384(20):1910–20.

29. Jovin TG, Li C, Wu L, et al. Trial of thrombectomy 6 to 24 hours after stroke due to basilar-artery occlusion. N Engl J Med. 2022;387(15):1373–84.
30. Tao C, Nogueira RG, Zhu Y, et al. Trial of endovascular treatment of acute basilar-artery occlusion. N Engl J Med. 2022;387(15):1361–72.
31. Qureshi AI, Lodhi A, Akhtar IN, Ma X, Kherani D, Kwok CS, Ford DE, Hanley DF, Hassan AE, Nguyen TN, Spiotta AM, Zaidi SF. Mechanical thrombectomy with intra-arterial thrombolysis versus mechanical thrombectomy alone in patients with acute ischemic stroke: a systematic review and meta-analysis. Int J Stroke. 2024;19(1):16–28.
32. Turc G, Tsivgoulis G, Audebert HJ, Boogaarts H, Bhogal P, De Marchis GM, et al. European Stroke Organisation (ESO)-European Society for Minimally Invasive Neurological Therapy (ESMINT) expedited recommendation on indication for intravenous thrombolysis before mechanical thrombectomy in patients with acute ischemic stroke and anterior circulation large vessel occlusion. J Neurointerv Surg. 2022;14(3):209.
33. Sentinel Stroke National Audit Programme. 2023. https://www.strokeaudit.org/.
34. Ramsay AIG, Morris S, Hoffman A, et al. Effects of centralizing acute stroke services on stroke care provision in two large metropolitan areas in England. Stroke. 2015;46:2244–51. https://doi.org/10.1161/STROKEAHA.115.009723.
35. Hill MD, et al. Efficacy and safety of nerinetide for the treat- ment of acute ischaemic stroke (ESCAPE-NA1): a multicentre, double-blind, randomised controlled trial. Lancet. 2020;395:878–87.
36. Wang Y, Wang Y, Zhao X, Liu L, Wang D, Wang C, et al. Clopidogrel with aspirin in acute minor stroke or transient ischemic attack. N Engl J Med. 2013;369(1):11–9.
37. Johnston SC, Easton JD, Farrant M, Barsan W, Conwit RA, Elm JJ, et al. Clopidogrel and aspirin in acute ischemic stroke and high-risk TIA. N Engl J Med. 2018;379(3):215–25.
38. Johnston SC, Amarenco P, Denison H, Evans SR, Himmelmann A, James S, et al. Ticagrelor and aspirin or aspirin alone in acute ischemic stroke or TIA. N Engl J Med. 2020;383(3):207–17.
39. Wang Y, Meng X, Wang A, Xie X, Pan Y, Johnston SC, et al. Ticagrelor versus clopidogrel in CYP2C19 loss-of-function carriers with stroke or TIA. N Engl J Med. 2021;385(27):2520–30.
40. Bereczki D, Fekete I, Prado GF, Liu M. Mannitol for acute stroke. Cochrane Database Syst Rev. 2007;3:CD001153. https://doi.org/10.1002/14651858.CD001153.pub2. PMID: 17636655; PMCID: PMC7032636.
41. Cruz-Flores S, Berge E, Whittle IR. Surgical decompression for cerebral oedema in acute ischaemic stroke. Cochrane Database Syst Rev. 2012;1:CD003435.
42. Jüttler E, Unterberg A, Woitzik J, Bosel J, Amiri H, Sakowitz OW, et al. Hemicraniectomy in older patients with extensive middle-cerebral-artery stroke. N Engl J Med. 2014;370(12):1091–100.
43. Stam J, De Bruijn SF, DeVeber G. Anticoagulation for cerebral sinus thrombosis. Cochrane Database Syst Rev. 2002;4:CD002005.
44. Coutinho J, de Bruijn SF, Deveber G, Stam J. Anticoagulation for cerebral venous sinus thrombosis. Cochrane Database Syst Rev. 2011;8:CD002005.
45. Steigleder T, Kollmar R, Ostgathe C. Palliative care for stroke patients and their families: barriers for implementation. Front Neurol. 2019;10:164. https://doi.org/10.3389/fneur.2019.00164. PMID: 30894836; PMCID: PMC6414790.
46. Gardiner C, Harrison M, Ryan T, Jones A. Provision of palliative and end-of-life care in stroke units: a qualitative study. Palliat Med. 2013;27(9):855–60.
47. Payne S, Burton C, AddingtonHall J, Jones A. End-of-life issues in acute stroke care: a qualitative study of the experiences and preferences of patients and families. Palliat Med. 2010;24(2):146–53.

Further Reading

Bhalla A, Patel M, Birns J. An update on hyper-acute management of ischaemic stroke. Clin Med. 2021;21:215–21.

National Clinical Guidelines for Stroke for the United Kingdom and Ireland 2023. https://www.strokeguideline.org

Venturelli PM, Appleton JP, Anderson CS, Bath PM. Acute treatment of stroke (except thrombectomy). Curr Neurol Neurosci Rep. 2018;18:77.

Chapter 4
Management of Haemorrhagic Stroke

Ngoc Huy Nguyen, Anthony Rudd, and Khanh Minh Tran

4.1 Introduction

Data are limited but it is evident that the incidence of primary intracerebral haemorrhage in Vietnam is much higher than in the USA and Europe. Venketasubramanian et al. [1] in a paper looking at stroke epidemiology in South Asia quoted a figure of haemorrhage being responsible for 47% of incident stroke. In 2016, a study from central Vietnam by Yamanashi et al. [2] called a population based study, although based only on hospital admissions gave a figure of about 38%. These figures compare with rates of 10–15% of strokes being due to haemorrhage in the UK [3]. The explanation for the difference is not known but may indicate the high prevalence and poor management of hypertension in these regions. Regional, cultural and dietary variations, such as increased salt and saturated fats use in these countries, could also be contributory as well as possible genetic factors.

The management of patients with stroke due to intracerebral haemorrhage (ICH) is different to ischaemic stroke and it is therefore essential that the diagnosis is made very rapidly after presentation so that the correct treatment can be implemented.

N. H. Nguyen (✉)
Phutho Department of Health, Phutho, Vietnam

VNU University of Medicine and Pharmacy, Hanoi, Vietnam
e-mail: ngochuynguyen8888@gmail.com

A. Rudd
King's College, London, UK

K. M. Tran
Phutho Department of Health, Phutho, Vietnam

A. Rudd et al. (eds.), *Stroke Management in Vietnam*,
https://doi.org/10.1007/978-981-96-0221-6_4

4.2 Clinical Features of ICH

It is not possible to diagnose ICH clinically with sufficient accuracy and therefore brain imaging is essential. Sudden onset headache at the same time or before the onset of the neurological symptoms, neck stiffness, vomiting and clouding of consciousness are all more likely in ICH than in ischaemic stroke. But equally ICH, especially small deep haemorrhages can just present with sudden onset focal neurological signs. And increasingly with increased access to MRI we are seeing patients with extensive microbleeds who have never presented with any neurological symptoms. About 85% of patients with ICH have an underlying structural abnormality such as an arteriovenous malformation or a cavernoma. By far, the most important risk factor is hypertension which typically causes bleeding from the deep perforating vessels resulting in deep haematomas, often in the basal ganglia or internal capsule. Elderly patients with large lobar haemorrhages may have underlying amyloid angiopathy. These patients have a high risk of rebleeding with between a 10% and 26% rebleeding risk annually.

4.3 Imaging

While MRI gives better information about the underlying cause of a haemorrhage than CT in the acute phase, the majority of patients will have a non contrast scan because it is easier and cheaper for both the hospital and the patient. It is very sensitive identifying haemorrhage although care does need to be taken where there are just small amounts of subarachnoid blood and where there is just a small amount of interventricular blood. The scan should try to identify:

- Is there haemorrhage and if so how much and where is it situated? Is it lobar or deep?
- Is there an underlying cause such as an arteriovenous malformation, primary or secondary malignancy or a cavernoma?
- Could the cause be due to a venous thrombosis?
- Are the images consistent with a vasculitis?
- How much background small vessel disease is there?
- Are there any signs which would indicate an increased likelihood of rebleeding such as the spot sign (Fig. 4.3) on angiography?

4.4 Typical Brain Imaging Features

Figures 4.1 and 4.2 illustrate the two typical types of primary intracerebral haemorrhage, basal ganglia bleed and lobar haemorrhage. Figure 4.3 illustrates the spot sign which can be predictive of recurrent bleeding. Figure 4.4 shows a typical bleed

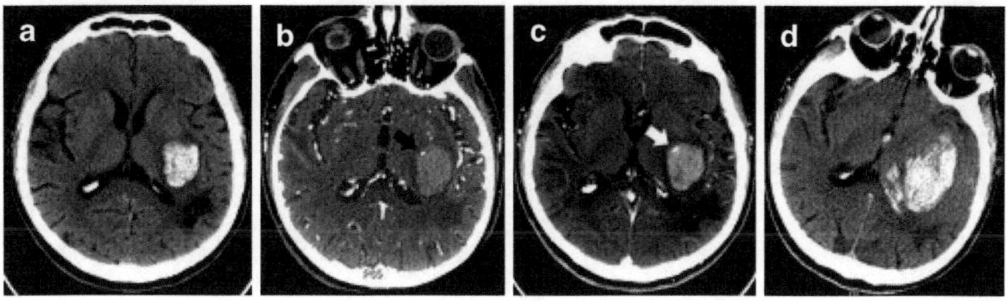

Fig. 4.3 Spot sign on CT angiogram, taken from the original paper Wada et al. [4]. (**a**) Unenhanced CT demonstrates left posterior putaminal and internal capsule hematoma with mild surrounding oedema. An old parieto-occipital infarct is seen posterior to this. (**b**) A small focus of enhancement is seen peripherally on CTA source images, consistent with the spot sign (black arrow). (**c**) Postcontrast CT demonstrates enlargement of the spot sign, consistent with extravasation (white arrow). (**d**) Unenhanced CT image 1 day after presentation reveals hematoma enlargement and intraventricular haemorrhage

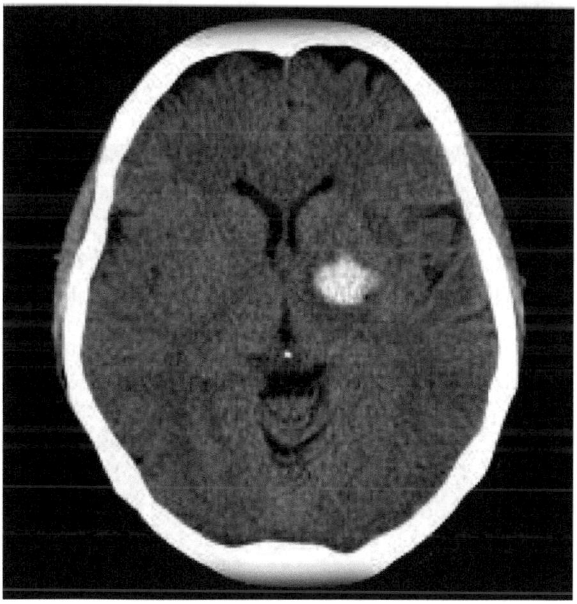

Fig. 4.1 Left basal ganglia haemorrhage secondary to hypertension in a 65-year-old man

secondary to an arteriovenous malformation and Fig. 4.5 a bleed secondary to a cavernoma. Figure 4.6 shows how haemorrhage in a patient on an anticoagulant can progress unless it is possible to reverse the anticoagulant rapidly.

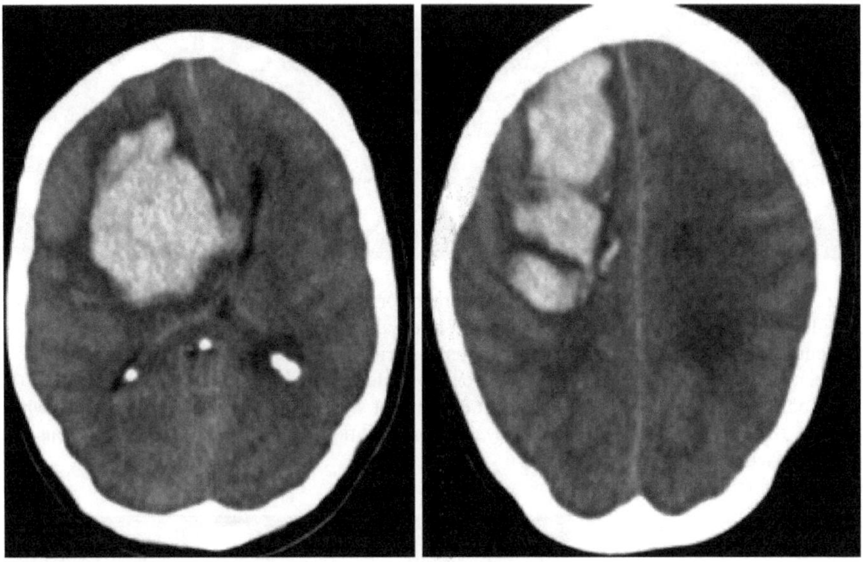

Fig. 4.2 Lobar haemorrhage in an 87-year-old woman; likely cause amyloid angiopathy

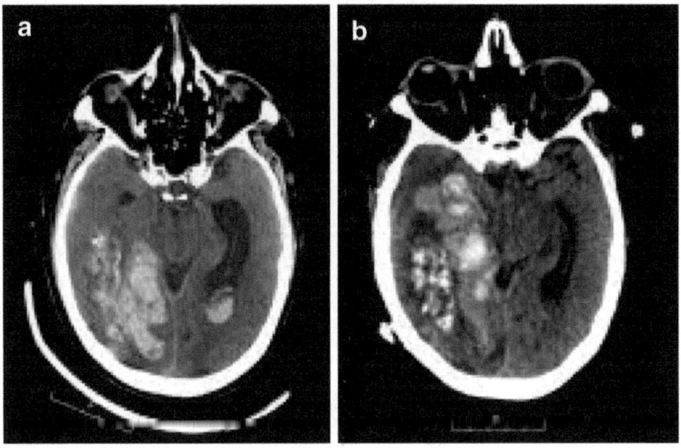

Fig. 4.4 Haemorrhage secondary to an AVM

4.5 Organisation of Care

ICH should be treated as a medical emergency, even in patients where the initial neurological deficit is small as there is a high risk of subsequent deterioration. Only a small proportion of patients will require surgery to evacuate the haematoma and our preference is for the patients to be initially managed on the stroke unit or if very severely ill with respiratory compromise on an intensive care unit. Both of these

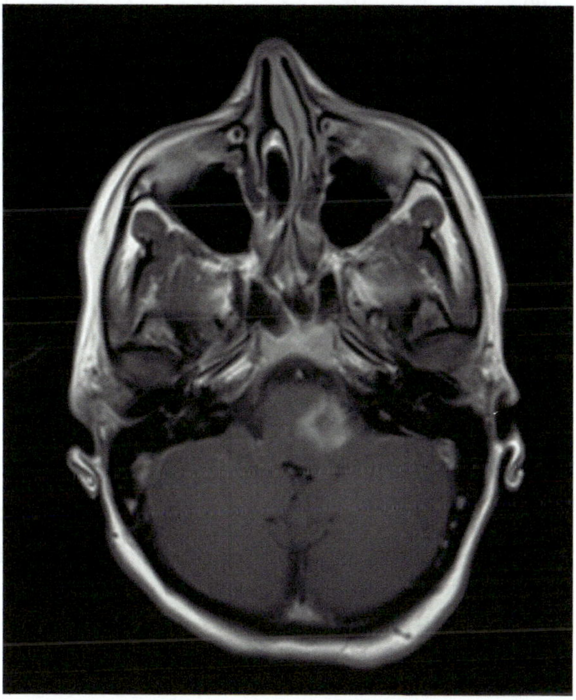

Fig. 4.5 Brainstem cavernoma in a 17-year-old woman

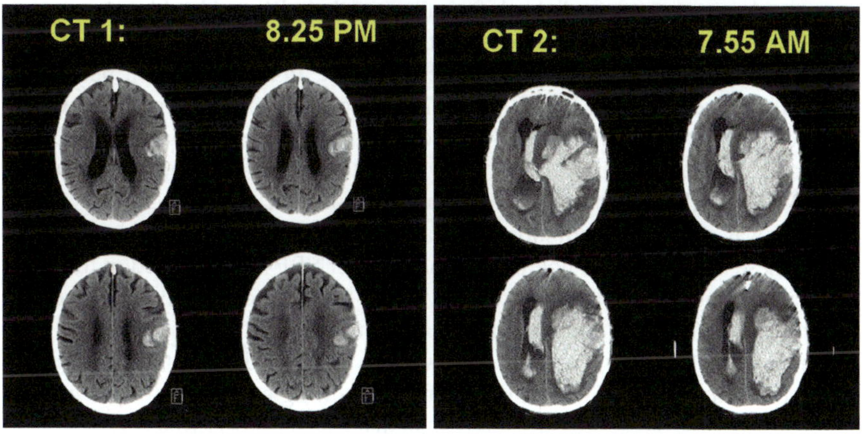

Fig. 4.6 Progression of an ICH ion a patient admitted on rivaroxaban

'medical' settings are likely to be better equipped to identify neurological deterioration early and also to have ready access to the full multidisciplinary team including physicians, nurses and therapists. If surgical intervention is then needed the patient can then be rapidly transferred to the operating theatre or neurosurgical unit. INTERACT3 [5] was a multicentre cluster randomised trial that enrolled more than

7000 patients from 10 countries that tested whether a bundle of care that involved early lowering of blood pressure, strict glucose control, anti-pyrexia treatment and rapid reversal of warfarin anticoagulation compared to standard care. The likelihood of poor functional outcome at 6 months was significantly reduced in the intervention group (OR 0.86 95%CI 0.76–0.97). This is an important study confirming that ICH is treatable provided it is treated as a medical emergency and all the components of care are delivered effectively.

4.6 Medical Management

4.6.1 *Blood Pressure Control*

The majority of patients with ICH will have prior hypertension and even those who do not may have had it undiagnosed or else have acutely raised blood pressure associated with the bleeding, as also happens with cerebral infarction. Whether and when blood pressure should be treated remains a difficult issue. The effect of reducing blood pressure in the first few hours after the onset of ICH has been evaluated in two multicentre RCTs. In INTERACT-2 [6], the rapid lowering of systolic blood pressure (SBP) to a target below 140 mmHg within 1 h in 2839 patients presenting within 6 hours of onset with mainly small, deep ICH did not reduce haematoma expansion or improve the primary outcome of death or major disability (mRS 3–6), but secondary outcomes (ordinal shift analysis of the mRS and health-related quality of life measures) were improved. Death (12% at 3 months) and institutionalisation (9%) were not affected by intensive treatment. In ATACH-2 [7], pursuing a lower SBP target of 110–139 mmHg within 2 h in 1000 patients presenting within 4.5 h of onset with small, deep ICH tended to reduce haematoma expansion but conferred no reduction in severe disability or death (mRS 4–6) compared to a target of 140–179 mmHg. Mortality (6.7%) was also not affected. More intensive SBP lowering was associated with more renal adverse events in the first 7 days. In comparing these two trials, it is noteworthy that a lower SBP was achieved in the acute phase in the standard treatment arm of ATACH-2 (all of whom received intravenous nicardipine) than in the intensive treatment arm of INTERACT2 (141 mmHg vs 150 mmHg, respectively). As the intensive arm of ATACH-2 led to a still greater SBP reduction, ATACH-2 can be interpreted as showing no additional benefit from a more aggressive blood pressure target than that tested in INTERACT2.

The evidence is therefore difficult to interpret and to draw conclusions. The UK National Clinical Guidelines [8] conclude that:

- Patients with acute spontaneous intracerebral haemorrhage with a systolic BP of 150–220 mmHg should be considered for urgent treatment within 6 h of symptom onset using a locally agreed protocol for BP lowering, aiming to achieve a systolic BP between 130 and 139 mmHg within one hour and sustained for at least 7 days, unless:

- The Glasgow Coma Scale is 5 or less;
- the haematoma is very large and death is expected;
- a macrovascular or structural cause for the haematoma is identified;
- immediate surgery to evacuate the haematoma is planned, in which case BP should be managed according to a locally agreed protocol.

The evidence largely applies to patients with deep haematomas. More research is need for all groups of patients but particularly those with lobar haemorrhages.

4.6.2 Haemorrhage Associated with Anticoagulants and Antiplatelet Treatment

Haemorrhage associated with anticoagulant use has a poor prognosis. About 15% of patients admitted with ICH in the UK have been taking either warfarin or one of the Direct Oral Anticoagulants (DOAC). It is vital that a drug history is obtained from the patient or relative and if not available then check clotting studies. The risk of haemorrhage is slightly lower with DOAC's than warfarin and the prognosis slightly better, but both are significantly worse than haemorrhage in patients not anticoagulated. Reversal of the agent where there is one available is urgent and systems should be in place in all hospitals for rapid testing (preferably near patient testing) and then rapid access to the antidotes. Patients with intracerebral haemorrhage in association with vitamin K antagonist treatment and with an INR of 1.4 or greater should have the anticoagulant reversed with a combination of prothrombin complex concentrate and intravenous vitamin K. Patients with intracerebral haemorrhage in association with direct oral anticoagulant. Patients taking dabigatran should receive idarucizumab. If idarucizumab is not available, 4-factor prothrombin complex concentrate may be considered. For those taking oral factor Xa inhibitors, it was reported at the World Stroke Organisation conference in 2023, although not yet published, that the trial of andexanet alfa was terminated early because of strongly favourable results. The ANNEXa-I [9] multicentre cohort open label study randomised 452 patients within 6 h of onset and within 15 h of taking either rivaroxaban, apixaban, or edoxaban. Excellent or good homeostasis was achieved in 63.9% of patients taking the andexanet compared to 52.4% of those on placebo. There were more thrombotic events in the treatment group and no functional outcome data were presented. It will be important to review all these data before use becomes routine.

About a quarter of patients admitted with ICH are taking antiplatelet agents and they have a worse outcome than those not taking them. This could, however, be in part due to the comorbidities associated with taking the antiplatelet drug in the first place. The drug should be stopped. A small trial of giving platelet transfusion showed worse outcomes in the treatment group.

4.6.3 *Tranexamic Acid*

The TICH-2 trial [10] tested whether tranexamic acid as a haemostatic agent could reduce the risk of rebleeding after ICH. This larger trial involving 2325 patients was negative for the primary outcome measure of functional status at 90 days although it did reduce 7 day mortality but not 90 day. Its use cannot be recommended at the moment.

4.6.4 *Surgery*

The benefits for surgery after ICH until recently has been uncertain following the negative trials coordinated by Mendelow et al from the UK (STICH) [11] involving craniotomy and minimally invasive surgery MISTIE III [12] with catheter drainage and the frequent instillation of a lytic in a delayed time window. Both these studies were based on the belief that intervention should be undertaken when both the haematoma and the clinical status of the patient were stable. The results of the Early Minimally Invasive Removal of Intracerebral Hemorrhage (ENRICH) trial [13, 14] were first reported at the 2023 annual meeting of the American Association of Neurological Surgeons, but the full results are, as yet, unpublished. ENRICH was undertaken at 37 hospitals in the USA and showed, for the first time, that functional recovery can be improved by surgical evacuation of the haematoma within 24 h of symptom onset. 300 patients were enrolled, including 93 (31%) with deep haematomas and 207 (69%) with lobar hemisphere haematomas. The primary endpoint at 6 months was the modified Rankin score, which was 0.46 for minimally invasive surgery and 0.37 for the non-surgery control (difference 0.084). The success of ENRICH may be attributed to the microinvasive endoscopic aspiration technique, which enabled the surgeon to perform early (median 17 h after symptom onset), and almost complete evacuation of the haematoma (volumes 30–80 mL) while also terminating any active bleeding. We await publication of the full results.

Where haemorrhage is in the posterior fossa causing raised intracranial pressure then evacuation and or shunting will be required. The same applies to hydrocephalus resulting from intraventricular haemorrhage.

4.7 Management of Complications

4.7.1 *Seizures*

The risk of seizures is high at about 10% after ICH. Prophylactic use of anticonvulsants is not advised because it is not known if the benefits outweigh the side effect of increased sedation. Clinicians need to be aware that seizures can be relatively hidden, just causing lowered conscious level, without evident convulsions. Where early seizures do occur treatment with an anticonvulsant for 3–6 months is recommended. Where the seizures occur late, they are likely to persist long term and therefore treatment should be continued indefinitely.

4.7.2 Venous Thrombosis Prevention

Anticoagulants, even low dose low molecular weight heparin (LMWH) used as prophylaxis against deep venous thrombosis (DVT) is likely to increase the risk of rebleeding after ICH. However, the risk of DVT and pulmonary embolism is high in immobile patients with hemiparetic limbs. The CLOTS3 trial [15] showed that intermittent pneumatic compression is an effective way of preventing DVT and should be used in preference to LMWH in both ICH and ischaemic stroke where there is a risk of haemorrhagic transformation of the infarct. The trials of compression stocKing's showed that they were ineffective or maybe even harmful [16].

References

1. Venketasubramanian N, Yoon BW, Pandian J, Navarro JC. Stroke epidemiology in South, East, and South-East Asia: a review. J Stroke. 2017;19(3):286–94.
2. Yamanashi H, Ngoc MQ, Huy TV, et al. Population-based incidence rates of first-ever stroke in Central Vietnam. PLoS One. 2016;11(8):e0160665.
3. Sentinel Stroke National Audit Programme. 2023. https://www.strokeaudit.org/.
4. Wada R, Aviv RI, Fox AJ, Sahlas DJ, Gladstone DJ, Tomlinson G, Symons SP. CT angiography "spot sign" predicts hematoma expansion in acute intracerebral hemorrhage. Stroke. 2007;38(4):1257–62.
5. Anderson CS. The third intensive care bundle with blood pressure reduction in acute cerebral haemorrhage trial (INTERACT3): an international, stepped wedge cluster randomised controlled trial. Lancet. 2023;402(10395):27–40.
6. Anderson CS, Heeley E, Huang Y, Wang J, Stapf C, Delcourt C, et al. Rapid blood-pressure lowering in patients with acute intracerebral hemorrhage. N Engl J Med. 2013;368(25):2355–65.
7. Qureshi AI, Palesch YY, Barsan WG, Hanley DF, Hsu CY, Martin RL, et al. Intensive blood-pressure lowering in patients with acute cerebral hemorrhage. N Engl J Med. 2016;375(11):1033–43.
8. National Clinical Guidelines for Stroke for the United Kingdom and Ireland. 2023. https://www.strokeguideline.org.
9. Connolly SJ. Randomized trial of andexanet alfa versus usual care in patients with acute intracranial hemorrhage while on an oral factor Xa inhibitor: ANNEXA-I. 15th World Stroke Congress Oct 10–12, 2023.
10. Sprigg N, Flaherty K, Appleton JP, et al. Tranexamic acid for hyperacute primary intra cerebral haemorrhage (TICH-2): an international randomised, placebo-controlled, phase 3 superiority trial. Lancet. 2018;391:2107–15.
11. Mendelow AD, Gregson BA, Fernandes HM, et al. Early surgery versus initial conservative treatment in patients with spontaneous supratentorial intracerebral haematomas in the

International Surgical Trial in Intracerebral Haemorrhage (STICH): a randomised trial. Lancet. 2005;365:387–97.
12. Hanley DF, Thompson RE, Rosenblum M, et al. Efficacy and safety of minimally invasive surgery with thrombolysis in intracerebral haemorrhage evacuation (MISTIE III): a randomised, controlled, open-label, blinded endpoint phase 3 trial. Lancet. 2019;393:1021–32.
13. Ma L, Hu X, Song L, et al. Early minimally invasive removal of intracerebral hemorrhage (ENRICH): study protocol for a multi-centered two-arm randomised adaptive trial. Front Neurol. 2023;14:1126958.
14. Pradilla G. Efficacy and safety of early minimally invasive removal of intracerebral hemorrhage (ENRICH): a multi-centered randomized adaptive trial. 91st AANS Annual Scientific Meeting April 21–24, 2023.
15. Dennis M, Sandercock P, et al. Effectiveness of intermittent pneumatic compression in reduction of risk of deep vein thrombosis in patients who have had a stroke (CLOTS 3): a multicentre randomised controlled trial. Lancet. 2013;382:516–24.
16. Dennis M, Sandercock PA, et al. Effectiveness of thigh-length graduated compression stocK-ing's to reduce the risk of deep vein thrombosis after stroke (CLOTS trial 1): a multicentre, randomised controlled trial. Lancet. 2009;373:1958–65.

Further Reading

Anderson CS. Stroke advances in 2023: a new horizon for the management of intracerebral haemorrhage. Lancet Neurol. 2024;23(1):12–3.

Cordonnier C, Demchuk A, Ziai W, Anderson CS. Intracerebral haemorrhage: current approaches to acute management. Lancet. 2018;392(10154):1257–68. https://doi.org/10.1016/S0140-6736(18)31878-6.

Greenberg SM, Ziai WC, Cordonnier C, et al. American Heart Association/American Stroke Association. 2022 guideline for the management of patients with spontaneous intracerebral hemorrhage: a guideline from the American Heart Association/American Stroke Association. Stroke. 2022;53(7):e282–361.

National Clinical Guidelines for Stroke for the United Kingdom and Ireland. 2023. https://www.strokeguideline.org.

Chapter 5
Rehabilitation of Stroke in Vietnam

Ngoc Huy Nguyen, Thong Van Nguyen, and Tan Van Phung

5.1 Introduction

The majority of people who have a stroke will need some rehabilitation. Up to 20% of patients may be suitable for intravenous thrombolysis acutely but with a number needed to treat to have one good outcome only 3% of stroke admissions will benefit from this treatment. May 10–15% of patients will be eligible for intra-arterial clot retrieval but with a number needed to treat for one good outcome of between 3 and 7, less than 5% of stroke admissions will benefit. Maybe 30% of patients will spontaneously make a good recovery but many of these will still be left with mild impairments both physical and psychological. And 20% of patients will have such severe strokes that they will die. So, for an average stroke population over 60% will have significant residual disability that they will need help recovering from. Rehabilitation services therefore are an essential part of every stroke service that need to be available to patients from the time of admission until discharge from hospital and then continuing in the community. Patients may continue to benefit from treatment for many months after their stroke and for some patients many years.

The evidence base for the efficacy of stroke is now strong in many areas but remains weak in many others. Trials of rehabilitation are much more complex to do

N. H. Nguyen (✉)
Phutho Department of Health, Phutho, Vietnam

VNU University of Medicine and Pharmacy, Hanoi, Vietnam
e-mail: ngochuynguyen8888@gmail.com

T. Van Nguyen
Vietnam Stroke Association, Hanoi, Vietnam

Stroke Center, Phutho General Hospital, Phutho, Vietnam

T. Van Phung
Phutho Department of Health, Phutho, Vietnam

A. Rudd et al. (eds.), *Stroke Management in Vietnam*,
https://doi.org/10.1007/978-981-96-0221-6_5

than drug trials or other acute interventions which is one of the reasons why acquiring the evidence has been slow. But a lack of evidence is not the same as evidence of ineffectiveness. Where there is a lack of evidence, we should be using our clinical experience to decide the best treatment for the person we are treating and where possible entering the patient in to clinical trials that will advance our knowledge for the future.

There are major differences in the way that rehabilitation is delivered in Vietnam both in traditional Vietnamese medical practice and in the 'Western' type of services, compared to the services provided in Europe and North America. The patients do not differ in terms of their disease and their post-stroke needs between Vietnam and other parts of the world, so the different methods of treatment are not justified by the setting or the patients. Studies are needed to establish which of the methods are most effective so that patients worldwide can be confident that they are getting access to the best evidence based care.

5.2 Principles of Rehabilitation

Recovery after stroke can happen in several ways. Neurones that have ceased working due to ischaemia in the area of the stroke termed the ischaemic penumbra, can recover if the cerebral circulation is re-established and the initial damage was not so severe that the neurones have died. There can be neuronal regeneration in the area of the stroke and there can be new axonal connections developed that enable parts of the brain not affected by the stroke to take over some of the lost functions i.e. neuronal plasticity. And then there is adaptive recovery which involves patients learning to change behaviour and find alternative ways to perform tasks that have been affected by the stroke. For example, learning to dress using just one arm. Our understanding of the mechanisms of recovery after stroke is increasing rapidly in part due to access to advanced imaging techniques such as functional MRI and Positron Emission Tomography and also as a result of in vitro techniques looking at mechanisms of neurogenesis. Good reviews of the mechanisms of brain recovery can be found reading Aderinto et al. [1] and Joy et al. [2]. But whatever the mechanism we know that the right staff and environment can influence how well a patient recovers. The human brain is capable of significant recovery after stroke, provided that the appropriate treatments and stimuli are applied in adequate amounts and at the right time.

5.3 Assessment of Function

Measurement of function is essential as a first step in the management of the stroke patient. The World Health Organization classification of functioning, disability and health (ICF) is the most widely accepted structure for examining the consequences of an illness such as stroke [3]. ICF has two parts, each with two components: Part 1 is functioning and disability divided into body functions and structures and secondly, activities and participation. Part 2 describes the contextual factors which are divided into the environmental and personal factors. It is essential to look at all of these factors in order to understand the impact of the stroke on a particular individual that has specific post-stroke impairments in the context of their personality, family network, previous fitness and health and environmental conditions. There are scales that have been developed to measure impairments, ability, participation and quality of life. The choice of scales will depend on what the measurements are being used for. If being used to monitor change then detailed evaluations may be needed in some of the domains. If populations are being followed for monitoring of quality of care or for research then well validated scales that have good inter-rater reliability should be chosen. These would include scales such as the Barthel Index, modified Rankin Score (mRS), Montreal Cognitive Assessment (MoCA), Hospital Anxiety and Depression Score (HAD) and the Short Form 12 (SF12). There are many others to choose from but not all will be suitable for stroke patients, not all will be available in Vietnamese or have been validated in a Vietnamese population.

5.4 Intensity and Duration of Rehabilitation

Recovery from stroke can continue for months or even years after the acute event. Some aspects of function seem to take longer to recover than others. So while the biggest improvements will occur in the early weeks and months further recovery can still occur folr much longer. For example, regaining speech after a stroke causing dysphasia has in our experience frequently continued for years. The key message is that there is huge variability between individuals that will depend on the size and site of the neurological damage, the quality of the brain away from the area of the stroke, the personality of the stroke victim and the quality and quantity of the rehabilitation. Given the variability it is a mistake to try and predict outcome too early in the course of the illness. Labelling someone as having no 'rehabilitation potential' soon after their stroke can become a self-fulfilling prophesy where clinical staff view the patient as untreatable and therefore don't treat them or do so half-heartedly. Likewise, the patient knowing that they are seen as being unlikely to recover will not be motivated to do the hard work necessary to overcome the impairments. However, there does come a time when acceptance that further recovery is not going to occur is important. Patients can put off restarting their lives in the mistaken belief that they will recover function when it would be more beneficial if they could learn to adapt their new situation and find ways around their impairments. Getting the balance right between optimism and realism is difficult, but one of the more important skills needed by rehabilitation staff.

Evidence about how much therapy is needed is scarce. No drug could be introduced into routine practice without being subjected to extensive testing for the best dose range. Enough to be effective but not so much that it is toxic. Very rarely is rehabilitation subjected to such rigorous evaluation. Our suspicion is that the vast majority of patients are given subtherapeutic doses of treatment both in terms of intensity and duration. Some studies have been done that show a clear link between increased intensity and improved outcome. In the UK, a standard has been in place for many years that all patients in hospital as a result of a stroke should receive at least 45 min of each therapy they need, so long as they can tolerate it, each day for 5 days a week. This standard applies to physiotherapy, occupational therapy and speech therapy Even this quite modest standard is often not met although there has been more progress in achieving higher intensity of therapy in some other countries such as Australia and Canada.

An analogy that is useful to use with professionals and patients is with learning new physical and intellectual skills such as developing skill at playing a musical instrument. It takes many hours of repetitive practice over many months or years to become proficient. The person may have a lesson from the teacher each week for perhaps an hour but then if they are to make progress they need to practice very regularly in between with the amount of practice to a large extent determining their success. Stroke patients may not be able physically or intellectually practice on their own, although this should be encouraged where possible, so a mixture of sessions with the therapist and with a therapy assistant to continue the exercises is usually the best arrangement. In the UK, the majority of treatment is given one to one rather than in groups. Again, there has been little research to show whether this is better than group therapy in terms of outcomes or use of scarce resources. One positive outcome from the COVID pandemic was that it was shown to be feasible to provide rehabilitation using telemedicine remotely. This is important particularly for patients after they have left hospital. The highest intensity of rehabilitation tends to occur while the patient is in hospital but as described above this is likely to be only a small period of time relative to the overall period during which recovery will occur. Systems must be in place to enable continued rehabilitation for as long as a patient is benefitting from it wherever they may be living. This can be face to face in the patient's home, as outpatients, in day hospitals or remotely using telemedicine.

5.5 Organization of Rehabilitation Services

In Vietnam, in common with many other countries, rehabilitation after stroke is often delivered by a different team to the one that provides the acute care. While this is understandable because the skills needed are different it can result in a situation where rehabilitation only starts properly when the acute team has finished their work. This is far from ideal as it is important that rehabilitation begins at the beginning of the patient journey. The ideal system is in our view one where the rehabilitation specialists are integrated with the acute team working on the same ward and as part of the multidisciplinary team. Rehabilitation should not just start when the neurologist has become bored with the patient or they have decided that they have done all they can!

Central to effective rehabilitation is teamwork. No one professional will have all the skills necessary to effectively treat a patient comprehensively. Most hospital stroke services will function best if they are delivered in a geographically defined area (see Chap. 16 on stroke units), have a range of staff including physicians with neurological and rehabilitation experience, stroke experienced nurses, physiotherapists, occupational therapists, speech and language therapists, psychologists, dietitians, pharmacists, as well as having access to experts in areas including psychiatry, foot health, orthoptics, orthotics, cardiology and gastro-enterology. The core members of the team should be meeting at least weekly to discuss and formulate plans for each of the patients. The patient's views must be taken into consideration as well as those of the patients family. Clear objectives must be set that are agreed by the whole team and this becomes especially important when it comes to planning for the discharge of the patient from the hospital.

Some patients will be transferred to lower level hospitals for their on-going rehabilitation. Where this happens it is vital that the team that is taking over the care of the patients should be involved in planning the transfer of their care and be provided with comprehensive documentation about the patient. This principal also applies where a patient is being transferred to a community team.

Working as a member of a multidisciplinary team requires special skills and training. An effective team also needs good leadership. This may come from the senior physician but equally there may be another person on the team who has more appropriate skills so the choice of leader should be made based not on a traditional hierarchical system but on one that recognizes where the strengths and weaknesses of the individual members of the team lies.

5.6 Specific Interventions

This chapter cannot cover all aspects of rehabilitation after stroke. Much of the evidence cited below comes from the recently published UK National Clinical Guidelines for Stroke [4], which we would recommend you use to get further information and references. This chapter summarizes interventions for some motor impairments, activities of daily living and communication problems but does not address important aspects of rehabilitation for psychological problems and many other less common issues that arise after stroke. We would highly recommend the textbook Stroke Recovery and Rehabilitation by Zorowitz et al. 2nd edition which although expensive is one of the definitive texts. https://www.springerpub.com/stroke-recovery-and-rehabilitation-9781620700068.html.

5.7 Motor Function

Hemiplegia is one of the most common impairments after a stroke and results in some of the most disabling effects ranging from loss of hand function to immobility and other problems with activities of daily living. Hemiplegia is usually the result of a combination of muscle weakness and changes in muscle tone. The degree of weakness is mainly determined by stroke severity, location and pre-morbid strength. Age and gender are not major factors in determining severity. Strengthening interventions increase strength, improve activity and do not increase spasticity [5], however, selection of appropriate exercises for an individual is important. Almost as important is to maintain and hopefully improve cardiorespiratory fitness through exercise. Low cardiorespiratory fitness can be seen at all times after stroke and can make it difficult for people with stroke to engage in rehabilitation and maintain basic mobility and daily activities [6]. This results in further inactivity, limits participation and increases the risk of recurrent stroke [7]. Cardiorespiratory fitness should therefore be an important target for rehabilitation to both maximize recovery and to reduce the risk of recurrence.

The recommendation from the guidelines is that 'people with weakness after stroke should be taught task-specific, repetitive, intensive exercises or activities to increase their strength. Exercise and repetitive task practice should be the principal rehabilitation approaches, in preference to other therapy approaches'. There is little evidence to show that passive movements or massage of either the arm or leg achieves is useful after stroke apart from preventing stiffness and contractures of the joints. Fitness training should aim to produce greater than 70% of maximum heart rate for 30–40 min, three to five times a week for at least 10 weeks. How this is achieved will depend on what the patient is capable of doing in terms of exercise and what their personal preferences are. But even chair bound patients can undertake fitness training. The evidence is summarized in a 2022 Cochrane review [8]. This provides high level of evidence that all types of exercise are safe and feasible for all stages of stroke recovery in people with all severities of stroke, even those with severe impairments who are unable to walk.

5.8 Arm Function

Approximately, 70% of stroke patients will have some degree of loss of arm function. Recovery can continue for months or years after the acute event so treatment should continue to be offered for as long as a patient is seen to be benefiting but even if treatment is halted continued review is necessary to ensure that the decision was correct and to ensure that the patient does not deteriorate. The objectives of the rehabilitation will vary according to the patient and degree of impairment. For some, the aim will be to regain normal or near normal function. At the other end of the spectrum, the aim may be just to maintain sufficient flexibility of the fingers to enable good hand hygiene.

Recovery of the upper limb is best achieved through training that involves repetition of functional tasks and exercises that follow motor learning principles. Components of functional tasks may be practiced but should then be incorporated into practice of the whole functional task. Training should be supplemented with aids and equipment as necessary to enable safe, intensive and functionally relevant practice. Electrical stimulation can be used as an adjunct to repetitive task practice and there is some evidence to support the use of vagal nerve stimulation [9].

Constraint-induced movement therapy (CIMT) has three components: Intensive graded practice of the paretic arm for 6 h a day for 2 weeks, constraining the non-paretic arm with a mitt to promote use of the weak arm for 90% of waking hours and a transfer training package to learn to use the paretic arm in a real-world environment completing functional tasks [10]. When all three of these components were use some benefit was found in functional outcomes [11].

Robotics are also being used although the evidence to support their use remains thin [12, 13]. They are expensive pieces of equipment but if they replace the need for one to one specialist therapy time then maybe they will be cost effective. More research is needed.

5.9 Balance

This can be a major problem after stroke contributed to by both leg and trunk weakness as well as sensory and cerebellar problems. As with other motor problems, the evidence supports repetitive task practice as the effective way of improving balance [14].

5.10 Independence in Daily Living

Personal activities of daily living (PADL) refer to a range of basic activities such as washing, dressing, bathing, going to the toilet, eating and drinking. These activities usually depend on the ability to transfer and the use of at least one hand. After a stroke PADL can be difficult due to both physical and cognitive impairments. The resultant loss of function can have implications on a person's ability to live independently at home and is therefore a key part of stroke rehabilitation. The main evidence is summarized in a Cochrane systematic review [15] which found that people with stroke who received occupational therapy targeting PADL performed better and had a reduced risk of a poor outcome (dependency in PADL, deterioration or death) compared to those without occupational therapy input.

However, there was limited information on the content of the therapy and research investigating the specific interventions that improve PADL is still required. A feasibility RCT has shown potential benefits of a systematic neuropsychological approach to dressing therapy after stroke but more robust evidence is required to guide practice.

5.11 Dysphagia

A number of treatments for dysphagia after stroke have been studied, including swallowing exercises, acupuncture, medicines, neuromuscular electrical stimulation (NMES), pharyngeal electrical stimulation (PES), thermal stimulation, transcranial direct current (tDCS), transcranial magnetic stimulation (TMS) and expiratory muscle strength training (EMST). The aim of treatment was to improve swallowing and to reduce the risk developing aspiration pneumonia. A Cochrane review of swallowing therapy, which included acupuncture, behavioural interventions, medication, NMES, PES, physical stimulation, tDCS and TMS concluded that swallowing therapy did not change outcomes of death or dependency/disability, case fatality or penetration aspiration score, but may have reduced length of hospital stay, dysphagia, chest infections and improved swallowing ability [16]. Non-invasive neurostimulation therapies may have some effect on swallowing recovery and improve quality of life but there is little evidence that they affect mortality, pneumonia, length of stay or feeding tube removal [17].

Two systematic reviews have suggested that respiratory muscle training may reduce the occurrence of respiratory complications and reduce laryngeal penetration in patients with dysphagia after stroke However, the time since stroke and the proportion of participants who had dysphagia were unclear, and the authors recommended that further research was needed [18].

5.12 Aphasia

A high-quality meta-analysis carried out by the RELEASE Collaborators (2022) [19] examined data from 25 published trials involving 959 people with aphasia across 10 different languages. This meta-analysis demonstrated a link between dose and outcome with people with aphasia who received more than 20–50 h of therapy making larger gains in language abilities and function, compared with those who received fewer hours. No functional communication gains were observed for people with aphasia receiving less than 5 h of therapy nor comprehension gains for those receiving less than 20 h.

Most of the evidence derives from people with chronic aphasia more than 6 months after stroke. People with aphasia should be offered therapy for as long as they continue to make meaningful gains in their language and communication abilities.

The greatest overall gains in language outcomes for people with aphasia after stroke are seen when therapy starts within 1 month of stroke.

Several trials of digital therapies for people with aphasia, have demonstrated large gains in naming in particular [20]. These therapies are not designed to replicate the interventions delivered by a speech and language therapist. Instead, they automate the repetitive based aspects of therapy.

5.13 Stroke Rehabilitation in Vietnam

Stroke rehabilitation has been a developing specialty in most hospitals and healthcare facilities in Vietnam since 2016. Before this time there was a lack of awareness of the importance of post-stroke rehabilitation. There was a need for education of standard knowledge, skills and abilities in stroke rehabilitation specialty for doctors and nurses.

A specialty training programme for nurses and doctors was supported by the World Stroke Organization and the Austrian government from 2017 to 2019 (Austrian Vietnamese Advancement Neurorehabilitation Treatment (AVANT)). Through 3 years of the specialty supported programme, the awareness and practical skills of doctor and nurse participants have been improved and changed positively in regards to their knowledge, skills and abilities. There was a total of 122 courses organized between 2017 and 2019 with courses aimed at four different groups. The course level A+ was for core trainers who were Vietnamese doctors and therapists selected from national central hospitals. All the courses for the core trainers were for 3 weeks in Salzburg, Austria.

There was a total of 32 core trainers trained from 2017 to 2019. After completing the training courses in Austria, those core trainers came back to Vietnam to organize training courses level A and level A1 to spread the standardized and systematized knowledge on neurorehabilitation for health professionals and patients' caregivers in Vietnam. The course level A and level A1 were for healthcare professionals. Participants in these courses were doctors and therapists working in the field of stroke, neurology, rehabilitation sent from 64 provincial hospitals in Vietnam. There was a total of 44 courses level A and level A1. The participants trained in knowledge and skills on the position of injuries, the method of early rehabilitation, early mobilization, exercises for daily activities and sensory exercises. About 3000 doctors and therapists participated between 2017 and 2019. All participants became the trainees after successfully doing a post-test and to be issued a certificate by the VNS AND WSO. After the course level A and level A1, the trainees were required to organize a course to share and educate the caregivers in their places of work.

There was a total of 73 courses for 4000 caregivers and patient's families in 64 provincial hospitals in Vietnam in 2017–2019. The caregivers received more than 20,000 booklets 'Essential Exercises for Neurohabilitation after stroke' and practical DVDs. The course level B had a significant effect on stroke caregivers and patient's families. They understood the importance of rehabilitation as well as how to help stroke survivors in daily life and patients' recovery.

This system of cascading the training from the international experts down to the carers of stroke patients has been highly successful and has helped to transform the delivery of stroke rehabilitation in Vietnam.

References

1. Aderinto N, AbdulBasit MO, Olatunji G, Adejumo T. Exploring the transformative influence of neuroplasticity on stroke rehabilitation: a narrative review of current evidence. Ann Med Surg. 2023;85(9):4425–32. https://doi.org/10.1097/MS9.0000000000001137. PMID: 37663728; PMCID: PMC10473303.
2. Joy MT, Carmichael ST. Encouraging an excitable brain state: mechanisms of brain repair in stroke. Nat Rev Neurosci. 2021;22(1):38–53. https://doi.org/10.1038/s41583-020-00396-7.
3. World Health Organisation Classification of functioning, disability and health. https://www.who.int/standards/classifications/international-classification-of-functioning-disability-and-health.
4. National Clinical Guidelines for Stroke. 2023. https://www.strokeguideline.org/app/uploads/2023/04/National-Clinical-Guideline-for-Stroke-2023.pdf?_gl=1*1nf120m*_up*MQ*_ga*MjQ3MDA0NTA0LjE3MTY1Nzg0MjI*_ga_EE3BZMVLRT*MTcxNjU3ODQyMS4xLjEuMTcxNjU3ODQyOS4wLjAuMA.
5. Ada L, Dorsch S, Canning CG. Strengthening interventions increase strength and improve activity after stroke: a systematic review. Austr J Physiother. 2006;52(4):241–8.
6. Kunkel D, Fitton C, Burnett M, Ashburn A. Physical inactivity post-stroke: a 3-year longitudinal study. Disabil Rehabil. 2015;37(4):304–10.
7. Billinger SA, Boyne P, Coughenour E, Dunning K, Mattlage A. Does aerobic exercise and the FITT principle fit into stroke recovery? Curr Neurol Neurosci Rep. 2015;15(2):519.
8. Saunders DH, Sanderson M, Hayes S, et al. Physical fitness training for stroke patients. Cochrane Database Syst Rev. 2020;3(3):Cd003316.
9. Engineer ND, Kimberley TJ, Prudente CN, et al. Targeted vagus nerve stimulation for rehabilitation after stroke. Front Neurosci. 2013;13:280–98.
10. Taub E, Uswatte G, Bowman MH, et al. Constraint-induced movement therapy combined with conventional neurorehabilitation techniques in chronic stroke patients with plegic hands: a case series. Arch Phys Med Rehabil. 2013;94(1):86–94.
11. Kwakkel G, Veerbeek JM, van Wegen EE, et al. Constraint-induced movement therapy after stroke. Lancet Neurol. 2015;14(2):224–34.
12. Chang WH, Kim YH. Robot-assisted therapy in stroke rehabilitation. J Stroke. 2013;15(3):174–81.
13. Mehrholz J, Pohl M, Platz T, et al. Electromechanical and robot-assisted arm training for improving activities of daily living, arm function, and arm muscle strength after stroke. Cochrane Database Syst Rev. 2018;9:CD006876.
14. Nindorera F, Nduwimana I, Thonnard JL, et al. Effectiveness of walking training on balance, motor functions, activity, participation and quality of life in people with chronic stroke: a systematic review with meta-analysis and meta-regression of recent randomized controlled trials. Disabil Rehabil. 2021;44(15):3760–71.
15. Legg LA, Drummond AE, Langhorne P. Occupational therapy for patients with problems in activities of daily living after stroke. Cochrane Database Syst Rev. 2006;4:CD003585.
16. Bath PM, Lee HS, Everton LF. Swallowing therapy for dysphagia in acute and subacute stroke. Cochrane Database Syst Rev. 2018;10:CD000323.
17. Dziewas R, Warnecke T, Stellato R, et al. Pharyngeal electrical stimulation for early decannulation in tracheotomised patients with neurogenic dysphagia after stroke (PHAST-TRAC): a prospective, single-blinded, randomised trial. Lancet Neurol. 2018;17(10):849–59.
18. Zhang W, Pan H, Zong Y, et al. Respiratory muscle training reduces respiratory complications and improves swallowing function after stroke: a systematic review and meta-analysis. Arch Phys Med Rehabil. 2022;103:1179–91.

19. RELEASE Collaborators. Precision rehabilitation for aphasia by patient age, sex, aphasia severity, and time since stroke? A prespecified, systematic review-based, individual participant data, network, subgroup meta-analysis. Int J Stroke. 2022;17(10):1067–77.
20. Braley M, Pierce JS, Saxena S, et al. A virtual, randomized, control trial of a digital therapeutic for speech, language, and cognitive intervention in post-stroke persons with aphasia. Front Neurol. 2021;12:626780.

Chapter 6
Prehospital Care for Stroke

Thanh Ngoc Le, Ngoc Huy Nguyen, Anthony Rudd, An Quang Nguyen, Viet Quoc Hoang, and RenYu Liu

6.1 Introduction

This is often the most neglected part of the stroke pathway but one that managed effectively has some of the greatest potential to enable effective treatment. Successful acute stroke care requires that treatment is started very early. Whether it is intravenous thrombolysis, endovascular thrombectomy, reversal of anticoagulation or control of high blood pressure in a patient with a hemorrhage or getting them to a stroke unit for high quality medical and nursing care, all are more effective when done soon after the stroke.

T. N. Le (✉)
VNU University of Medicine and Pharmacy, Hanoi, Vietnam

N. H. Nguyen
VNU University of Medicine and Pharmacy, Hanoi, Vietnam

Phutho Department of Health, Phutho, Vietnam
e-mail: lengocthanh61@gmail.com

A. Rudd
King's College, London, UK

A. Q. Nguyen
Phutho Medical College, Phutho, Vietnam

V. Q. Hoang
Stroke Center, Phutho General Hospital, Phutho, Vietnam

R. Liu
Departments of Anesthesiology and Critical Care, and Neurology, Perelman School of Medicine, University of Pennsylvania, Philadelphia, PA, USA

A. Rudd et al. (eds.), *Stroke Management in Vietnam*,
https://doi.org/10.1007/978-981-96-0221-6_6

The importance of ensuring that all the stages of stroke care are coordinated is summarized in what is called the "Chain of Survival" (Fig. 6.1). A group of clinicians including paramedics, stroke physicians and neurologists and emergency physicians in 2018 to produce a consensus document summarizing the key components of the prehospital stroke pathway [1]. This paper is being used as the basis of this chapter.

The ten key aspects that every prehospital stroke service needs to consider are summarized in Fig. 6.2 again taken from the paper and will be discussed in more detail in this chapter.

6.1.1 *Stroke Registry*

Data are essential to improve care and outcomes. It is difficult to know how to improve a service without data giving information about what is working well and what needs to improve. Data collection should be kept to a minimum and preferably obtained from routine data sources so as not to get in the way of delivering care. Ideally data should be collected at a national level including all potential stroke patients, but very few countries have been able to do this. The UK has started collecting prehospital data and linking it to the national hospital based audit. But it has proved difficult to collect the information consistently and then link it to the in-patient dataset. Registries require appropriate resource allocation from hospitals, Emergency Medical Services (EMS) and government funding and built in to any audit should be some way of assessing data quality. In many areas, regions and countries the EMS transport a minority of stroke patients. In these areas it is important to record how the patient arrived at hospital and how long it took from the onset of symptoms to arrival.

6.1.2 *Public Awareness*

The principal reasons why so many patients internationally arrive at the hospital so late is that the stroke is not recognized by either the patient or people who witness it and even if they do they do not realize that stroke is potentially treatable if it is treated as an emergency and the patient is taken to the right hospital. In a summary of 22 studies that surveyed the public's knowledge of the symptoms of stroke only a few participants could name more than two risk factors with a substantial proportion not knowing a single sign of stroke [2]. Lower socio-economic groups and people with less education were less knowledgeable than higher socio-economic groups and people with higher education. Having identified that stroke is a possibility, where there is an EMS, it has been shown that patients brought to the hospital by EMS arrive sooner after onset of their symptoms than those transported by other means and receive more rapid evaluation and treatment [3]. A survey of access to

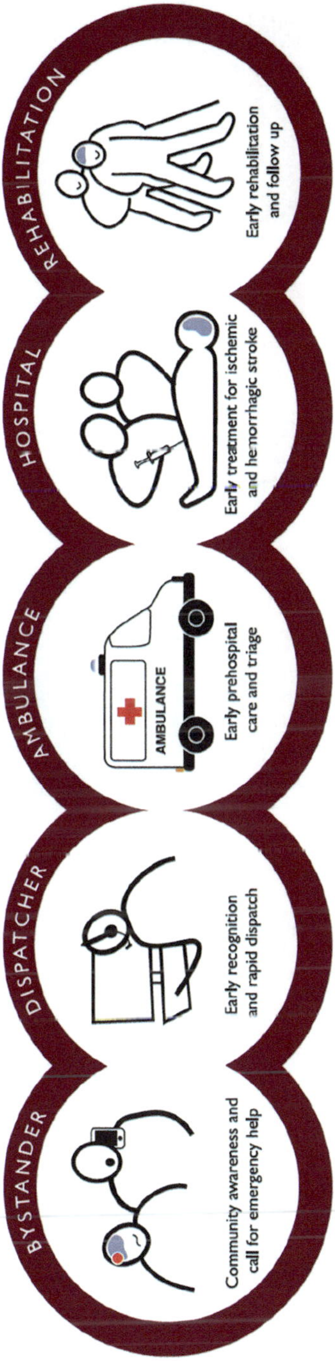

Fig. 6.1 Chain of Survival for Acute Stroke

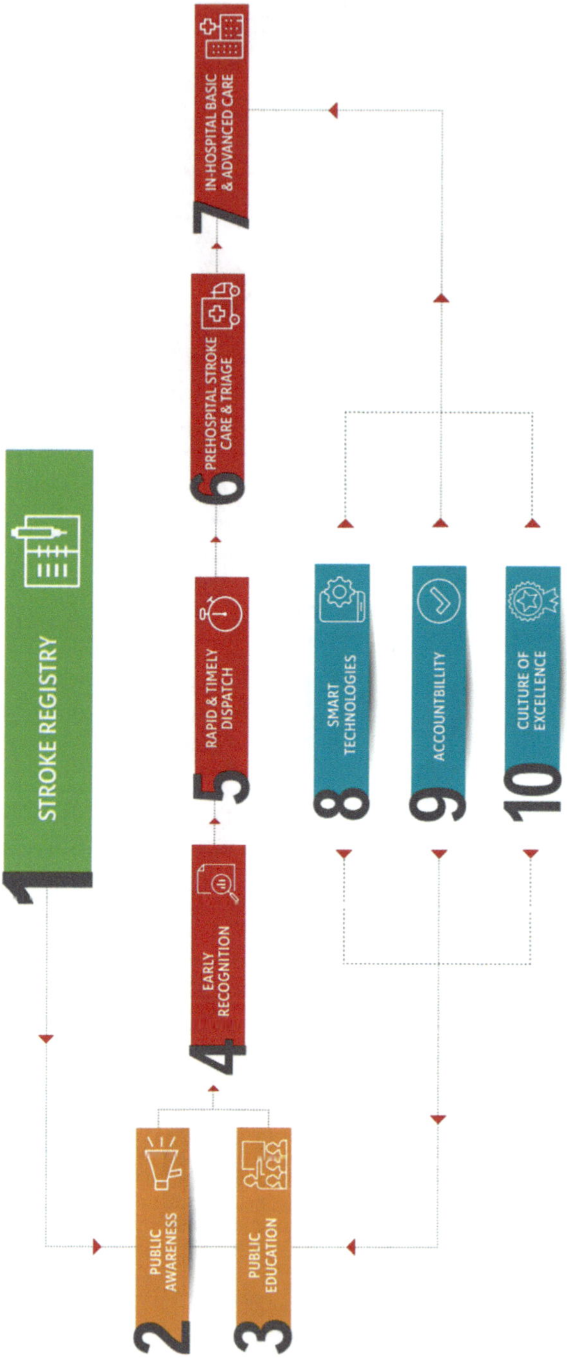

Fig. 6.2 Ten Stages for Prehospital Care

prehospital care published in 2023[4] shows very variable access to EMS predictably with greater access in high income countries compared to low and middle income countries. But, even in high income countries, there are still often unnecessary delays. Studies have shown that in countries with well-developed EMS systems, people with stroke use EMS about 60% of the time for transportation to the hospital [5]. Individuals showing signs of major stroke such as paresis, aphasia, or altered level of consciousness are more likely to use EMS than those with symptoms such as vision disturbance, ataxia, or vertigo [6, 7]. Patients transported by EMS receive more sophisticated prehospital care and evaluation [7] and are treated more quickly at the stroke center [8].

6.1.3 Start Public Education

Educational efforts should be broad-based and built upon advertising success in other domains. These can include mass media campaigns, targeted programs in schools, ambassadors, and social media. Regardless of approach, one challenge is maintaining the durability of the education initiative, and this may require repeat messaging in various media formats and recurring reminders using testimonials of success.

Unfortunately, there is only limited evidence to support any particular approach to raising public awareness of symptoms and appropriate response. A paper from Canada [9] reported five Face, Arm, Speech, Time (FAST) public awareness campaigns and four periods of surveying knowledge among 2451 patients in Quebec province between 2016 and 2019 (Fig. 6.3). FAST is one of the most widely used systems to educate people, first developed in Newcastle in the UK about 30 years ago and since translated into many different languages (Figs. 6.4 and 6.5).

The Canadian study is one of the few that has evaluated effectiveness of a public awareness campaign over a long period of time. Overall, there was a significant improvement of 26% in FAST stroke sign knowledge between survey waves 1 and 4 but after the last campaign, 30.5% were still unable to name a single FAST sign. Factors associated with worse performance were male sex and whether the

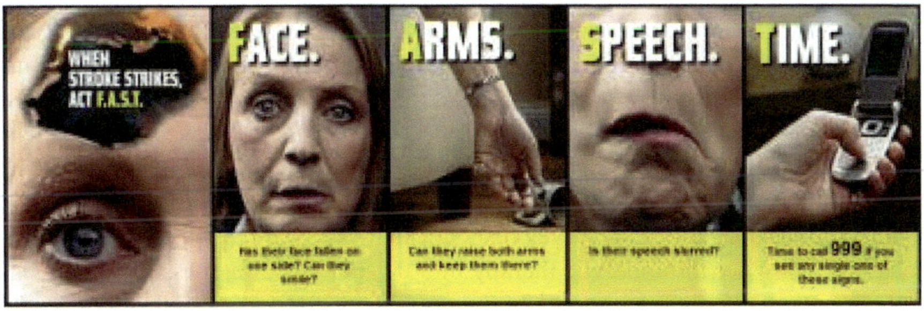

Fig. 6.3 Images from the UK FAST campaign

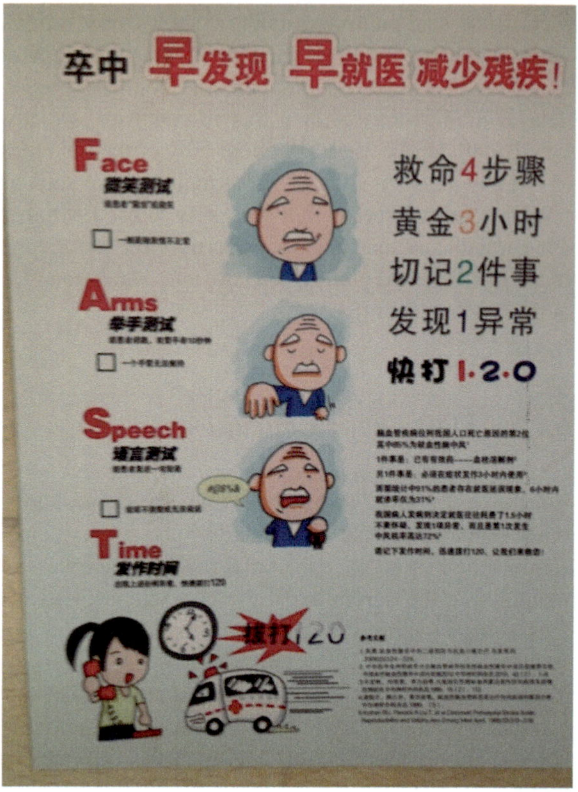

Fig. 6.4 Images from FAST campaign in China

respondent was retired. These findings confirm the findings from an older paper from the UK [10] on impact of FAST campaigns where the key findings did show raised awareness but poorest penetration particularly into the black minority groups.

One novel approach recognizes that using FAST in countries where English is not commonly understood and where the Western alphabet is not used is unlikely to be successful, particularly in groups with only a few years of education. Instead, they have based their prompt to act quickly on the emergency phone number, whether it is 911 or 120 as in China (Fig. 6.6).

Using this tool, the group used massive media coverage and community-based educational sessions with videos to promote the message. They surveyed the response on two occasions during the programme [12]. A total of 3066 participants responded to the first survey in 2016, and 15,207 participants responded in 2018 across China. The acceptance rate for Stroke 1-2-0 versus FAST was 50.2% versus 19.1% in 2016 and changed significantly to 82.2% versus 8.0% in 2018 ($p < 0.001$). Stroke 1-2-0 was well accepted by all ages and by people with different academic qualifications. Only 6.5% of survey respondents were aware that there was a therapeutic window for thrombolytic therapy in 2016, but this awareness increased significantly to 32.8% in 2018. Only 12.6% of people in 2016 indicated that they would

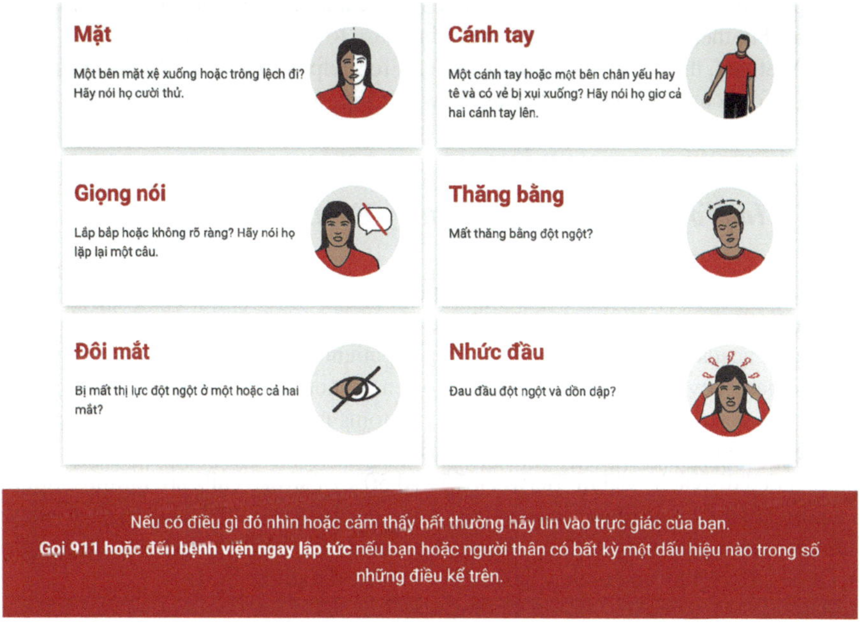

Fig. 6.5 Stroke Awareness Campaign Information from Vietnam

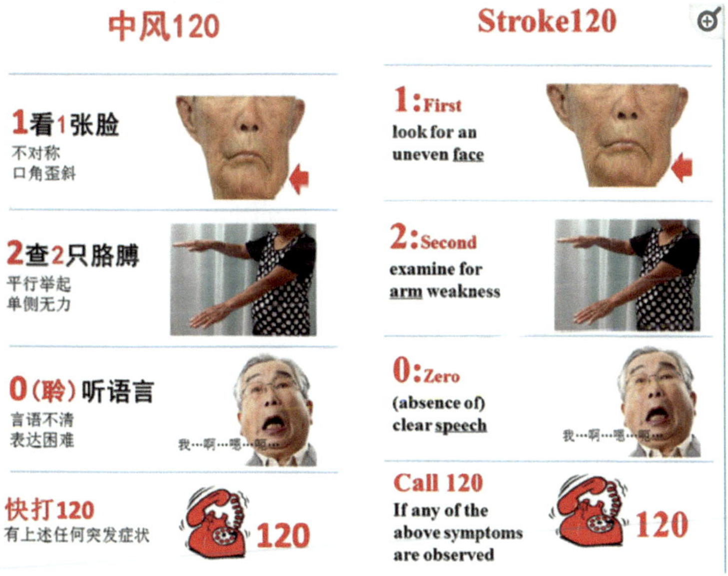

Fig. 6.6 Stroke 120 Campaign for China [11]

send patients with stroke to the nearest hospital capable of performing thrombolytic therapy, but there was a nearly threefold increase to 52.5% in 2018.

In Vietnam, the emergency number to call for help is 112. The 120 idea has been adapted for countries that use 112 as shown in Fig. 6.7.

6.1.4 Improve Early Recognition by First Responders

Early recognition of potential stroke symptoms by emergency dispatchers is critical to activating emergency stroke care. Once a call to an emergency center occurs, the call-taker needs to differentiate the 1–2% of patients with stroke from the range of other emergency conditions. As patients often do not recognize their symptoms as being due to stroke, their description of symptoms may be unclear. Emergency call centers often use a predefined guideline for prioritizing stroke as part of their computer aided dispatch system. Between 25 and 50% of stroke calls are mimics. Some identification strategies are insensitive, detecting between 40% and 65% of acute strokes with variable specificity. There is no evidence favoring any one diagnostic scale or strategy by emergency call takers to identify stroke [13].

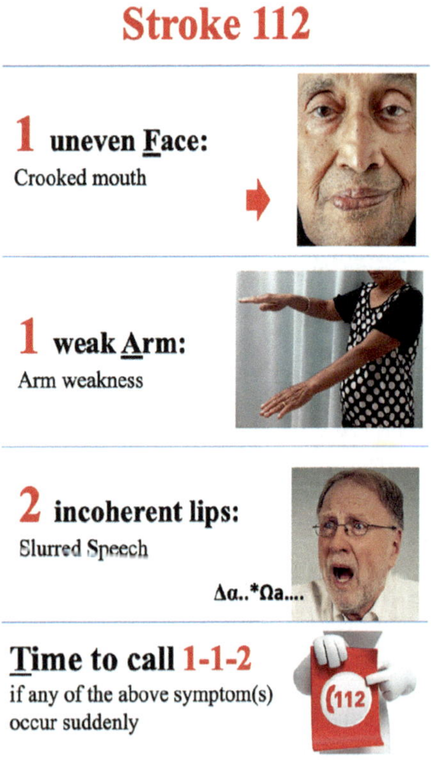

Fig. 6.7 Public Awareness message for countries that use 112 as their emergency number

Relatively little stroke specific training is given to most paramedic students in most countries and the World Stroke Association survey [4] reported that less than half of the people responding reported that any training on stroke was given to call handlers and paramedics.

Training has been shown to be effective. A study done in Lithuania [14] that provided just two, 1 h sessions to a maximum of 20 paramedics at a time showed that knowledge improved after the training and transport times were significantly shorter.

6.1.5 Practice Rapid and Timely Dispatch

Having recognized the possibility that stroke is a possibility, it is then vital that there are systems in place to ensure that they dispatch an ambulance as quickly as possible. In a Norwegian study [15], when the emergency call-taker suspected a diagnosis of stroke, ambulance services were dispatched as high priority response to 92% of patients. But if the call-taker missed the diagnosis, the ambulance was dispatched as high priority response in only about 55% of cases. Even patients with transient stroke symptoms should have an acute EMS response. But to achieve this, the ambulance service must have sufficient vehicles and staff available 24 h a day and the paramedics must have been given sufficient training to know what to do when they get to the patient. Having a governmental instruction that stroke is medical emergency and setting some standards for timely response can be very effective at making sure that stroke is given the correct priority.

6.1.6 Optimize Prehospital Stroke Care and Triage

There are three phases of a prehospital stroke care program: field screening and assessment, treatment in the field and in transit, and notification of the receiving hospital. During the screening phase, emergency personnel should use validated stroke identification tools [16, 17]. Once stroke is suspected, other tools may be employed aiming to identify strokes due to large vessel occlusion (LVO) [18, 19]. The tool needs to correctly identify all LVO patients so that they can be taken to the thrombectomy center and excludes the majority of those without LVO so that the thrombectomy center is not overwhelmed with patients it cannot treat. In other words what is needed is a scale with high sensitivity and specificity. A paper by Nguyen et al [20] reconstructed seven prediction scales from paramedic documentation in 2007 cases including the Los Angeles Motor Scale (LAMS), the Rapid Arterial Occlusion Evaluation (RACE), the Cincinnati Stroke Triage Assessment Tool, the prehospital Acute Stroke Severity (PASS), the gaze-face-arm-speech-time, the Field Assessment Stroke Triage for Emergency Destination and the gaze, facial asymmetry, level of consciousness, extinction/inattention.

Outcomes were LVO and feasibility rates—the proportion of acute stroke codes for which the prehospital scale could be reconstructed. 158 (7.9%) of the sample had LVO. The accuracy of the scales ranged between 0.79 and 0.89, with LAMS and RACE scales having highest scores. Sensitivity ranged from 38% to 62%, and specificity from 80% to 93%. The scale feasibility rates varied between 78% and 88%, with the highest rate for the PASS scale. All seven prediction scales had high specificity, but low sensitivity and fairly low feasibility rates.

So, no clinical tool yet meets the needs to accurately triage patients to a thrombectomy center. There are some pieces of new technology being developed, particularly small light CT scanners that might prove to be useful in this situation. Ultrasound to identify LVO can be useful for some patients but has not yet been tested in real life at the roadside. Furthermore, training paramedics to use ultrasound and equipping ambulances may not prove practicable for many services. It is also important not to delay transfer to hospital where definitive tests and decisions can be made.

Essential vital sign assessment should include heart rate, blood pressure, blood glucose, and pulse oximetry measurements [21, 22]. The pre-arrival notification phase is the critical link between prehospital and hospital care to shorten the time interval from hospital arrival to treatment initiation. In addition to notifying that a suspected stroke patient is on the way, provision of key information will allow the hospital to prepare for appropriate prompt assessment and treatment [23, 24]. There is an important balance between adequate assessment and treatment in the prehospital environment and rapid transport to definitive hospital care. The patient should be triaged to a predefined facility for intravenous thrombolysis and potential EVT based on the local stroke system of care.

It is key for effective acute stroke services to have regional planning of a stroke system of care and clear pathways to minimize delays in therapeutic decision-making and delivery of care. This requires transportation to a center that will minimize treatment time. Optimizing these transport decisions requires modeling based on factors such as population density, stroke incidence, hospital capabilities and performance metrics, and transport times. An ideal acute stroke service is one that is reached quickly, with immediate access to stroke specialist care either on site or via telemedicine, capable of advanced brain imaging including angiography and perfusion with a dedicated stroke unit, expertise in intravenous thrombolysis and EVT, and all organized to provide expert care with minimal delay [25].

6.1.7 *Optimize in-Hospital Triage and Acute Care*

This topic is covered in other chapters but it bears repeating that without coordination between the EMS and the hospital and efficient care in the emergency department valuable time will be lost and patients who otherwise may walk out of the hospital a few hours later may remain disabled for the rest of their lives.

6.1.8 Use Smart Technologies

New technologies are emerging and have been successful in other areas of emergency care and may assist with recognition and early treatment of stroke. Machine Learning and artificial intelligence are being evaluated to assist dispatchers in recognizing possible cases of stroke and are already used to aid in interpretation of neuroimaging. Smartphones are available in most communities, including low resource countries and can be used to communicate between the hospital specialists and the ambulance crew. Telemedicine is invaluable in providing expert advice in the acute setting, particularly in hospitals in rural areas where 24/7 on site specialists availability is not feasible (43). Mobile stroke units have been shown to shorten assessment and treatment times compared to conventional hospital care and improve outcomes. They are further discussed in the chapter on stroke units.

6.1.9 Demonstrate Accountability

One of the hallmarks of excellent stroke care is an ongoing quality improvement program with transparent public reporting of data. Regular monitoring of the metrics allows the public to identify the best-performing centers while motivating improvement amongst hospitals at the lower end of the performance spectrum to improve (46).

6.1.10 Create a Culture of Excellence

The secret of moving a system from its current performance level to a "Culture of Excellence" requires an environment that empowers, focuses, and engages staff and equips teams with the right mindset and skills necessary to achieve the best results. A culture of excellence has a system and staff that use a combination of best practice evidence and performance data to continually review their practices and identify opportunities to improve patient care. To achieve a culture of excellence, every staff member must understand not only the organization's vision, but also know their own roles, responsibilities, and the specific actions they need to implement to achieve this vision.

6.2 Conclusions

There needs to be as much effort designing, delivering, and monitoring prehospital stroke services as there is for in-patient services. Involving stroke specialists in this process together with paramedics and healthcare planners is necessary for truly effective services to be provided.

References

1. Rudd AG, Bladin C, Carli P, et al. Utstein recommendation for emergency stroke care. Int J Stroke. 2020;15(5):555–64.
2. Stroebele N, Müller-Riemenschneider F, Nolte CH, Müller-Nordhorn J, Bockelbrink A, Willich SN. Knowledge of risk factors, and warning signs of stroke: a systematic review from a gender perspective. Int J Stroke. 2011;6(1):60–6.
3. Ekundayo OJ, Saver JL, Fonarow GC, et al. Patterns of emergency medical services use and its association with timely stroke treatment: findings from get with the guidelines-stroke. Circ Cardiovasc Qual Outcomes. 2013;6:262.
4. Rudd AG, Zhao J, Ford G, et al. Results of an international survey on the status of prehospital care. Int J Stroke. 2023;18(9):1084–91.
5. Mochari-Greenberger H, Xian Y, Hellkamp AS, et al. Racial/ethnic and sex differences in emergency medical services transport among hospitalized US stroke patients: analysis of the National get with The Guidelines–Stroke Registry. J Am Heart Assoc. 2015;4(8):e002099.
6. Kleindorfer D, Lindsell CJ, Moomaw CJ, et al. Which stroke symptoms prompt a 911 call? A population-based study. Am J Emerg Med. 2010;28(5):607–12.
7. Oostema JA, Chassee T. Reeves M, vol. 22. Emergency Dispatcher Stroke Recognition: Associations with downstream care: Prehosp Emerg Care; 2018. p. 1–6.
8. Caceres JA, Adil MM, Jadhav V, et al. Diagnosis of stroke by emergency medical dispatchers and its impact on the prehospital care of patients. J Stroke Cerebrovasc Dis. 2013;22(8):e610–e4.
9. Rioux B, Brissette V, Marin FF, et al. The impact of stroke public awareness campaigns differs between sociodemographic groups. Can J Neurol Sci. 2022;49(2):231–8.
10. Robinson TG, Reid A, Haunton VJ, et al. The face arm speech test: does it encourage rapid recognition of important stroke warning symptoms? Emerg Med J. 2013;30(6):467–71.
11. Zhao J, Liu R. Stroke 1-2-0: a rapid response programme for stroke in China. Lancet Neurol. 2017;16(1):27–8.
12. Zhao J, Li X, Liu X, et al. Changing the strategy and culture of stroke awareness education in China: implementing stroke 1-2-0. Stroke Vasc Neurol. 2020;5(4):374–80.
13. Rudd M, Buck D, Ford GA, Price CI. A systematic review of stroke recognition instruments in hospital and prehospital settings. Emerg Med J. 2016;33(11):818–22.
14. Sveikata L, Melaika K, Wiśniewski A, et al. Interactive training of the emergency medical services improved prehospital stroke recognition and transport time. Front Neurol. 2022;13:765165.
15. Viereck S, Møller TP, Iversen HK, et al. Medical dispatchers recognise substantial amount of acute stroke during emergency calls. Scand J Trauma Resusc Emerg Med. 2016;24(1):89.
16. Kidwell CS, Starkman S, Eckstein M, et al. Identifying stroke in the field: prospective validation of the Los Angeles prehospital stroke screen (LAPSS). Stroke. 2000;31(1):71–6.
17. Bray JE, Martin J, Cooper G, et al. Paramedic identification of stroke: community validation of the Melbourne ambulance stroke screen. Cerebrovasc Dis. 2005;20(1):28–33.
18. Richards CT, Huebinger R, Tataris KL, et al. Cincinnati prehospital stroke scale can identify large vessel occlusion stroke. Prehosp Emerg Care. 2018;22(3):312–8.

19. Perez de la Ossa N, Carrera D, Gorchs M, et al. Design and validation of a prehospital stroke scale to predict large arterial occlusion the rapid arterial occlusion evaluation scale. Stroke. 2014;45:87–91.
20. Nguyen TTM, van den Wijngaard IR, Bosch J, et al. Comparison of prehospital scales for predicting large anterior vessel occlusion in the ambulance setting. JAMA Neurol. 2021;78(2):157–64.
21. Jauch EC, Saver JL, Adams, et al. Guidelines for the early management of patients with acute ischemic stroke: a guideline for healthcare professionals from the American Heart Association/American Stroke Association. Stroke. 2013;44(3):870–947.
22. Slavin SJ, Sucharew H, Alwell K, et al. Prehospital neurological deterioration in stroke. Emerg Med J. 2018;35:507.
23. Hsieh M-J, Tang S-C, Chiang W-C, et al. Effect of prehospital notification on acute stroke care: a multicenter study. Scand J Trauma Resusc Emerg Med. 2016;24(1):57.
24. Higashida R, Alberts MJ, Alexander DN, et al. Interactions within stroke systems of care: a policy statement from the American Heart Association/American Stroke Association. Stroke. 2013;44(10):2961–84.
25. Norrving B, Barrick J, Davalos A, et al. Action plan for stroke in Europe 2018–2030. Eur Stroke J. 2018;3:2396987318808719.

Chapter 7
Prevention of Stroke

Ngoc Huy Nguyen, Thong Van Nguyen, Anthony Rudd, and Trung Dinh Tran

7.1 Introduction

Worldwide vascular disease is the most common cause of death and one of the most important causes of adults developing long-term disability. Ischaemic heart disease is the number one cause with cerebrovascular disease taking second position. The Global Burden of Disease (GBD) study data [1] are summarised in Fig. 7.1 showing that as a cause of disability little will have changed between the early 2010 and 2020. Stroke is largely a preventable disease. It is estimated that if hypertension and hyperlipidaemia were controlled at a whole population level about 80% of all strokes would be prevented.

A more detailed study of predicted changes in Europe published by King's College, London and the Stroke Alliance for Europe [2] suggests that the number of strokes will increase by 25% between 2015 and 2025 with a 45% increase in the number of stroke deaths. These data are summarised in Fig. 7.2. The increases are largely the result in the ageing population in Europe.

N. H. Nguyen (✉)
Phutho Department of Health, Phutho, Vietnam

VNU University of Medicine and Pharmacy, Hanoi, Vietnam
e-mail: ngochuynguyen8888@gmail.com

T. Van Nguyen
Vietnam Stroke Association, Hanoi, Vietnam

Stroke Center, Phutho General Hospital, Phutho, Vietnam

A. Rudd
King's College, London, UK

T. D. Tran
Faculty of Public Health, Danang University of Medical Technology and Pharmacy, Danang, Vietnam

A. Rudd et al. (eds.), *Stroke Management in Vietnam*,
https://doi.org/10.1007/978-981-96-0221-6_7

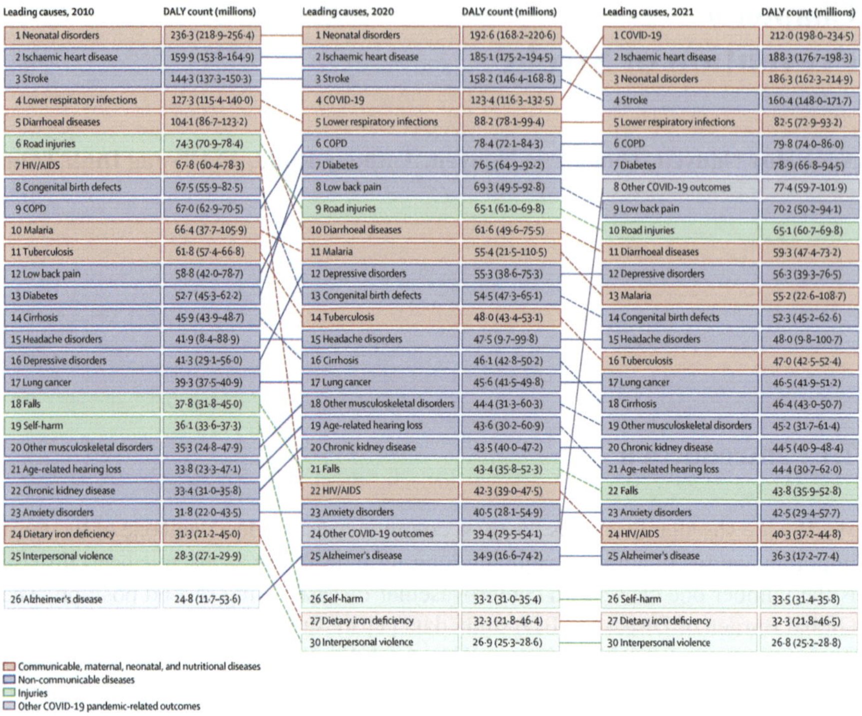

Fig. 7.1 Global burden of disease study predicted change in cause of disability worldwide

7.2 Vietnamese CVD Mortality and Morbidity

More information on cardiovascular disease morbidity is given in Chap. 1 on the epidemiology of stroke. In Vietnam, according to the World Health Organisation, cardiovascular diseases were responsible for 31% of all deaths in 2016 [3]. The prevalence of hypertension among adults 18–69 years was 18.9%, according to Viet Nam STEPWise approach to Surveillance (STEPS) 2015 with only 13.6% of hypertensive patients reported to be managed at a health facility. The World Heart Foundation published in 2019 a useful summary of cardiovascular risk factor prevalence in Vietnam, reproduced in Fig. 7.3 [4].

Over a quarter of the population are estimated to have hypertension, half of the female population are overweight and over a third have raised total cholesterol. Nearly half of the male population smoke although very few women were smoking at the time of the study. However, as Vietnam increases its per capita income, which it is doing very fast the concern is that 'western' risk factor patterns will become even more prevalent with increasing rates of obesity, type 2 diabetes, hypercholesterolaemia and hypertension and increasing rates of smoking in the female population.

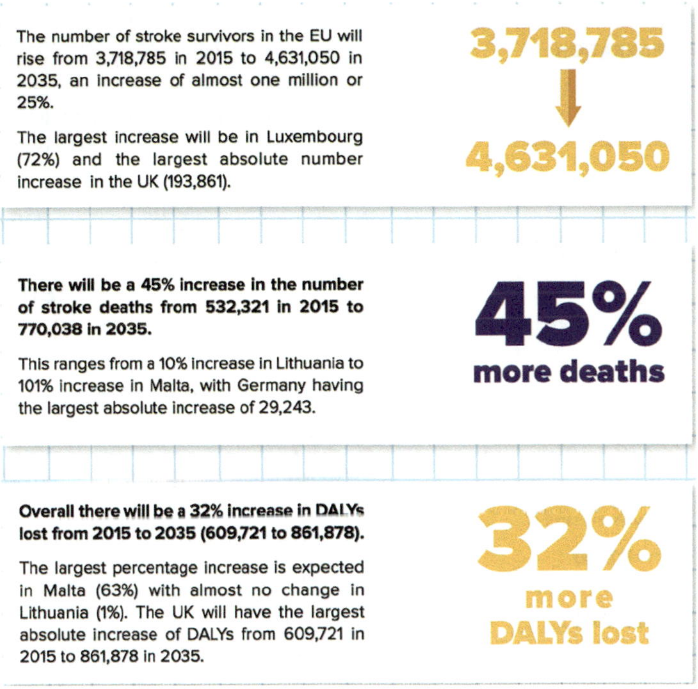

Fig. 7.2 Predicted changes in stroke related deaths and disability 2015–2025

All these data show that if effective primary and secondary cardiovascular risk reduction strategies were successful, they could have a huge impact on reducing the rates of death and disability in Vietnam.

7.3 Stroke Risk Factors

Stroke is not a single disease but all the subtypes share some of the risk factors with each also having specific risks. A simplified graphic that does not take into consideration the variation in risk factors for ischaemic stroke subtypes is shown in Fig. 7.4.

Risk factors can also be divided into those that are modifiable and those that are not. We can do little about age, which is one of the strongest risk factors for stroke, likewise gender, ethnicity and our genes. This chapter will focus on the modifiable risk factors and most of what is included in each of the sections is equally applicable to both primary prevention (the prevention of stroke before the onset of any cardiovascular disease) and secondary prevention (the prevention of recurrent vascular disease. Primary prevention usually focusses on population based risk reduction

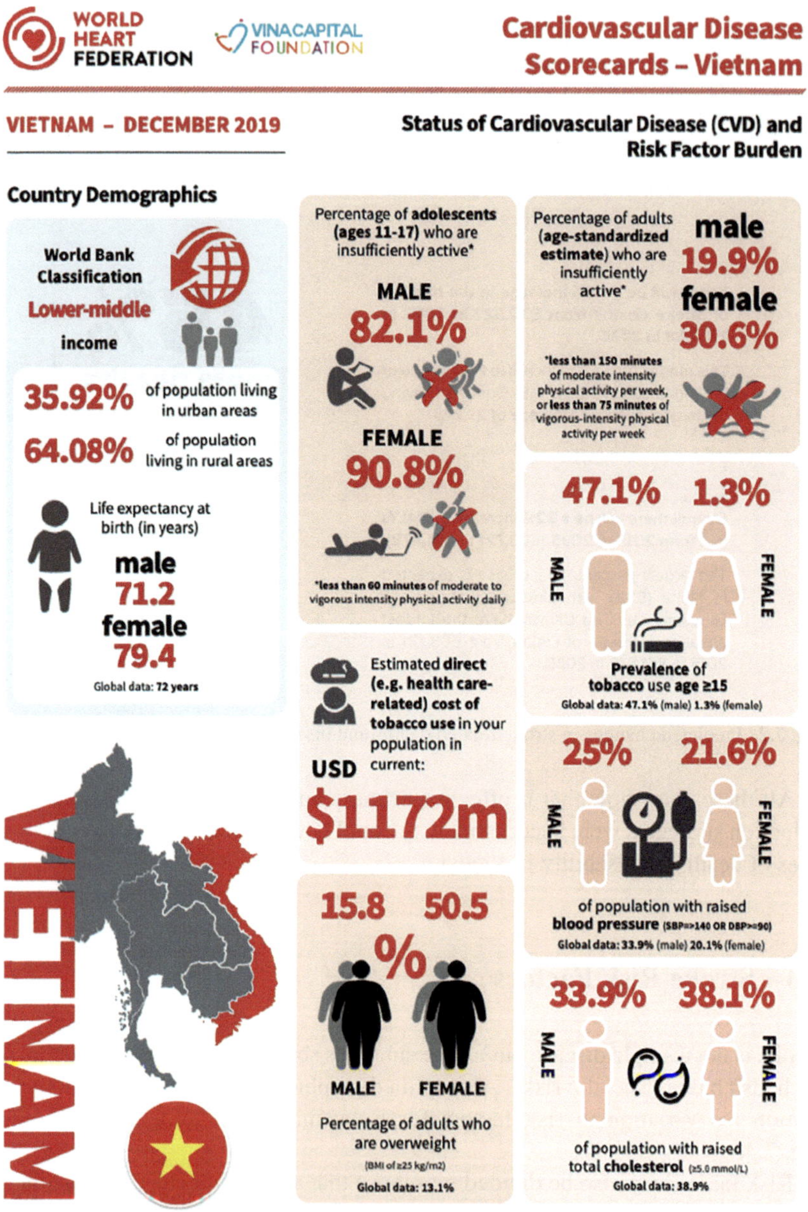

Fig. 7.3 World Heart Foundation infographic on cardiovascular disease in Vietnam

strategies or focussing on particularly high risk groups while secondary prevention is likely to focus on the individual patient who is by definition high risk.

Effective strategies for stroke prevention require a comprehensive multidisciplinary approach to identify and manage major risk factors and to promote adherence

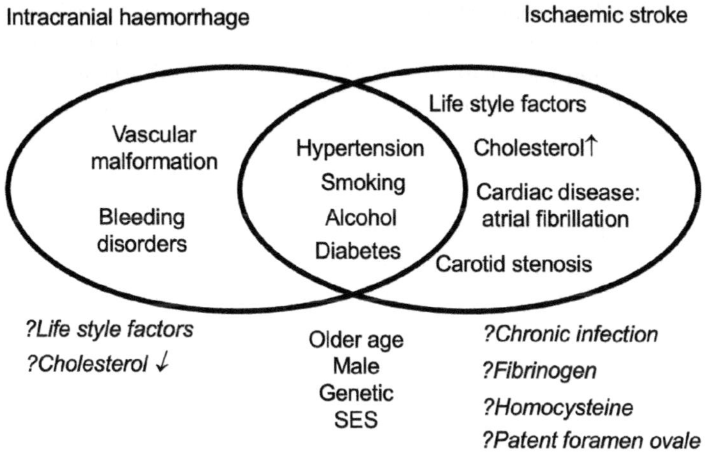

Fig. 7.4 Stroke risk factors

to preventive protocols. Despite the availability of stroke risk assessment tools for identification of individuals at sufficiently increased risk of stroke, and clinical guidelines providing an evidence base to guide modern stroke prevention and treatment, considerable gaps have been reported in the translation of recommendations into practice, particularly for risk factors that are asymptomatic such as hypertension, hypercholesterolaemia and most patients with atrial fibrillation. Uptake of stroke prevention strategies remains low in most populations especially in low and middle income countries and countries with national health services or insurance schemes without coverage that extends to the whole population. The challenge remains to identify strategies for effective implementation for the benefits of primary and secondary prevention of stroke in different population groups. Few data on the risk factor profile for stroke in Vietnam have been published but a papers from Ngoc NH et al. [5, 6] suggests that most of the risk factors reported from other countries are also found in Vietnam but with high levels of smoking and alcohol useage.

7.4 Hypertension

Hypertension is the most prevalent treatable risk factor in Vietnam and worldwide, for the prevention of stroke and its recurrence [7]. The higher the blood pressure, the greater the chances of developing both ischaemic and haemorrhagic stroke [8]. Evidence from the combined results of nine well conducted prospective observational studies demonstrate positive, continuous and apparently independent associations between diastolic blood pressure (DBP) and stroke, with no evidence of any 'threshold' below which lower levels of DBP were not associated with lower risk of stroke [9]. Data from the Framingham study demonstrated a fivefold increase in the probability of developing an ischaemic stroke in those with BP ≥160/95 mmHg compared to those with BP <140/90 mmHg [10]. Information obtained from one million adults in 61 prospective observational studies also demonstrated a strong positive association between usual BP and stroke mortality at all ages, without any evidence of a threshold down to at least 115/75 mmHg [11]. A 10 mmHg lower than usual SBP or 5 mmHg lower than usual DBP from this review was estimated to be associated in the long term with about 40% lower risk of stroke death. A meta-analyses of randomised controlled trials of BP lowering and stroke suggests a dose–response relationship with a 10 mmHg reduction in systolic blood pressure (SBP) being associated with a 31% reduction in stroke risk [12].

The prevalence of hypertension increases with advancing age with more than half of people aged 60–69 years, and approximately 75% of people aged 70 years and older being affected [13]. The risk of hypertension is higher in black men and women as well as South Asian men compared to their white counterparts [14]. Treatment and control of hypertension eliminates the excess cardiovascular disease mortality risk observed among the hypertensive population [15]. However, even in developed countries, many patients with hypertension remain undetected or untreated and a large proportion of patients who do receive treatment do not achieve target blood pressure levels [16, 17]. Blood pressure is adequately controlled in only 20% of the 50 million hypertensives in the USA and in <10% of hypertensives in most European countries [18]. Possible explanations for this finding included the use of low-dose prescriptions, inadequate adjustment of doses and poor patient compliance [19]. Unfortunately, there is no magic solution to this problem, particularly poor patient compliance. But rates may be better when patients receive proper information about why control of hypertension is important, where there is a well-developed and pro-active primary healthcare system and where drug treatment is affordable.

7.5 Diabetes

An increase in stroke risk, independent of other cardiovascular disease risk factors, has been reported in those with diabetes [20, 21]. A systematic overview of epidemiological studies and surveys found that 13% of all deaths from stroke worldwide were attributable to high blood glucose [22]. The relative risk of stroke among Swedish men with diabetes in the Multifactor Primary Prevention Study during a 28 year follow-up period was 2.42 (CI 1.94–3.02) [23]. Among Japanese-American men in the Honolulu Heart Program, participants with diabetes had an increased risk of thromboembolic stroke of 2.45 (CI 1.73–3.47), compared to those without diabetes over a 22 year follow-up period [21].

The prevalence of diabetes in Vietnam was reported to be 6% in 2017 [24] compared to about 9% in the US People with type 2 diabetes often have additional stroke risk factors, including hypertension, dyslipidemia and obesity, and a meta-analysis of 27 trials found that antihypertensive regimens provided significant benefit on fatal/nonfatal stroke in patients with type 2 diabetes compared to placebo [25]. Tight control of glucose levels probably does reduce macrovascular events although with the risk of more episodes of hypoglycaemia [26].

7.6 Smoking

Cigarette smoking is a potent risk factor for stroke [27]. Smoking possibly contributes to increased stroke risk through both acute effects on the risk of thrombus generation in narrowed arteries and chronic effects related to an increased burden of atherosclerosis. A meta-analysis of 32 studies including 17 cohort, 14 case-control and 1 hypertension intervention found an overall relative risk of stroke associated with cigarette smoking of 1.5 (95% CI: 1.4–1.6) [28]. The pooled relative risk estimates indicate a dose response from 1.37 (CI: 1.24–1.52) in those smoking <10/day to 1.82 (CI: 1.70–1.96) in those smoking >20/day. Cessation of cigarette smoking reduces stroke risk. In the British Regional Heart Study [29], current smokers were demonstrated to have a fourfold relative risk of stroke compared to never smokers (3.7; CI: 2.0–6.9) during an average follow-up period of 12.75 years after full adjustment of other risk factors. Ex-cigarette smokers showed lower risk than current smokers but showed excess risk compared with never smokers (RR 1.7; CI 0.9–3.3). The benefit of giving up smoking completely was seen within 5 years of quitting, with no further consistent decline in risk thereafter but this was dependent on the amount of tobacco smoked [30]. Those who smoked <20 cigarettes/day reverted to the risk level of those who had never smoked while heavy smokers retained a more than twofold risk compared with never smokers (RR2.2; 95% CI 1.1–4.3). A Cochrane review [31] of 78 studies with over 150,000 people came to the following conclusions:

- Nicotine e-cigarettes, varenicline and cytisine are the stop-smoking aids most likely to help people quit smoking.
- On average, for every 100 people trying to quit, around 14 are likely to succeed using an e-cigarette, varenicline or cytisine in any given quit attempt. This is compared to 6% who are likely to quit without using any aids.
- Dual nicotine replacement therapy (NRT) methods, like combining a patch with gum, may be almost as effective, with approximately 12% likely to successfully quit. However, this estimate is less certain than those for the other stop-smoking aids.
- Using only one form of NRT, such as a patch alone, leads to around 9% people successfully quitting.
- Cytisine, a highly effective smoking cessation medicine, is highlighted but is unavailable in most countries.

7.7 Lipids

A meta-analysis of prospective studies from the Asia-Pacific region, a 1 mmol/l increase in total cholesterol was associated with a 25% (95% CI: 13–40%) increased risk of fatal or nonfatal ischaemic stroke and a 20% (95% CI: 8–30%) decreased risk of fatal haemorrhagic stroke over 2 million person-years of follow-up demonstrating an association between total cholesterol and ischaemic but not haemorrhagic strokes [32]. During a mean follow-up period of 16.8 years in the British Regional Heart Study, higher levels of HDL cholesterol were associated with a significant decrease in the risk of nonfatal stroke even after adjustment for potential confounders (adjusted relative risk = 0.59, 95% CI 0.39–0.90) [33]. Total cholesterol showed no graded association with fatal strokes, but men with levels ≥8.1 mmol/L showed a non-significant increased risk of nonfatal stroke (adjusted RR = 1.46, 95% CI 0.91–2.32).

A meta-analysis of 62 prospective cohort studies [34] containing nearly a million patients overall however showed that higher HDL-C levels were associated with a 24% reduced risk of fatal and nonfatal ischaemic stroke but a 21% increased risk of primary intracerebral haemorrhage per 1 mmol/l increase in HDL-C level.

Data from the UK reported that 64.6% of adults had a total cholesterol ≥5 mmol/l [35]. The mean total cholesterol in 2002 was 5.4 (5.2–5.5) mmol/l in high income countries and 4.3 (4.2–4.8) mmol/l in low-income countries [36, 37]. Despite the lack of clear association between serum total cholesterol and risk of stroke in observational epidemiological studies, the results of lipid-lowering trials with statins suggest some benefit for stroke reduction. An overview of 16 published randomised trials of statins, following up subjects for an average of 3.3 years, demonstrated large reductions in total and low-density lipoprotein cholesterol (22% and 30% respectively) and significant reductions in risks of stroke of 29% (95% CI: 14–41%) in those assigned to statin drugs [38]. The Stroke Prevention by Aggressive Reduction in Cholesterol Levels (SPARCL) trial [39] randomised patients with a recent TIA or stroke, who had no known coronary heart disease and had a baseline LDL cholesterol between 100 and 190 mg/dl (2.6–4.9 mmol/l), to atorvastatin 80 mg daily or placebo. The trial demonstrated a 16% reduced relative risk of fatal or nonfatal strokes in the treatment group compared to the placebo group, during a median follow-up of 4.9 years (adjusted hazard ratio 0.84; CI 0.71–0.99). A meta-analysis of 11 randomised clinical trials [40] with over 20,000 patients to evaluate the association between more intensive vs less intensive LDL-C–lowering statin-based therapies with outcomes for patients with ischemic stroke showed that over a mean of 4 years follow-up higher dose regimes were more effective than lower dose (absolute risk, 8.1% vs 9.3%; RR, 0.88; 95% CI, 0.80–0.96). More intensive LDL-C–lowering statin-based therapies were associated with a reduced risk of major cardiovascular events, but with an increased risk of haemorrhagic stroke, compared with less intensive LDL-C–lowering statin-based therapies.

7.8 Physical Activity

Regular physical activity has well-established benefits for reducing the risk of premature death and cardiovascular disease and the beneficial effects of physical activity have been documented for stroke [41, 42]. Over a follow-up period of up to 32 years, the Framingham study investigators reported an increased risk of stroke associated with the lowest levels of physical activity in men. Among men included in this analysis, the crude risk ratios for medium levels of physical activity was 0.36 (95% CI; 0.22–0.59) and 0.33 (95% CI: 0.22–0.50) for high levels of physical activity compared with the lowest level of physical activity. A strong inverse association between physical activity and the risk of stroke was demonstrated in the British Regional Heart Study after 9.5 years of follow-up that was independent of age, social class, smoking, heavy drinking, SBP and pre-existing ischaemic heart disease or stroke (RR 1.0 for inactivity, 0.6 for moderate activity and 0.3 vigorous activity; test for trend $p = 0.008$) [43].

7.9 Obesity

Evidence from large-scale prospective studies has documented that increased weight is associated with an increased risk of stroke [44]. In the Physician's Health Study, a prospective cohort study of US male physicians, participants with BMI ≥30 kg/m^2 had an adjusted relative risk of 2.0 (95% CI: 1.48–2.71) for total stroke, 1.95 (95% CI: 1.39–2.72) for ischaemic strokes and 2.25 (95% CI: 1.01–5.01) for haemorrhagic stroke compared to participants with BMI <23 kg/m^2 during 12.5 years of follow-up. Each unit increase of BMI was associated with a significant 6% increase in the adjusted relative risks of total, ischaemic and haemorrhagic strokes. Similar finding have been reported for women. Obesity is an increasing problem in nearly all countries, particularly high income countries and those transitioning from middle to high income. The WHO estimates that globally there are more than one billion overweight adults (BMI ≥25 kg/m^2) [45]. Until recently there has been little evidence that traditional weight loss strategies resulted in a reduction in cardiovascular or cerebrovascular risk. But an important trial published in 2023 in the New England Journal of Medicine showed that Semaglutide can reduce stroke and cardiac events [46]. Semaglutide is a glucagon-like peptide-1 receptor agonist, that has been shown to reduce the risk of adverse cardiovascular events in patients with diabetes. This study was a multicentre, double-blind, randomized, placebo-controlled trial that enrolled 17,604 patients, 45 years of age or older with pre-existing cardiovascular disease and a body-mass index of 27 or greater but no history of diabetes. They were randomised to weekly subcutaneous semaglutide at a dose of 2.4 mg or placebo. A primary cardiovascular end-point event occurred in 6.5% in the semaglutide group and 8.0% in the placebo group (hazard ratio, 0.80; 95% confidence interval, 0.72–0.90; $P < 0.001$) showing that semaglutide was superior to placebo in reducing the incidence of death from cardiovascular causes, nonfatal myocardial infarction, or nonfatal stroke at a mean follow-up of 39.8 months.

7.10 Atrial Fibrillation

The attributable risk of stroke for AF increased significantly with age, from 1.5% for those aged 50–59 years, to 23.5% for those aged 80–89 years [47]. The reported prevalence of AF in England and Wales in 1998 increased from 1/1000 in under 35 year olds to 10% in those aged 85 years and over [48]. Studies in Southeast Asia recorded an AF rate in a lower range from 5.8% to 23.4%. A cross-sectional study conducted on 2038 consecutive patients with TIA or ischemic stroke admitted to Bach Mai Hospital, Hanoi found AF on standard electrocardiogram or Holter monitor in 18.1% (95% CI: 16.46–19.85) [49]. Randomised controlled trials have demonstrated warfarin therapy to be highly efficacious in reducing risk of ischaemic stroke in patients with AF, with relatively low rates of bleeding [50, 51]. Analysis of data from five randomised trials comparing warfarin or aspirin with control in patients with AF, demonstrated warfarin consistently decreasing the risk of stroke in patients with AF (a 68% reduction in risk) with virtually no increase in the frequency of major bleeding [52]. The efficacy of aspirin in this study was less consistent, and patients younger than 65 years with AF and without a history of hypertension, previous stroke or transient ischaemic attack, or diabetes were at very low risk of stroke even when untreated (annual rate of stroke = 1% compared to 4.5% for the control group and 1.4% for the warfarin group). More recent studies using Direct Oral Anticoagulants (DOAC) has found that they are as effective as warfarin, may have fewer haemorrhagic side effects, have better patient compliance and are preferred by patients [53] (see Chap. 21).

7.11 Carotid Stenosis

A carotid stenosis of greater than 50% (diameter reduction) is reported in 5–9% of men and women 65 years or older [54, 55]. Natural history studies reflect an annual stroke risk between 1% and 3.4% among persons with an asymptomatic carotid artery stenosis between 50% and 99% [56, 57]. Results from the North American Symptomatic Carotid Endarterectomy Trial (NASCET) that randomised patients with TIA or a nondisabling stroke to surgery or to medical care, demonstrated a significant advantage of carotid endarterectomy in patients with high-grade stenosis (70–99% narrowing in the luminal diameter) and a moderate reduction in stroke risk in patients with symptomatic moderate carotid stenosis (50–69% narrowing) [58, 59]. There was a 17% absolute risk reduction of ipsilateral stroke at 18 months in the surgical group ($p < 0.001$) and the risk of any severe stroke or death from any cause was reduced in the surgical group (absolute risk reduction of 7% $p < 0.01$). In patients with high moderate stenosis (50–69%) in the NASCET trial, the 5-year risk of ipsilateral stroke or death for the medical group was 22.2% and was 15.7% for the surgical group (absolute risk reduction of 6.5%). In a pooled analysis of data from NASCET, the European Carotid Surgery Trial (ECST) and Veterans Affairs trial 309 during 35,000 patient-years of follow-up, surgery was reported to increase the 5 year risk of ipsilateral ischaemic stroke in patients with less than 30% stenosis (absolute risk reduction −2.2%, $p = 0.05$), have no effect in patients with 30–49% stenosis (3.2%, $p = 0.6$), of marginal benefit in those with 50–69% stenosis (4.6%, $p = 0.04$) and highly beneficial in those with 70% stenosis or greater without near occlusion (16%, $p < 0.001$) [60].

Trials of surgery for asymptomatic carotid stenosis show a very small decrease in the absolute risk of stroke Surgery for asymptomatic carotid stenosis has been shown relative reductions in the risk of stroke (about 50%) but, with a low overall risk of stroke in this population, the absolute risk reductions are small (about 5% over 10 years) [61]. The benefit appears to be restricted to those less than 75 years of age and may be smaller in women than in men. On the basis of these data, the number needed to undergo surgery to prevent one extra stroke over 10 years is about 20 and roughly twice this to prevent one extra disabling or fatal stroke. There have been significant developments in medical secondary prevention since the asymptomatic carotid surgery trials recruited their patients. It seems highly likely that the risk of stroke and other vascular outcomes for patients would be less if these trials were conducted now. With small absolute benefits, likely made smaller still or negated by modern medical management surgery for asymptomatic stenosis cannot be considered a cost or clinically effective intervention.

7.12 Transient Ischaemic Attack

The risk of further stroke is highest early after stroke or TIA and may be as high as 10% within the first week, 20% within the first month and increases to 29% at 5 years (see Chap. 8). Patients with recurrent stroke have on average, poorer outcomes than those with first stroke with 24-month survival reported to be 48.3% versus 56.7%, respectively [62]. It is important for appropriate secondary prevention to be implemented as soon as possible and continued in the long term. The non randomised Early use of eXisting PREventive Strategies for Stroke (EXPRESS) study [63] showed that urgent assessment and treatment after the onset of TIA or minor stroke reduced the 90-day risk of recurrent stroke by about 80%. Effective implementation of secondary stroke preventive measures will not only reduce the rate of recurrent stroke, but also potentially reduce the morbidity and mortality related to coronary heart disease.

7.13 Strategies to Implement Risk Factor Reduction

Interventions to reduce the risk of stroke reported in a review included those to change professional behaviours in preventing and managing stroke, interventions targeted at patients and the public and interventions targeted at health services [64].

Positive associations were found between skills training and improvements in professional attitude to stroke patients and stroke care. Patient decision making aids were associated with increased patient choice which did not necessarily enhance subsequent adherence to treatment. A review of randomised controlled trials assessing the effectiveness of multiple risk factor intervention using counselling and/or educational approaches with or without pharmacological interventions found modest reductions in smoking prevalence, systolic blood pressure and blood cholesterol level in the intervention groups [65]. In a review of community interventions to manage hypertension among black ethnic groups, health education combined with individualised support for patients to self-manage hypertension were associated with reductions in blood pressure levels and improvements in blood pressure control [66].

Although data on secondary prevention of stroke has shown excellent adherence to stroke prevention strategies in some populations with 84% of patients on aspirin one year after their strokes, lower rates (50–70%) have been achieved in others populations [67, 68]. The use of antihypertensives for patients with hypertension and appropriate antiplatelet and anticoagulation therapy for patients with atrial fibrillation are similarly low. The Euroaspire surveys conducted in several centres in Europe demonstrates the difficulty in reducing smoking, obesity and cholesterol and controlling blood pressure at the population level in patients with coronary heart disease even in high income countries [19]. As the number of medications that a patient requires increases, adherence and compliance to therapy are likely to decrease [69]. It has been proposed that a single daily pill (polypill) combining half-doses (to minimise toxicity) of a beta-blocker, thiazide diuretic and an ACE-inhibitor, together with a statin, folic acid and aspirin administered to people with known cardiovascular disease and everyone aged 55 years and over, would reduce the incidence of stroke by 80% [70]. The use of the 'polypill' which concomitantly reduce multiple risk factors without increasing the pill burden has the potential to improve cardiovascular disease risk management, thereby reducing the incidence of cardiovascular disease (see Chap. 21).

References

1. GBD 2021 Diseases and Injuries Collaborators. Global incidence, prevalence, years lived with disability (YLDs), disability-adjusted life-years (DALYs), and healthy life expectancy (HALE) for 371 diseases and injuries in 204 countries and territories and 811 subnational locations, 1990-2021: a systematic analysis for the Global Burden of Disease Study 2021. Lancet. 2024;403(10440):2133–61.
2. Kings College London and the Stroke Alliance for Europe. Burden of stroke in Europe. https://www.safestroke.eu/wp-content/uploads/2020/06/The-Burden-Of-Stroke-In-Europe-Report-Main-Document_ENG_All-references.pdf.
3. WHO. Cardiovascular diseases in Vietnam. https://www.who.int/vietnam/health-topics/cardiovasculardiseases#:~:text=However%2C%20currently%20CVDs%20are%20the,to%20more%20than%20170%20000.

4. World Heart Foundation Vietnam Country Report. 2019. https://world-heart-federation.org/world-heart-observatory/resource/vietnam-country-report/.
5. Ngoc NH, Thong NV, Hien LX et al. Predictors of ischaemic stroke in elderly patients in Vietnam. Genet Mol Res 2021;20(1) gmr 18741.
6. Ngoc NH, An NQ. Risk factors of ischemic cerebral vascular accident. Genet. Mol. Res 2021;20(1) gmr 18742.
7. Williams B, Poulter NR, Brown MJ, et al. Guidelines for management of hypertension: report of the fourth working party of the British Hypertension Society, 2004-BHS IV. J Hum Hypertens. 2004;18(3):139–85.
8. Chobanian AV, Bakris GL, Black HR, et al. Seventh report of the Joint National Committee on prevention, detection, evaluation, and treatment of high blood pressure. Hypertension. 2003;42(6):1206–52.
9. MacMahon S, Peto R, Cutler J, et al. Blood pressure, stroke, and coronary heart disease. Part 1, prolonged differences in blood pressure: prospective observational studies corrected for the regression dilution bias. Lancet. 1990;335(8692):765–74.
10. Kannel WB, Dawber TR, Cohen ME, et al. Vascular disease of the brain–epidemiologic aspects: the Framingham study. Am J Public Health Nations Health. 1965;55:1355–66.
11. Lewington SR, Clarke N, et al. Age-specific relevance of usual blood pressure to vascular mortality: a meta-analysis of individual data for one million adults in 61 prospective studies. Lancet. 2002;360(9349):1903–13.
12. Lawes CM, Bennett DA, Feigin VL, et al. Blood pressure and stroke: an overview of published reviews. Stroke. 2004;35(3):776–85.
13. Burt VL, Whelton P, Roccella EJ, et al. Prevalence of hypertension in the US adult population. Results from the Third National Health and Nutrition Examination Survey, 1988-1991. Hypertension. 1995;25(3):305–13.
14. Primatesta P, Bost L, Poulter NR. Blood pressure levels and hypertension status among ethnic groups in England. J Hum Hypertens. 2000;14(2):143–8.
15. Gu Q, Burt VL, Paulose-Ram R, et al. High blood pressure and cardiovascular disease mortality risk among U.S. adults: the third National Health and Nutrition Examination Survey mortality follow-up study. Ann Epidemiol. 2008;18(4):302–9.
16. Hajjar I, Kotchen TA. Trends in prevalence, awareness, treatment, and control of hypertension in the United States, 1988-2000. JAMA. 2003;290(2):199–206.
17. Wolf-Maier, Cooper RS, Kramer H, et al. Hypertension treatment and control in five European countries, Canada, and the United States. Hypertension. 2004;43(1):10–7.
18. Wolf PA, Grotta JC. Cerebrovascular disease. Circulation. 2000;102(Suppl 4):75–80.
19. Kotseva K, Wood D, De Backer G, et al. Cardiovascular prevention guidelines in daily practice: a comparison of EUROASPIRE I, II, and III surveys in eight European countries. Lancet. 2009;373(9667):929–40.
20. Wolf PA, D'Agostino RB, Belanger AJ, et al. Probability of stroke: a risk profile from the Framingham Study. Stroke. 1991;22(3):312–8.
21. Burchfield CM, Curb JD, Rodriguez BL, et al. Glucose intolerance and 22-year stroke incidence. The Honolulu Heart Program. Stroke. 1994;25(5):951–7.
22. Danaei G, Lawes CM, Vander Hoorn S, et al. Global and regional mortality from ischaemic heart disease and stroke attributable to higher-than-optimum blood glucose concentration: comparative risk assessment. Lancet. 2006;368(9548):1651–9.
23. Harmsen P, Lappas G, Rosengren GA, et al. Long-term risk factors for stroke: twenty-eight years of follow-up of 7457 middle-aged men in Goteborg, Sweden. Stroke. 2006;37(7):1663–7.
24. Ton TT, Tran ATN, Do IT, et al. Trends in prediabetes and diabetes prevalence and associated risk factors in Vietnamese adults. Epidemiol Health. 2020;42:e2020029.
25. Turnbull F, Neal B, Algert C, et al. Effects of different blood pressure-lowering regimens on major cardiovascular events in individuals with and without diabetes mellitus: results of prospectively designed overviews of randomized trials. Arch Intern Med. 2005;165(12):1410–9.

26. Aldafas R, Crabtree T, Vinogradova Y, et al. Efficacy and safety of intensive versus conventional glucose targets in people with type 2 diabetes: a systematic review and meta-analysis. Expert Rev Endocrinol Metab. 2023;18(1):95–110.
27. Rodriguez BL, D'Agostino R, Abbott RD, et al. Risk of hospitalized stroke in men enrolled in the Honolulu Heart Program and the Framingham Study: a comparison of incidence and risk factor effects. Stroke. 2002;33(1):230–6.
28. Shinton R, Beevers G. Meta-analysis of relation between cigarette smoking and stroke. BMJ. 1989;298(6676):789–94.
29. Wolf PA, D'Agostino RB, Kannel WB, et al. Cigarette smoking as a risk factor for stroke. The Framingham Study. JAMA. 1988;259(7):1025–9.
30. Wannamethee SG, Shaper AG, Whincup PH, et al. Smoking cessation and the risk of stroke in middle-aged men. JAMA. 1995;274(2):155–60.
31. Lindson N, Theodoulou A, Ordóñez-Mena JM, et al. Pharmacological and electronic cigarette interventions for smoking cessation in adults: component network meta-analyses. Cochrane Database Syst Rev. 2023;9:CD015226. https://doi.org/10.1002/14651858.CD015226.pub2.
32. Zhang X, Patel A, Horibe H, et al. Cholesterol, coronary heart disease, and stroke in the Asia Pacific region. Int J Epidemiol. 2003;32(4):563–72.
33. Wannamethee SG, Shaper AG, Ebrahim S. HDL-cholesterol, total cholesterol, and the risk of stroke in middle-aged British men. Stroke. 2000;31(8):1882–8.
34. Qie R, Liu L, Zhang D, et al. Dose response association between high density lipoprotein cholesterol and stroke. A systematic review and meta-analysis of prospective cohort studies. Prev Chronic Dis. 2021;18:200278.
35. Primatesta P, Poulter NR. Lipid levels and the use of lipid-lowering agents in England and Scotland. Eur J Cardiovasc Prev Rehabil. 2004;11(6):484–8.
36. Johnston SC, Mendis S, Mathers CD. Global variation in stroke burden and mortality: estimates from monitoring, surveillance, and modelling. Lancet Neurol. 2009;8(4):345–54.
37. WHO. WHO global infobase. Geneva: World Health Organisation; 2008. http://www.who.int/infobase/comparestart.aspx.
38. Hebert PR, Gaziano JM, Chan KS, et al. Cholesterol lowering with statin drugs, risk of stroke, and total mortality. An overview of randomized trials. JAMA. 1997;278(4):313–21.
39. Amarenco P, Bogousslavsky J, Callahan JA, et al. High-dose atorvastatin after stroke or transient ischemic attack. N Engl J Med. 2006;355(6):549–59.
40. Lee M, Cheng CY, Wu YL, et al. Association between intensity of low-density lipoprotein cholesterol reduction with statin-based therapies and secondary stroke prevention: a meta-analysis of randomized clinical trials. JAMA Neurol. 2022;79(4):349–58.
41. Kiely DK, Wolf PA, Cupples LA, et al. Physical activity and stroke risk: the Framingham Study. Am J Epidemiol. 1994;140(7):608–20.
42. Sacco RL, Gan R, Boden-Albala B, et al. Leisure-time physical activity and ischemic stroke risk: the Northern Manhattan Stroke Study. Stroke. 1998;29(2):380–7.
43. Wannamethee G, Shaper AG. Physical activity and stroke in British middle aged men. BMJ. 1992;304(6827):597–601.
44. Kurth T, Gaziano JM, Berger K, et al. Body mass index and the risk of stroke in men. Arch Intern Med. 2002;162(22):2557–62.
45. WHO. Obesity and overweight fact sheet. 2006. http://www.who.int/dietphysicalactivity/publications/facts/obesity/en/.
46. Lincoff AM, Brown-Frandsen K, Colhoun HM, et al. Semaglutide and cardiovascular outcomes in obesity without diabetes. N Engl J Med. 2023;389(24):2221–32.
47. Wolf PA, Abbott RD, Kannel WB. Atrial fibrillation as an independent risk factor for stroke: the Framingham Study. Stroke. 1991;22(8):983–8.
48. Majeed A, Moser K, Carroll K. Trends in the prevalence and management of atrial fibrillation in general practice in England and Wales, 1994-1998: analysis of data from the general practice research database. Heart. 2001;86(3):284–8.

49. Phong PD, Tung BN, Hung PM, et al. Prevalence and factors associated with atrial fibrillation in patients with transient ischemic attack or ischemic stroke in Northern Vietnam. J Clin Med. 2023;12(17):5516.
50. The Boston Area Anticoagulation Trial for Atrial Fibrillation Investigators. The effect of low-dose warfarin on the risk of stroke in patients with nonrheumatic atrial fibrillation. N Engl J Med. 1990;323(22):1505–11.
51. Author. Adjusted-dose warfarin versus low-intensity, fixed-dose warfarin plus aspirin for high-risk patients with atrial fibrillation: stroke prevention in atrial fibrillation III randomised clinical trial. Lancet. 1996;348(9028):633–8.
52. Author. Risk factors for stroke and efficacy of antithrombotic therapy in atrial fibrillation. Analysis of pooled data from five randomized controlled trials. Arch Intern Med. 1994;154(13):1449–57.
53. Khouja C, Brunton G, Richardson M, et al. Oral anticoagulants: a systematic overview of reviews on efficacy and safety, genotyping, self-monitoring, and stakeholder experiences. Syst Rev. 2022;11:23.
54. O'Leary DH, Polak JF, Kronmal RA, et al. Distribution and correlates of sonographically detected carotid artery disease in the cardiovascular health study. The CHS Collaborative Research Group. Stroke. 1992;23(12):1752–60.
55. Fine-Edelstein JS, Wolf PA, O'Leary DH, et al. Precursors of extracranial carotid atherosclerosis in the Framingham Study. Neurology. 1994;44(6):1046–50.
56. Autret A, Pourcelot L, Saudeau D, et al. Stroke risk in patients with carotid stenosis. Lancet. 1987;1(8538):888–90.
57. Nadareishvili ZG, Rothwell PM, Beletsky V, et al. Long-term risk of stroke and other vascular events in patients with asymptomatic carotid artery stenosis. Arch Neurol. 2002;59(7):1162–6.
58. North American Symptomatic Carotid Endarterectomy Trial (NASCET) Investigators. Benefit of carotid endarterectomy for patients with high-grade stenosis of the internal carotid artery. National Institute of Neurological Disorders and Stroke, Stroke and Trauma Division. Stroke. 1991;22(6):816–7.
59. Barnett HJ, Taylor DW, Eliasziw M, et al. Benefit of carotid endarterectomy in patients with symptomatic moderate or severe stenosis. N Engl J Med. 1998;339(20):1415–25.
60. Rothwell PM, Eliasziw M, Gutnikov SA, et al. Analysis of pooled data from the randomised controlled trials of endarterectomy for symptomatic carotid stenosis. Lancet. 2003;361(9352):107–16.
61. Halliday A, Harrison M, Hayter E, et al. 10-year stroke prevention after successful carotid endarterectomy for asymptomatic stenosis (ACST-1): a multicentre randomised trial. Lancet. 2010;376(9746):1074–84.
62. Samsa GP, Bian J, Lipscomb J, et al. Epidemiology of recurrent cerebral infarction: a medicare claims-based comparison of first and recurrent strokes on 2-year survival and cost. Stroke. 1999;30(2):338–49.
63. Rothwell PM, Giles MF, Chandratheva A, et al. Effect of urgent treatment of transient ischaemic attack and minor stroke on early recurrent stroke (EXPRESS study): a prospective population-based sequential comparison. Lancet. 2007;370(9596):1432–42.
64. Redfern J, McKevitt C, Rudd A, et al. Review of interventions to change patient and professional behaviors in stroke management and prevention. In: Trafton J, Gordon WP, editors. Best practices in the behavioural management of chronic disease, vol. 1. Los Banos: Institute for Brain Potential; 2006.
65. Ebrahim S, Beswick A, Burke M, et al. Multiple risk factor interventions for primary prevention of coronary heart disease. Cochrane Database Syst Rev. 2006;4:CD001561.
66. Connell P, Wolfe C, McKevitt C. Preventing stroke: a narrative review of community interventions for improving hypertension control in black adults. Health Soc Care Community. 2008;16(2):165–87.
67. Hamann GF, Weimar C, Glahn J, et al. Adherence to secondary stroke prevention strategies–results from the German Stroke Data Bank. Cerebrovasc Dis. 2003;15(4):282–8.

68. Rundek T, Sacco RL. Risk factor management to prevent first stroke. Neurol Clin. 2008;26(4):1007–45.
69. Sleight P, Pouleur H, Zannad F. Benefits, challenges, and registerability of the polypill. Eur Heart J. 2006;27(14):1651–6.
70. Wald NJ, Law MR. A strategy to reduce cardiovascular disease by more than 80%. BMJ. 2003;326(7404):1419.

Chapter 8
Unusual Causes of Stroke

Christopher Pieri, Thong Van Nguyen, Ngoc Huy Nguyen, An Quang Nguyen, Viet Quoc Hoang, and Anthony Rudd

8.1 Introduction

Up to 30% of strokes are labelled as being cryptogenic (unknown or obscure origin) after the usual investigations have failed to identify a cause. There are many unusual causes of stroke which may be missed potentially leading to major consequences both in overall outcome and risk of recurrence, that need to be known about and considered in the differential diagnosis of these patients. Many of the diagnoses mentioned in this chapter are rare and may never be seen by an individual clinician during their clinical practice, but they certainly won't be found unless the clinician recognises the possibility and knows how they present. Some of the diagnoses however, such as extracranial arterial dissection, stroke secondary to patent foramen ovale and posterior reversible encephalopathy syndrome are not so rare and are

C. Pieri (✉)
Stroke Medicine, St Thomas' Hospital, London, UK
e-mail: Christopher.Pieri@gstt.nhs.uk

T. Van Nguyen
Vietnam Stroke Association, Hanoi, Vietnam

Stroke Center, Phutho General Hospital, Phutho, Vietnam

N. H. Nguyen
Phutho Department of Health, Phutho, Vietnam

VNU University of Medicine and Pharmacy, Hanoi, Vietnam

A. Q. Nguyen
Phutho Medical College, Phutho, Vietnam

V. Q. Hoang
Stroke Center, Phutho General Hospital, Phutho, Vietnam

A. Rudd
King's College, London, UK

A. Rudd et al. (eds.), *Stroke Management in Vietnam*,
https://doi.org/10.1007/978-981-96-0221-6_8

diagnosed much more easily with the routine use of advanced imaging. Others are much more frequently seen in some parts of the world compared to others, such as sickle cell disease and Takayasu arteritis.

The list of possible causes is long. This chapter only covers a relatively small number of the multitude of causes. Only a brief description is given for each condition mentioned and readers are advised to read the references for more detail. The classification presented here is based on one used in an excellent review by Hurford et al. [1].

8.2 Cardiac Causes

8.2.1 *Patent Foramen Ovale*

Approximately, 25% of the population will have a patent foramen ovale (PFO) that has persisted into adult life. The incidence in patients with cryptogenic stroke is up to 40%. The difficulty for the stroke physician is therefore to identify those patients where the PFO is the cause of the stroke and not just an epi-phenomenon. Under normal conditions if there is blood flow across the PFO, it will be from the high pressure left atrium to the right atrium, therefore not putting a patient at risk of a venous thrombus entering the arterial system. However, if the patient increases their intrathoracic pressure by doing a Valsalva manoeuvre or straining hard, then flow can reverse, allowing thrombi to enter the arterial system from the venous side. There are three possible mechanisms by which a PFO may cause a stroke, paradoxical embolism, thrombus forming at the site of the PFO or the PFO increasing the risk of atrial fibrillation.

A meta-analysis [2] suggests that certain features of stroke associated with a PFO increase the likelihood that the PFO is clinically relevant:

- Large size with evidence of significant reverse flow with or without a Valsava manoeuvre
- The presence of an atrial septal aneurysm (ASA)
- Young age of the patient
- The lesion appears on brain imaging as being likely to be embolic, e.g., a wedge cortical infarct
- Multiple infarcts, potentially of different ages, in different vascular territories
- A history that suggests that the stroke occurred following an episode of increased thoracic pressure.

Case history: a 48-year-old previously fit man with no known vascular risk factors had flown from the USA to the UK. After landing, he struggled to remove a heavy bag from the overhead locker. A few moments later he collapsed with a dense right hemiplegia and aphasia. He was taken to the nearest stroke centre where he had a thrombectomy for an M1 occlusion performed 2 h after the onset of symptom. He made a full recovery within 48 h. Investigations revealed a large PFO with an

ASA. No thrombus was identified in the leg veins and no other possible cause of the stroke was identified. It seems likely that he developed a deep venous thrombosis on the flight and while straining to remove his bag the thrombus embolized and entered the arterial circulation through the PFO.

Where a PFO is suspected investigations should include a transthoracic echocardiogram followed by a trans-oesophageal echocardiogram with air injected to show how many bubbles are crossing from the right side to the left and under what circumstances. Our practice is to always review these cases in a multidisciplinary case conference including the stroke physician/neurologist, haematologist and cardiologist.

Management has become clearer following the publication of three major trials comparing medical treatment with closure of the PFO; CLOSE, REDUCE and RESPECT. All these studies showed better outcomes for closure compared to antiplatelet therapy alone. However, compared to the previous negative trials all of these had much stricter entry criteria, excluding those patients with other stroke risk factors and with CLOSE requiring the presence of an ASA or greater right to left shunting. No trial has so far reported a comparison between closure and anticoagulation.

8.2.2 Endocarditis and Atrial Myxoma

Early diagnosis is essential as the prognosis for these two conditions without treatment is poor [3, 4]. Any acute stroke patient known to have valvular heart disease or in whom cardiac auscultation indicates the possibility of an abnormality should have an urgent transthoracic echocardiogram. Likewise, this should also be done for any patient with evidence of sepsis associated with acute stroke where there is no clear cause for the sepsis. Endocarditis is an unusual cause of stroke with an incidence of about 3–10 cases per 100,000 population [5]. The cause is most commonly infective endocarditis but can also be associated with non-bacterial thrombotic endocarditis and Libman-Sacks endocarditis seen in association with lupus erythematosus and antiphospholipid syndrome. Symptomatic stroke occurs in about a third of patients with endocarditis although the rate is much higher for asymptomatic embolism. Diagnosis is made by having a high clinical suspicion, careful clinical examination looking for the peripheral signs of endocarditis, with blood cultures and echocardiography, sometimes requiring both transthoracic and trans-oesophageal echocardiography. The appearance of the stroke on brain imaging can be that of an infarct or haemorrhage with the mechanism for haemorrhage being bleeding into infarcts, rupture of a vessel wall affected by septic arteritis, or rupture of a mycotic aneurysm. While treatment with intravenous antibiotics may be sufficient to effect a cure some patients will require surgery to replace the infected valve.

Case history: A 30-year-old man presents to his local emergency department with progressive exertional dyspnoea worsening over the last 2 weeks. He states that while he could previously walk as far as he wanted, he is now acutely short of breath on walking just short distances. He has a background of active intravenous drug use, untreated chronic hepatitis C infection and alcohol dependency. On admission, the clerking doctor notices that he has a loud pan-systolic murmur alongside a low-grade fever and raised inflammatory markers. A subsequent trans-thoracic echocardiogram confirms the presence of a large mobile mass attached to the posterior leaflet of the mitral valve with significant regurgitation across the valve. He is started on intravenous antibiotics, and a cardiothoracic opinion is sought. However, a couple of days later, he is found to be difficult to rouse and is observed to not be moving his left side. His GCS is calculated to be 9 (E2V3M4) and he is rushed for an urgent CT brain. This unfortunately demonstrates a large embolic left sided infarct with evidence of bleeding within the infarcted core.

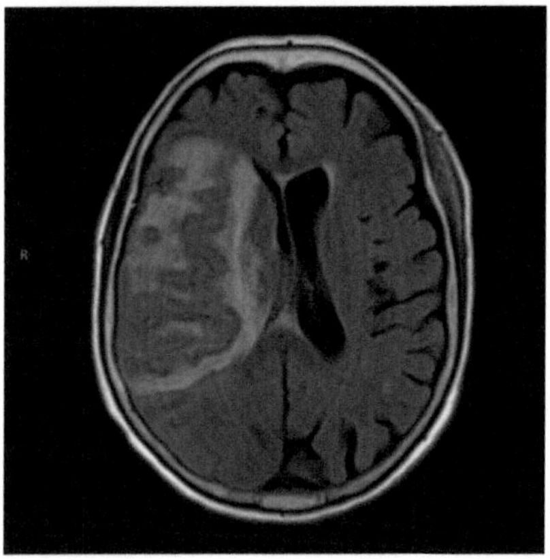

Axial flair MRI sequence demonstrating large wedge-shaped right MCA territory infarct of embolic aeology with scattered hyperdensity demonstrating haemorrhagic transformation within the ischaemic core.

Axial flair MRI sequence demonstrating large wedge-shaped right MCA territory infarct of embolic aetiology with scattered hyperdensity demonstrating haemorrhagic transformation within the ischaemic core

8.3 Haematological Causes [6]

There are multiple haematological causes of stroke with any condition resulting in either an increased thrombotic tendency such as polycythaemia rubra vera or thrombocystosis increasing the risk of cerebral ischaemic damage and any condition causing increased bleeding tendency such as von Willebrand's disease, haemophilia and thrombocytopaenia, increasing the risk of intracerebral haemorrhage. Hypercoagulable states may result from malignancy especially lung, colorectal and pancreatic. One report suggested that as many as 5–10% of cryptogenic ischaemic strokes may be the result of previously undiagnosed malignancy [7].

8.3.1 Sickle Cell Disease [8]

As the prognosis of sickle cell disease (SCD) has improved so it has become a more important cause of stroke in adults. Eleven percent of patients have a clinically evident stroke by 20 years of age and 24% by 45 years of age. Symptomatic and asymptomatic ischaemic stroke as well as haemorrhagic stroke are all more common in patients with SCD than in the general population. Ischaemic strokes are secondary to vasculopathy and intracranial large artery stenosis. Haemorrhages account for one third of SCD related stroke and may be subarachnoid, intraparenchymal, intraventricular, or any combination of the three. Acute management of the ischaemic strokes should be the same as for patients without sickle disease. Although there is sparse data on the use of thrombolytics there seems little reason to suppose that it would not have similar efficacy and likewise for patients with large vessel occlusion, thrombectomy should be considered. Haemoglobin S levels should be reduced to less than 30% by exchange transfusion and there is evidence to support maintaining regular exchange transfusions after a stroke to prevent further events.

8.3.2 Antiphospholipid Syndrome (APLS) [6]

Diagnosing antiphospholipid syndrome requires a combination of clinical features together with laboratory findings. The clinical criteria include recurrent foetal miscarriage and venous or arterial ischaemia and the laboratory findings of anticardiolipin antibodies and/or anti-ß2 glycoprotein-1 on at least two sets of tests several months apart. A single isolated positive antibody is relatively common especially in the context of acute illness such as stroke, but the true prevalence is only about 5 per 100,000. APLS can co-exist with systemic lupus erythematosus. The presence of the antibodies interferes with the endogenous anticoagulant mechanisms resulting in a procoagulant state.

The ischaemic damage is most commonly embolic in appearance, although it can present with features more typical of small vessel disease. Management is with long term anticoagulation using a vitamin K antagonist such as warfarin aiming for an INR of between 2 and 3. A trial (TRAPS) comparing the efficacy of a direct oral anticoagulant with warfarin in a high-risk group was stopped early because of an excess of clinical end points in the rivaroxaban group [9].

8.4 Inflammatory Causes [10]

8.4.1 Primary Angiitis of the Central Nervous System (PACNS)

PACNS is defined by an autoimmune vasculitis confined to the CNS and not secondary to any other condition. The underlying aetiology is not known and given the range of clinical and radiological features may be a syndrome with several underlying mechanisms. It can occur at any age but is seen predominantly in the middle aged. The estimated incidence is 2.4 cases per million. Clinical presentation is varied but may present with an acute ischaemic event combined with progressive cognitive and/or psychiatric problems. Headache is common feature which is unusual in more common causes of cerebral ischaemia. MRI appearances are heterogenous but nearly always show ischemic change, sometimes with enhancement with gadolinium and in about three quarters of cases, abnormalities of the arterial wall on MRA. Usually, multiple vascular territories are involved. Definitive diagnosis is difficult and even brain biopsy may not be confirmatory. Histological confirmation is only obtained in one third of patients who have a biopsy with changes ranging from granulomatous to lymphocytic or acute necrotising vasculitis.

No randomised controlled trials of treatment have been reported and given the rarity of the condition are unlikely to be performed. Immunosuppression with high dose steroids and/or cyclophosphamide are the most usual treatments although there have been case reports of treatment using rituximab and infliximab. Most patients recover with treatment although with a relapse rate of about 30%. It is suggested that patients are kept on low dose maintenance treatment long term.

8.4.2 Secondary Vasculitides Including Giant Cell Arteritis

There are multiple conditions that can cause a generalised vasculitis leading to cerebral ischaemia. Vessel wall involvement can occur in small, medium and large vessels so the clinical presentation can be very varied. The aetiologies include malignancy, autoimmune disease and drug usage. Because of the systemic nature of the vascular inflammation when cerebral ischaemia occurs there may be other generalised symptoms such as weight loss, malaise, joint pain and skin rashes. When giant cell arteritis is suspected, a history of visual loss and jaw claudication should be sought. Bechet's syndrome may present with stroke and genital ulceration. Diagnosis can be difficult. It is essential to ensure that infective causes are excluded before starting immunosuppression.

8.4.3 *Takayasu Disease [11, 12]*

This is a rare vasculitis affecting the aorta and its main branches that occurs predominantly in young people, particularly women. It is rare after the age of 40 years. The aetiology is unknown but there seem to be some genetic factors that predispose to the disease. A genetic relationship with the HLA-B*52 allele, which is more prevalent in Asian populations, has been reported and may explain why the disease is more common in some Asian populations. The course of the disease is very variable and may progress over many years. As the disease can affect any of the major branches of the aorta, physical findings may be very varied including ischaemic upper limbs, different blood pressures in the two arms, seizures, syncope, vertigo and ischaemic heart disease. Aortic arteriography (CT or MR) using contrast may show areas of stenosis with vascular inflammation. Because of the rarity of the disease there are no large trials of treatment. Steroids are most commonly used in combination with antiplatelet drugs sometimes in combination with other immunosuppressive drugs. Surgery or stenting of vessels may be needed to relieve ischaemia.

8.5 Non Inflammatory Vasculopathies

8.5.1 *Moyamoya Angiopathy [10]*

This is a chronic disorder characterised by progressive stenosis of both internal carotid arteries and their branches leading to the development of fine collateral vessels in the deep areas of the brain. It can occur as a primary disease or occasionally secondary to other conditions such as sickle cell disease, neck radiotherapy and Downs syndrome. The incidence is approximately ten times higher in Asian countries, particularly Japan than in Europe and the USA. The aetiology is unknown but the association with the gene RNF213 suggests at least a partial genetic component. Presentation occurs in both children and adults and can be with ischaemic stroke or haemorrhagic, secondary to rupture of collateral vessels. Headache is a common associated symptom as are movement disorders secondary to basal ganglia involvement. Diagnosis requires angiography of the cerebral vessels. Treatment of the acute strokes is difficult as intravenous thrombolysis is relatively contraindicated because the high risk of intracerebral haemorrhage. Surgery using extracranial, intracranial bypass procedures has been shown to be effective at improving vascularization and reducing the risk of recurrent ischaemia and haemorrhage.

8.5.2 Reversible Cerebral Vasoconstriction Syndrome (RCVS) and Posterior Reversible Encephalopathy Syndrome (PRES) [10]

These are overlapping syndromes with similar presentations and radiographic findings. The pathophysiology is hypothesised to be vasoconstriction and endothelial dysfunction precipitated by some vasoactive trigger including some drugs (e.g., cocaine, ecstasy, over the counter cold medications containing adrenaline or noradrenaline, migraine medications containing triptans, some psychotropic drugs and antiparkinsonian medications). It has also been reported in association with pregnancy, COVID-19 and neuroendocrine tumours. In RCVS seizures occur in about 20% of cases with haemorrhage in 40% and ischaemia in 40%. Treatment should focus on removing the possible precipitating factors and giving calcium channel blockers. Prognosis is usually good with complete resolution within 3 months. PRES shares many of the risk factors but also includes hypertension. Radiographic findings are of oedema in the posterior circulation, although there have also been reports of abnormalities in the anterior circulation as well. It is important to control the blood pressure. Again, prognosis is good although long term neurological sequalae occur in about 10–20% of cases.

8.5.3 Cervical Artery Dissection including Connective Tissue Diseases Such as Marfans and Ehlers-Danlos [13]

As acute imaging using CT or MRI of the cervical arteries becomes more of a routine and higher quality, the diagnosis is made much more frequently, especially in younger patients; some reports suggest that it accounts for 10–20% of strokes in patients under the age of 50 years. In the majority of cases, no underlying cause is found although trauma such as experienced on fairground rides, neck manipulation by people practicing osteopathy and attempted strangulation have all been reported. A minority of cases are due to underlying connective tissue disorders such as Marfan's syndrome and Ehlers-Danlos syndrome. In many cases, there are no specific clinical features, but dissection can be accompanied by neck or retro-orbital pain and Horner's syndrome on the ipsilateral side to the damaged artery associated with contralateral ischaemic changes. There have been few randomised controlled trials of treatment due to the rarity of the condition but an underpowered study (CADISS trial), showed no benefit for anticoagulants over antiplatelet drugs. Our preference is to use antiplatelets and to continue until imaging shows complete resolution of the arterial abnormality.

8.5.4 Radiation Induced Vasculopathy [14]

Radiotherapy given to the neck for the treatment of head and neck carcinoma increases the risk of carotid stenosis over subsequent years. One study followed up 96 patients who had received such treatment showing internal carotid artery stenosis of 70% or more in 12 patients (12.5%) and common carotid artery stenosis of 70% or more in 9 patients at a mean of 80 months following the end of treatment. Stenting of the artery is preferred to carotid endarterectomy in these patients which is contrary to the stenting trials in patients with atheromatous disease. Given the high rate of stenosis consideration should be given to screening these patients on an annual basis using Doppler ultrasound.

8.6 Infections [15]

8.6.1 Bacterial Infections

8.6.1.1 Bacterial Meningitis

15–25% of cases of bacterial meningitis are complicated by ischaemic stroke with the rate of stroke being higher from Streptococcus pneumoniae at 36% and lower with Neisseria meningitides at 9%. Bacterial pathogens can stimulate the formation and release of inflammatory cytokines that damage the vascular endothelium. Angiography can show arterial narrowing, focal dilatation and vessel wall irregularities suggesting that vasculitis may be one of the mechanisms. The infection can also result in coagulopathies which increase the risk of thrombus formation.

8.6.1.2 Syphilis

The incidence of syphilis is increasing particularly in association with HIV infection with cerebral infarction occurring in approximately 15% of neurosyphilis cases, typically 5–12 years after the initial infection. It can cause an obliterative endarteritis of medium- and large-sized blood vessel walls.

8.6.1.3 Tuberculosis

Tuberculosis remains a major cause of morbidity and mortality in low- and middle-income countries, and with increasing flows of migration is also a significant issue in high income areas of the world. Tuberculous meningitis is associated with ischaemic stroke in 15–60% of patients. Ruptured tubercles in the subarachnoid space cause an inflammatory reaction which is most pronounced at the base of the brain.

Local arteries and veins may be encased and subsequently develop intimal proliferation and fibrinoid necrosis resulting in cerebral ischaemia.

8.6.2 *Viral Infections*

8.6.2.1 HIV [16]

HIV infection increases the risk of ischaemic stroke both during the acute phase of the illness when viral load is high and CD4 counts low and also in the longer term when the disease is well controlled with antiretroviral therapy. A systematic review showed the prevalence of stroke was nearly one per hundred among people with HIV aged 15 years and over and reached four per hundred for those aged more than 50 years, rates that are about 1.5 times higher than in the general population. There are several postulated mechanisms of stroke in the context of HIV, including cardio-thromboembolism, opportunistic infections, HIV-associated vasculopathy, coagulopathy, concomitant drug use and for patients on long- term treatment metabolic syndrome caused by antiretroviral drugs.

8.6.2.2 Varicella Zoster

Primary infection or reactivation of varicella zoster can cause a small and large vessel vasculitis, with the potential to cause cerebral infarctions. A history of a rash, either zoster (shingles) or varicella (chicken pox), is found in about two-thirds of those with VZV vasculopathy. Although the rash and stroke may occur concomitantly, the average time from rash to stroke symptoms is 4 months. Imaging studies usually show infarction typically with lesions in the grey-white matter junction. Vessel imaging typically shows beading with areas of narrowing and post-stenotic dilatation.

8.6.2.3 COVID-19

COVID-19 is associated with hypercoagulable states and endothelial abnormalities resulting in infarction in both venous and arterial territories. Ischaemic stroke is reported to occur in about 2% of infections with the virus, but up to 50% of cases with critically severe infections. COVID-19 has also been associated with vasculitis, including in children and teenagers, where a Kawasaki like presentation of multisystem abnormalities originating from medium-sized vessel inflammation has been implicated.

8.6.3 Fungal Infections

These are rare and mainly occur in association with immunosuppressed patients including those treated for malignancy, after organ transplants, and in HIV infection. The most common is infection with the yeast Cryptococcus, mainly affecting the meninges but can also produce abscesses in the brain parenchyma. Other fungi that can occasionally be associated with stroke are *Aspergillus* spp., Rhinocerebral mucormycosis, Histoplasma capsulatum, and in the southern United States Coccidioides immitis.

8.7 Drugs and Stroke

8.7.1 Recreational Drugs [17]

Recreational drug use is an important cause of stroke especially in the young. Not only may substances themselves increase the risk, but injecting drugs may also cause infections such as septicaemia, hepatitis, HIV and endocarditis, which, in turn, can cause both ischemic and haemorrhagic stroke.

Cannabis is most widely used and frequent use of it may increase the risk of stroke substantially although it is difficult to know whether this a true independent effect or a reflection of confounding factors such as smoking.

Amphetamine and related substances. The use of amphetamine is associated with a fivefold increase in the risk of stroke, both ischemic and haemorrhagic. This may be due to inducing acute severe hypertension or an increased thrombotic tendency.

Cocaine is the recreational drug most commonly associated with stroke. There is evidence that the use of cocaine within the last 24 h is strongly associated with an increased risk of stroke, especially with crack cocaine, with increased risk also being shown among habitual users. (OR 7.9; 95% CI, 1.8–35.0). Possible mechanisms include acute hypertensive crisis or platelet activation and aggregation.

8.7.2 Therapeutic Drugs [18]

A good systematic review of the association between stroke and therapeutic drugs examined 81 drugs or drug classes [18]. While there are clear well known associations between anticoagulants and antiplatelet drugs and the risk of intracerebral haemorrhage, for many drugs there is relatively poor quality evidence. The drugs where there is strong evidence are oral contraceptives containing oestrogen with a dose relationship shown between the risk of stroke and the amount of oestrogen. The effect is augmented for older women and smokers. However, although there is a clear increased relative risk, the absolute risk is quite small given that the risk of stroke in women of reproductive age is low. The estimate is that 5165 women needed to be treated per year for there to be one additional stroke. There is good evidence linking antipsychotic drugs such as haloperidol, quetiapine and risperidone with an increased risk of stroke. Bevacizumab is a monoclonal antibody licenced for the use of colorectal cancer and some other solid tumours. In a meta-analysis, there was a clear relationship, especially when used in higher doses, between its use and the risk of ischaemic stroke. Tamoxifen is approved for treatment of oestrogen receptor–positive breast cancer and ductal carcinoma in situ and to reduce the incidence of breast cancer in women at high risk. Meta-analysis of RCTs showed an increased risk of ischaemic stroke.

8.8 Hereditary Causes [10]

8.8.1 Cerebral Autosomal Dominant Arteriopathy with Subcortical Infarcts and leukoencephalopathy (CADASIL)

Associated with abnormalities of the NOTCH-3 gene on chromosome 19 this is a vasculopathy characterised by migraine, usually with aura, and recurrent cerebral ischaemic events and early progressive cognitive decline. Onset is usually in early or middle adulthood with a prevalence of 2–5/100,000. Radiological findings include characteristic white matter hyperintensities, extending to the external capsules and the anterior temporal lobe. It is a progressive disorder for which there is currently no proven treatment.

8.8.2 Fabry's Disease

Fabry's disease is an X linked lysosomal storage disease caused by alpha galactosidase A deficiency. The incidence varies around the world from 1 per 40,000 births to 1 per 120,000. It is associated with dermatological and eye abnormalities. The risk of stroke is increased about 12-fold with onset particularly in women under the age of 45 years. It can cause strokes due to small, middle and large vessel occlusion and is often associated with microbleeds seen on MR imaging. There are multiple other systems that can be involved. Early diagnosis is important as enzyme replacement therapy can slow or halt the progression of the disease.

8.9 Migraine [10]

Although the data are not perfect, it does seem likely that migraine with aura, particularly in women under the age of 45 and who smoke, increases the relative risk of ischaemic stroke, perhaps by a factor of about seven. The more frequent the migraine the higher the risk. However, given the low risk of stroke in this age group, the absolute risk of stroke in young women remains low. It should be regarded as a diagnosis of exclusion, only to be made once other possibilities have been excluded. Migraine is associated with a brief period of hyperperfusion followed by hypoperfusion, and it is this period of hypoperfusion that occasionally results in infarction. Migraine is associated with patent foramen ovale (PFO) which is also associated with stroke, which can make establishing a definitive diagnosis difficult. While closure of the PFO might reduce the risk of stroke there is little evidence to suggest that it reduces the frequency or severity of migraine.

8.10 Venous Stroke [19]

Cerebral sinus venous thrombosis (CSVT) accounts for about 1% of all strokes. It is a potentially fatal condition but if recognised early and treated appropriately, usually with anticoagulants, the outcome is often good even when the brain imaging appears to show extensive damage and haemorrhage. There are multiple potential risk factors including prothrombotic conditions, both hereditary and acquired, infections, particularly mastoiditis and meningitis, trauma, including neurosurgical procedures and jugular vein catheterisation, intracranial tumours and arteriovenous malformations, dehydration, disseminated malignancy and some drugs including tamoxifen. It can present in multiple ways depending on the location and extent of the thrombosis. Headache is present in over 80% of patients which is much higher than in arterial stroke. As well as the focal neurological deficits, seizures and disturbance of consciousness are frequent. Diagnosis can be difficult and is very dependent on the clinician considering the diagnosis. Unless venous phase CT or MRI is requested or the radiologist is informed about the possible diagnosis, they may not identify thrombus in the venous sinuses. Treatment should be with therapeutic doses of heparin even if there is intracranial haemorrhage. The bleeding will have come from capillaries which rupture because of the raised pressure secondary to venous obstruction. Although there are no clinical trials that we are aware of, our usual practice is to continue with anticoagulation until the venous sinuses appear normal on venography or after 6 months. The American Heart Association guidelines recommend anticoagulation for 3–6 months in provoked CSVT, 6–12 months in unprovoked CSVT, and potentially lifelong in recurrent CSVT, VTE following CSVT, or CSVT associated with severe thrombophilia with target international normalised ratio of 2–3.

Case history: A 52-year-old lady currently undergoing treatment of metastatic breast cancer with chemoradiotherapy reports to her oncology team that she has been recently troubled by a persistent headache. She describes a stubborn frontal headache that has been present for the last 2 weeks which she notices especially when she first wakes up each morning. She feels it is slowly getting more prominent and resistant to simple analgesia and in the last 48 h has noted that her right-hand grip strength is diminished. She undergoes extensive investigation including MR venography which reveals a large venous sinus thrombosis in the superior sagittal sinus with a filling defect noted on administration of contrast, the 'empty delta sign'. She is immediately commenced on therapeutic anticoagulation with low molecular weight heparin with gradual improvement in symptoms and weakness observed over ensuing weeks.

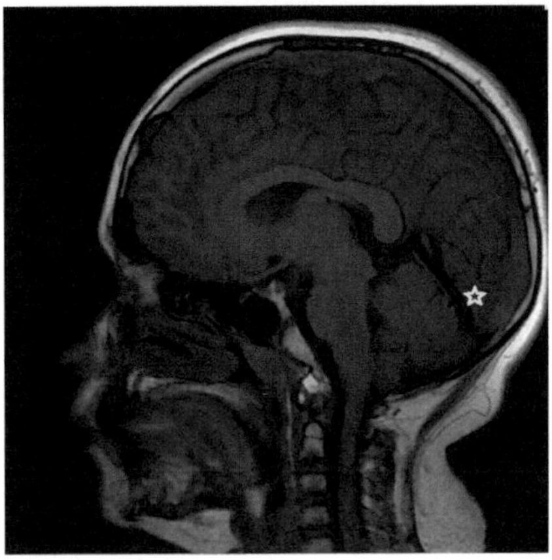

MRI venogram demonstrating a large acute cerebral venous thrombosis in the superior sagittal sinus. The clot can be noted to be isodense on this T1-weighted sequence

8.11 Stroke in Pregnancy [20, 21]

A systematic review of 11 studies of stroke in pregnancy reported an incidence of all types of strokes in 30 people per 100,000; three times the expected incidence in an age matched population. Most occur prepartum or in the early perinatal period. The independent risk factors found were maternal age over 35 years, gestational diabetes mellitus, migraine, pre-eclampsia and pre-existing hypertension. When comparing the ratio between infarct, haemorrhagic and venous strokes, it is noted that haemorrhagic and venous stroke are much more frequent in pregnancy compared to the general population. While many of the risk factors for stroke are the same in pregnancy as in the non-pregnant populations, there are a number of causes that are specific to pregnancy that need to be considered. Pregnancy can produce a hypercoagulable state due to hyperemesis, pre-eclampsia and ovarian hyperstimulation syndrome. The hypertensive syndromes of pregnancy, particularly pre-eclampsia and eclampsia are major risk factors for both haemorrhage and ischaemic stroke. Amniotic fluid embolism, while rare, can cause stroke. Labour can precipitate extracranial vessel dissection. And co-existing prothrombotic conditions such as antiphospholipid syndrome, sickle cell disease, mechanical heart valves can be exacerbated by pregnancy, while treatment with anticoagulants for atrial fibrillation or other causes of cardioembolic stroke may be more difficult and result in either under or over coagulation.

Management of stroke in pregnancy need not differ from management in non-pregnant patients. Pregnancy is not a reason to withhold alteplase or intravenous thrombolysis or thrombectomy, although it is vital to ensure that the diagnosis is correct. In our experience in the UK, it is not uncommon to have non organic stroke symptoms presenting late in pregnancy.

References

1. Hurford R, Siripurapu R, Emsley HCA, Lovett J, Werring D, Punter MNM. Uncommon causes of ischaemic stroke: how to approach the diagnosis. Pract Neurol. 2023;23(1):35–45. https://doi.org/10.1136/pn-2022-003449. Epub 2022 Jul 21.
2. Krittanawong C, Virk HU, Kumar A, Wang Z, Mahtta D, Khalid U, Denktas AE, Volpi JJ, Jneid H. Meta-analysis comparing percutaneous closure versus medical therapy for patent foramen ovale. Am J Cardiol. 2022;172:174–7. https://doi.org/10.1016/j.amjcard.2022.03.013. Epub 2022 Apr 5.
3. Mayfield JJ, Otto CM. Stroke and noninfective native valvular disease. Curr Cardiol Rep. 2023;25(5):333–48. https://doi.org/10.1007/s11886-023-01855-0. Epub 2023 Mar 27.
4. Lee VH, Connolly HM, Brown RD Jr. Central nervous system manifestations of cardiac myxoma. Arch Neurol. 2007;64(8):1115–20. https://doi.org/10.1001/archneur.64.8.1115.
5. Greco N, Tiu C, Terecoasa E, Bajenaru O. Endocarditis and stroke. Maedica. 2014;9(4):375–81. PMID: 25705308; PMCID: PMC4316883.
6. Osteraas ND, Dafer RM. Advances in management of the stroke etiology one-percenters. Curr Neurol Neurosci Rep. 2023;23(6):301–25. https://doi.org/10.1007/s11910-023-01269-z. Epub 2023 May 29. PMID: 37247169; PMCID: PMC10225785.
7. Sener U, Keser Z. Ischemic stroke in patients with malignancy. Mayo Clin Proc. 2022;97(11):2139–44. https://doi.org/10.1016/j.mayocp.2022.09.003.
8. Howard J. Sickle cell disease: when and how to transfuse. Hematol Am Soc Hematol Educ Program. 2016;2016(1):625–31. https://doi.org/10.1182/asheducation-2016.1.625. PMID: 27913538; PMCID: PMC6142434.
9. Pengo V, Hoxha A, Andreoli L, Tincani A, Silvestri E, Prisco D, Fierro T, Gresele P, Cafolla A, De Micheli V, Ghirarduzzi A, Tosetto A, Falanga A, Martinelli I, Testa S, Barcellona D, Gerosa M, Denas G. Trial of rivaroxaban in antiphospholipid syndrome (TRAPS): two-year outcomes after the study closure. J Thromb Haemost. 2021;19(2):531–5. https://doi.org/10.1111/jth.15158. Epub 2020 Nov 29.
10. Bersano A, Kraemer M, Burlina A, Mancuso M, Finsterer J, Sacco S, Salvarani C, Caputi L, Chabriat H, Oberstein SL, Federico A, Lasserve ET, Hunt D, Dichgans M, Arnold M, Debette S, Markus HS. Heritable and non-heritable uncommon causes of stroke. J Neurol. 2021;268(8):2780–807. https://doi.org/10.1007/s00415-020-09836-x. Epub 2020 Apr 21.
11. Adams HP. Takayasu disease and stroke. Pract Neurol. 2020;1:58–61.

12. Bhandari S, Butt SRR, Ishfaq A, Attaallah MH, Ekhator C, Halappa Nagaraj R, Mulmi A, Kamran M, Karski A, Vargas KI, Lazarevic S, Zaman MU, Lakshmipriya Vetrivendan G, Shahzed SMI, Das A, Yadav V, Bellegarde SB, Ullah A. Pathophysiology, diagnosis, and management of takayasu arteritis: a review of current advances. Cureus. 2023;15(7):e42667. https://doi.org/10.7759/cureus.42667. PMID: 37525862; PMCID: PMC10386905.
13. Liu S, Zhang X, Bai X, Yang Y, Wang T, Xu X, Xu R, Li L, Feng Y, Yang K, Wang X, Guo X, Chen J, Ma Y, Jiao L. Antiplatelet vs. anticoagulation in cervical artery dissection: a systematic review and meta-analysis of randomized controlled trials. Front Neurol. 2021;12:745106. https://doi.org/10.3389/fneur.2021.745106. PMID: 34899569; PMCID: PMC8651981.
14. Cheng SWK, Ting ACW, Lam LK, Wei WI. Carotid stenosis after radiotherapy for nasopharyngeal carcinoma. Arch Otolaryngol Head Neck Surg. 2000;126:517–21.
15. Fugate JE. Infectious causes of stroke. Pract Neurol. 2020;1:47–5.
16. Du M, Wang Y, Qin C, Mi D, Liu M, Liu J. Prevalence and incidence of stroke among people with HIV. AIDS. 2023;37(11):1747–56. https://doi.org/10.1097/QAD.0000000000003632.
17. Martinez-Majander N. https://eso-stroke.org/illicit-drug-use-and-the-risk-of-stroke/.
18. Marto JP, Strambo D, Livio F, Michel P. Drugs associated with ischemic stroke: a review for clinicians. Stroke. 2021;52(10):e646–59. https://doi.org/10.1161/STROKEAHA.120.033272. Epub 2021 Aug 18.
19. Idiculla PS, Gurala D, Palanisamy M, Vijayakumar R, Dhandapani S, Nagarajan E. Cerebral venous thrombosis: a comprehensive review. Eur Neurol. 2020;83(4):369–79. https://doi.org/10.1159/000509802. Epub 2020 Sep 2.
20. Cauldwell M, Rudd A, Nelson-Piercy C. Management of stroke and pregnancy. Eur Stroke J. 2018;3(3):227–36. https://doi.org/10.1177/2396987318769547. Epub 2018 Apr 12. PMID: 31008353; PMCID: PMC6453206.
21. Khalid A, Hadbavna A, Williams D, Byrne B. A review of stroke in pregnancy: incidence, investigations and management. Obstet Gynaecol. 2020;22:21–33. https://doi.org/10.1111/tog.12624.

Chapter 9
Diagnosis and Management of TIA

Christopher Pieri, Thanh Ngoc Le, Anthony Rudd, and Khanh Minh Tran

9.1 Definition of Transient Ischaemic Attack (TIA) [1]

Transient ischemic attack is traditionally defined by the World Health Organisation as an acute focal cerebrovascular event lasting less than 24 h. It was originally seen as the equivalent of angina pectoris, chest pain due to ischaemia but without any permanent tissue damage. However, the introduction of increasing sensitive brain imaging has shown that differentiating TIA from stroke simply using a time definition is entirely arbitrary. Symptoms resolving after a few minutes or hours can often be associated with structural damage visible on an MRI scan. Between 30 and 50% of traditionally defined TIAs are associated with abnormalities seen on diffusion weighted magnetic resonance imaging. For this reason, a new definition is now widely accepted that TIA is a transient episode of neurological dysfunction caused by focal brain, retinal or spinal cord ischemia that is not associated with acute infarction.

C. Pieri (✉)
Stroke Medicine, St Thomas' Hospital, London, UK
e-mail: Christopher.pieri@nhs.net

T. N. Le
VNU University of Medicine and Pharmacy, Hanoi, Vietnam

A. Rudd
King's College, London, UK

K. M. Tran
Phutho Department of Health, Phutho, Vietnam

A. Rudd et al. (eds.), *Stroke Management in Vietnam*,
https://doi.org/10.1007/978-981-96-0221-6_9

9.2 Epidemiology of TIA [2, 3]

There are few high quality population-based studies on the frequency and aetiology of TIA, largely because of the changing definitions of TIA and the need for acute access to MRI imaging which is still not available to all clinical services worldwide. Even using the old clinical definition was problematic as the clinical diagnosis of TIA is difficult. There are many mimics of TIA that can make definitive diagnosis uncertain even for experienced clinicians. Furthermore, even in societies with well-educated populations and easy access to clinical services, many patients experiencing transient neurological symptoms will ignore them and therefore not be included in surveys of the frequency of the condition. Given these limitations reports cite figures of between 0.6 and 1.1 per thousand per year. For the Vietnamese population that would mean between 66,000 and 110,000 cases annually.

Of patients who present with stroke between 7% and 40% will have had a prior TIA, most frequently in the month before the stroke, and according to data from the Oxford Community Stroke Project, 26% will have had a TIA either on the day of the stroke or the previous day. These data therefore highlight the importance of treating TIA as a medical emergency and implementing very rapid stroke prevention measures.

9.3 Making the Diagnosis of TIA Clinically [4]

If a patient is seen while still having focal neurological symptoms, then it should be assumed that they are having a stroke. The vast majority of patients with TIA will be normal when first seen by a clinician and diagnosis will be entirely dependent upon taking a good history from the patient and ideally from any witness to the event. Just as with stroke TIA can result in focal neurological symptoms of a very wide variety.

Data from the Oxford Community Stroke Project from 184 consecutive TIA patients on the frequency of symptoms is given in Table 9.1. Unilateral weakness or hemisensory loss are the most frequent symptoms, followed by slurred speech and monocular blindness (amaurosis fugax). Vertigo and dysphagia were very unusual and there were no cases of patients presenting with faintness, non-specific dizziness, confusion or disorientation, incontinence or syncope without any associated focal symptom.

We teach our clinicians that differentiating TIA from stroke mimics can often be achieved by asking the four questions given in Table 9.2.

In this chapter covers stroke and TIA mimics and should be read in conjunction with this chapter.

Case History 1

A 58-year-old gentleman is referred to the Emergency Department with right sided weakness and speech disturbance. He has a past medical background of

Table 9.1 Presenting clinical symptoms of patients with TIA

Neurological symptoms during TIA	% of 184
Unilateral weakness, heaviness, clumsiness	50
Unilateral sensory symptoms	35
Slurred speech (dysarthria)	23
Transient monocular blindness	18
Difficulty speaking (dysphasia)	18
Unsteadiness (ataxia)	12
Vertigo	5
Homonymous hemianopia	5
Diplopia	5
Bilateral limb weakness	4
Crossed motor and sensory loss	1
Dysphagia	1

Table 9.2 Is it a vascular event or something else?

1. Are the neurological symptoms *focal* rather than *non-focal*?
2. Are the focal neurological symptoms *negative* rather than *positive*?
3. Was the *onset* of the focal neurological symptoms *sudden*?
4. Were the focal neurological symptoms *maximal at onset* rather than progressing over a period?

If *YES* to all questions, the symptoms are almost certainly caused by vascular pathology (cerebral ischaemia or haemorrhage). If the answer to even one is NO then TIA is unlikely Is it a vascular event or not?

hypertension and type 2 diabetes mellitus. On review, he reported sudden onset weakness occurring 6 h previously whilst at work which has now fully resolved. He described his right leg being heavy and numb suddenly, coinciding with slurred speech and word-finding difficulties. He also stated that a similar episode occurred the week before but was much more short-lived. He undergoes a CT brain in A&E which shows no haemorrhage and commenced on aspirin 300 mg once daily. He is referred to the local TIA team for urgent review.

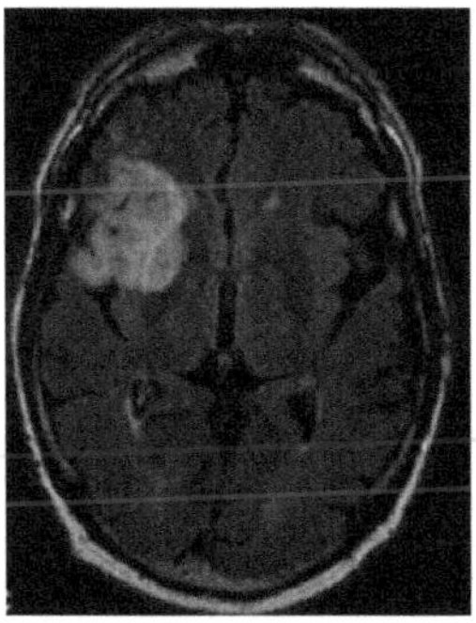

MRI diuffsion weighted imaging demonstrating a subacute left middle cerebral artery infarction. Imaging was performed within two weeks of symptom onset.

MRI diffusion weighted imaging demonstrating a subacute left middle cerebral artery infarction. Imaging was performed within 2 weeks of symptom onset.

Case History 2
A 68-year-old male was reviewed in the TIA clinic after being referred by his GP with a 3 month of transient monocular right visual loss. His background is significant for a long heavy smoking history and hypercholesterolaemia for which he takes a statin. He reports recurrent episodes of right eye visual loss which he describes as like a black curtain coming down his vision. These episodes usually last for less than a minute at a time and have been occurring more frequently recently. His neurological examination is normal. A carotid Doppler is arranged which shows a critical 90% narrowing in his right internal carotid artery. He is commenced on an antiplatelet agent and referred to the Vascular team for urgent carotid artery intervention.

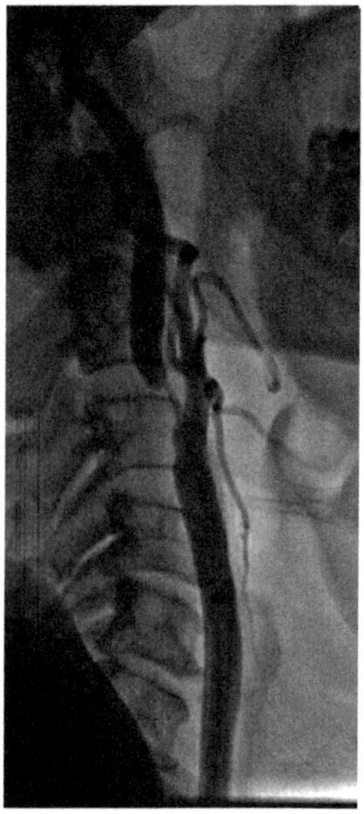

MRI angiography (MRA) demonstrating focal stenosis affecting the left internal carod artery just beyond the bifurcation of the common carotid artery.

MRI angiography (MRA) demonstrating focal stenosis affecting the left internal carotid artery just beyond the bifurcation of the common carotid artery.

9.4 Investigating TIA [3, 5–7]

The most important process in establishing the diagnosis is taking a very careful history. Examination of the patient is necessary with a neurological examination to establish whether there are any residual asymptomatic neurological signs that would suggest stroke rather than TIA and a cardiovascular examination looking for hypertension, peripheral vascular disease, atrial fibrillation, other causes of cardioembolic disease and evidence of carotid disease.

In many cases, presenting as possible TIA to primary care, the emergency department of the hospital or to the specialist clinic, the history and examination will enable TIA to be excluded and a diagnosis made that requires no further investigation. Where TIA is clearly the diagnosis brain imaging is often needed but not in all cases. If it will not change management, then we usually will not scan the patient. Where it is essential to know the size and site of a lesion then the imaging of choice is MRI with diffusion weighted images (DWI) included. It is important for getting the most value from MRI that it is done within a few days of the symptoms as DWI abnormalities can resolve after that time, especially for small lesions. When patients are at risk of intracerebral bleeds because they are on anticoagulants or have a bleeding diathesis then immediate CT brain scan is appropriate to exclude haemorrhage. However, if the patient has presented more than 7 days after the symptom, then small haematomas may no longer be visible on a CT, so MRI with SWI is the imaging modality of choice.

If MRI is not available or the patient presents late, then CT scanning is much less valuable and should only be used if alternative intracerebral pathology is being considered or there is the possibility that the symptoms could have been caused by intracerebral haemorrhage.

The other investigations that will be needed for a patient with probable TIA include tests of renal and hepatic function, full blood count including platelets, serum lipids, 12 lead electrocardiogram with consideration being given to performing more prolonged cardiac monitoring if a cardioembolic source is considered as a possibility, carotid ultrasound (if carotid endarterectomy would be considered if there was significant stenosis). Some patients may require an echocardiogram.

9.5 Risk Stratification [8]

The most widely used risk stratification score to identify those patients with the greatest chance of developing stroke is the ABCD [2] score(Table 9.3).

Pooled stroke risks for ABCD [2] dichotomised score for the nine studies that reported data at both 7 days and 90 days.

$ABCD^2$ score	Percentage	95% CI
At 7 days		
≥4	4.7	2.4–8.7
<4	1.6	1.0–3.4
At 90 days		
≥4	8.2	4.7–14.0
<4	2.7	1.5–4.7

Table 9.3 ABCD [2] Score

Clinical feature	Score
Age > 60 years	1
Blood pressure systolic >140 or diastolic >90	1
Unilateral weakness	2
Speech disturbance without weakness	1
Duration of symptoms (minutes)	
>60	2
10–59	1
Diabetes	1

The message from these studies is that a score of 4 and above does mean that the patient has a higher risk of proceeding to stroke over the 3 months following the TIA; the highest risk being in the first month. However, even with a lower score the risk is there. So, while it might be reasonable to triage patients based on their score, in clinical services with very limited resources, the best solution is to treat all patients with possible TIA as medical emergencies. The score was introduced and used widely in the UK for a number of years while TIA services were being established. It was also misused particularly by primary care and emergency department clinicians as a diagnostic tool for TIA for which it was never intended and is inappropriate for. The diagnosis of TIA needs to be made first and only then should the ABCD [2] be calculated.

9.6 Management

The following information is largely taken from the 2023 edition of UK National Clinical Guidelines for Stroke [5] which is the most recent high quality review of the evidence. For much of the background behind the recommendations and the references go to https://www.strokeguidelines.org

9.6.1 Organisation of Care

TIA should be regarded as a medical emergency that needs to be managed by clinicians with expertise in cerebrovascular disease and neurology. As stated above, the highest risk of developing a completed stroke is within the first few days after a TIA and therefore services should be organised in a way that enables patients to be seen preferably within 24 h of the initial event regardless of the day of the week [9, 10]. Different models have been developed depending on how stroke services are organised. In our hospital, a stroke specialist nurse carries a mobile phone that primary care, emergency department clinicians, ophthalmologists and any others can phone and speak directly to her. She has sufficient expertise to be able to provide initial advice on the basis of the history given by the referring physician and then to arrange to see the patient, usually with a stroke specialist physician the same day, either in the outpatient department or on the stroke unit.

Alternative models are to arrange to have specialists seeing the patient in the emergency department or to conduct the initial assessment remotely using telemedicine. Whoever sees the patient should have easy access to radiology, preferably for the same day MRI scanning or alternatively for CT scanning as well as the other investigations outlined in the previous section.

When the patient for whatever reason presents more than 7 days after the TIA, then management is less urgent and the standard set for specialist assessment in the UK is within the following week.

9.6.2 Immediate Treatment

All patients and any friends or family accompanying them should be given information about what to do if any symptoms recur. They should be advised to immediately call for an emergency ambulance or get to the nearest stroke specialist hospital as quickly as possible.

9.6.3 Antiplatelet Therapy

The CHANCE trial [11] showed in a Chinese population of patients with TIA or minor ischaemic stroke (NIHSS 0–3) that dual antiplatelet therapy started within 24 h of onset for 21 days resulted in a significant reduction in ischaemic stroke from 11.7% (aspirin group) to 8.2% (aspirin-clopidogrel group) with no significant difference in haemorrhagic stroke. A 300 mg loading dose of clopidogrel was used in this trial. The POINT trial (Johnston et al., 2018) showed in patients with TIA or minor ischaemic stroke (NIHSS 0–3) that dual antiplatelet therapy started within 12 h of onset and continued for 90 days resulted in a significant reduction of ischaemic stroke from 6.5% (aspirin group) to 5.0% (aspirin-clopidogrel group). The trial was stopped early because of effectiveness and a significant increase in major haemorrhage in the dual antiplatelet group with an absolute risk increase of 0.5%. A 600 mg loading dose of clopidogrel was used in this trial. Pooled analysis of these trials demonstrated the benefit of dual antiplatelet therapy up to at least 21 days.

So the recommendations of the UK Stroke guideline development group are:

1. If TIA is considered likely the patient should immediately be given aspirin 300 mg. This should be done by the first clinician seeing the patient unless there is a high chance that the symptoms could be due to haemorrhage.
2. The following antiplatelet regimens should be considered as soon as possible:
   (a) For patients within 24 h of onset of TIA or minor ischaemic stroke and with a low risk of bleeding, clopidogrel (initial dose 300 mg followed by 75 mg

per day) plus aspirin (initial dose 300 mg followed by 75 mg per day for 21 days) followed by monotherapy with clopidogrel 75 mg once daily.
(b) OR Ticagrelor (initial dose 180 mg followed by 90 mg twice daily) plus aspirin (300 mg followed by 75 mg daily for 30 days) followed by antiplatelet monotherapy with ticagrelor 90 mg twice daily or clopidogrel 75 mg once daily.

3. For patients with TIA or minor ischaemic stroke who are not appropriate for dual antiplatelet therapy, clopidogrel 300 mg loading dose followed by 75 mg daily should be given.
4. A proton pump inhibitor should be considered for concurrent use with dual antiplatelet therapy to reduce the risk of gastrointestinal haemorrhage.
5. For patients with recurrent TIA or stroke whilst taking clopidogrel, consideration should be given to clopidogrel resistance and the appropriate test performed.

9.6.4 Lipid Management

A high intensity statin should be started immediately for all patients unless clear contraindications, e.g., atorvastatin 20–80 mg.

9.6.5 Anticoagulation

If the patient with TIA has atrial fibrillation a rapid onset anticoagulant should be started as soon as intracerebral haemorrhage has been excluded by brain imaging.

There is no indication to anticoagulate patients unless there is evidence of a cardioembolic cause for the TIA. That includes patients who have had recurrent TIA despite being on an antiplatelet regime.

9.6.6 Management of Blood Pressure

When patients have a presenting blood pressure of over 140/90 at presentation with a TIA antihypertensive medication should be started in the clinic.

9.6.7 Lifestyle Advice

All patients should be given lifestyle advice as appropriate to their risk factors. All smokers should be strongly encouraged to stop immediately. Diabetics with poorly controlled blood glucose should be managed with diet and medication as appropriate to get rapid normoglycaemia. Dietary advice, preferably from a specialist dietitian should be provided to all patients and advice should be given about the importance of improving cardiorespiratory fitness.

9.6.8 Carotid Surgery

Patients with TIA who after specialist assessment are considered candidates for carotid intervention should have carotid imaging performed within 24 h of assessment. This includes carotid duplex ultrasound or either CT angiography or MR angiography. If stenosis of 50–99% as measured using theNorth American Symptomatic Carotid Endarterectomy Trial (NASCET) method, then the patient should be referred for carotid endarterectomy to be performed as soon as possible. Ideally within 7 days of the onset of symptoms in a vascular surgical centre experienced in the procedure and one that audits its outcomes, preferably comparing them to other national or international centres.

Patients with lesser degrees of carotid stenosis should not have carotid surgery but be managed with best medical treatment.

Patients who meet the criteria for carotid intervention but who are unsuitable for open surgery (e.g., inaccessible carotid bifurcation, re-stenosis following endarterectomy, radiotherapy-associated carotid stenosis) should be considered for carotid angioplasty and stenting.

9.6.9 Psychological Support

Even though the patient will have no residual neurological deficits after the TIA, it is very likely that they will be anxious. For many, it will be the first experience of a potentially life changing illness and all the advice given will inevitably increase their level of anxiety that they may have a disabling or fatal stroke anytime. While it is important that the patient understands the seriousness of the diagnosis of TIA, they also need to be reassured that if they follow the advice given then their risks are low.

9.7 Management of Recurrent TIA [12]

Recurrent neurological events presenting with the same symptoms each time are unlikely to be due to TIA. It can happen where there is a localised area of intracranial cerebral artery stenosis but that is unusual. Alternative diagnoses should be sought including migraine, epilepsy and psychiatric causes. Where the diagnosis is recurrent TIA, then risk factor management should be reviewed, checking that the patient is complying with treatment. Where the patient is on clopidogrel, check for clopidogrel resistance and if present switch to an alternative antiplatelet agent. There is no evidence to support using multiple antiplatelet drugs for the longer term; if anything this strategy will just increase side effects without enhancing efficacy. Likewise, there is no indication to try anticoagulation in the absence of a cardioembolic source for the emboli.

References

1. Easton JD, Saver JL, Albers GW, et al. Definition and evaluation of transient ischemic attack. Stroke. 2009;40(6):2276–93.
2. Degan D, Ornello R, Tiseo C, De Santis F, Pistoia F, Carolei A, Sacco S. Epidemiology of Transient ischemic attacks using time-or tissue-based definitions: a population-based study. Stroke. 2017;48(3):530–6. https://doi.org/10.1161/STROKEAHA.116.015417. Epub 2017 Jan 31.
3. Amarenco P. Transient ischemic attack. N Engl J Med. 2020;382(20):1933–41. https://doi.org/10.1056/NEJMcp1908837.
4. Amin HP, Madsen TE, Bravata DM, Wira CR, Johnston SC, Ashcraft S, Burrus TM, Panagos PD, Wintermark M, Esenwa C. American Heart Association emergency neurovascular Care Committee of the Stroke Council and Council on peripheral vascular disease. Diagnosis, workup, risk reduction of Transient ischemic Attack in the emergency department setting: a scientific statement from the American Heart Association. Stroke. 2023;54(3):e109–21. https://doi.org/10.1161/STR.0000000000000418. Epub 2023 Jan 19.
5. National Clinical Guideline for Stroke. 2023. https://www.strokeguidelines.org
6. Coutts SB, Goyal M. Emergent neurovascular imaging: a necessity for the work-up of minor stroke and TIA. AJNR Am J Neuroradiol. 2015;36(12):2194–5. https://doi.org/10.3174/ajnr.A4553. Epub 2015 Sep 24. PMID: 26405088; PMCID: PMC7964267.
7. Wardlaw J, Brazzelli M, Miranda H, et al. An assessment of the cost-effectiveness of magnetic resonance, including diffusion-weighted imaging, in patients with transient ischaemic attack and minor stroke: a systematic review, meta-analysis and economic evaluation. In: Health Technology Assessment, No. 18.27. Southampton (UK): NIHR Journals Library; 2014.
8. Yu AY, Coutts SB. Stroke: risk assessment to prevent recurrence after mild stroke or TIA. Nat Rev Neurol. 2015;11(3):131–3. https://doi.org/10.1038/nrneurol.2015.16. Epub 2015 Feb 17
9. Rothwell PM, Coull AJ, Giles MF, Howard SC, Silver LE, Bull LM, Gutnikov SA, Edwards P, Mant D, Sackley CM, Farmer A, Sandercock PA, Dennis MS, Warlow CP, Bamford JM, Anslow P, Oxford Vascular Study. Change in stroke incidence, mortality, case-fatality, severity, and risk factors in Oxfordshire, UK from 1981 to 2004 (Oxford vascular study). Lancet. 2004;363(9425):1925–33. https://doi.org/10.1016/S0140-6736(04)16405-2.
10. Rothwell PM, Giles MF, Chandratheva A, Marquardt L, Geraghty O, Redgrave JN, Lovelock CE, Binney LE, Bull LM, Cuthbertson FC, Welch SJ, Bosch S, Alexander FC, Silver LE, Gutnikov SA, Mehta Z. Early use of existing preventive strategies for stroke (EXPRESS) study. Effect of urgent treatment of transient ischaemic attack and minor stroke on early recurrent stroke (EXPRESS study): a prospective population-based sequential comparison. Lancet. 2007;370(9596):1432–42. https://doi.org/10.1016/S0140-6736(07)61448-2. Erratum in: Lancet 2008 Feb 2;371(9610):386. Carasco-Alexander, Faye [corrected to Alexander, Faye C].

11. Wong KS, Wang Y, Leng X, Mao C, Tang J, Bath PM, Markus HS, Gorelick PB, Liu L, Lin W, Wang Y. Early dual versus mono antiplatelet therapy for acute non-cardioembolic ischemic stroke or transient ischemic attack: an updated systematic review and meta-analysis. Circulation. 2013;128(15):1656–66. https://doi.org/10.1161/CIRCULATIONAHA.113.003187. Epub 2013 Sep 12.
12. Coutts SB, Hill MD, Campos CR, Choi YB, Subramaniam S, Kosior JC. Demchuk AM; VISION study group. Recurrent events in transient ischemic attack and minor stroke: what events are happening and to which patients? Stroke. 2008;39(9):2461–6. https://doi.org/10.1161/STROKEAHA.107.513234. Epub 2008 Jul 10.

Chapter 10
Stroke Mimics and Stroke Chameleons: Causes and Management

Christopher Pieri, Anthony Rudd, and Quan Hong Nguyen

10.1 Introduction

Up to 50% of calls to emergency medical services with suspected stroke are due to stroke mimics and about 10% of patients assessed in the emergency department as having ischaemic stroke will subsequently be found to have an alternative diagnosis after further investigation. It is essential that mimics are recognised early to avoid administering potentially dangerous acute stroke treatments such as intravenous thrombolysis, providing the correct treatment for the condition and avoid overloading specialist stroke services with patients who would be better managed in alternative settings. There is also the issue of 'stroke chameleons'. Strokes that present atypically, initially appearing to be more likely to be due to an alternative diagnosis. It is essential that these are also diagnosed promptly to provide an opportunity for acute revascularisation where appropriate.

10.2 Recognising Mimics by Paramedics

The most important role for the prehospital clinical staff is to identify stroke as a possibility and then transport the patient as quickly as possible to a place where definitive treatment can be given. Time spent identifying possible stroke should be

C. Pieri (✉)
Medicine, St Thomas' Hospital, London, UK
e-mail: Christopher.pieri@nhs.net

A. Rudd
King's College, London, UK

Q. H. Nguyen
Department of Neurology, 108 Military Central Hospital, Hanoi, Vietnam

A. Rudd et al. (eds.), *Stroke Management in Vietnam*,
https://doi.org/10.1007/978-981-96-0221-6_10

as short as possible, so taking a detailed history from the patient or observers is inappropriate and also unlikely to be productive unless the person taking the history is a skilled clinician. Screening tests such as the FAST (**F**ace, **A**rm, **S**peech, **T**ime) [1] have been shown to be fairly sensitive for anterior circulation stroke but much less so for posterior territory lesions. But it is less specific. It cannot, for example, differentiate between facial weakness due to a Bell's palsy and a stroke. Likewise, it won't help separate dysarthria secondary to intoxication or local causes from central causes such as stroke. But it is quick and easy to administer and can be taught to prehospital clinical staff and the public with little difficulty. More complex scores such as the ROSIER (**R**ecognition **O**f **S**troke **I**n the **E**mergency **R**oom) take longer, are more difficult to teach and offer very little additional sensitivity and specificity.

10.3 Recognising Mimics in the Emergency Department

Even with a highly effective prehospital emergency medical service, there will, therefore, be a high number of patients delivered to the hospital with suspected stroke who have other diagnoses. It is therefore essential that suspected stroke patients are met on arrival by clinicians experienced in making the diagnosis. The most important skill is in taking the history and understanding where symptoms are atypical. A thorough clinical examination of both the neurological system and the cardiovascular system is required. It is insufficient simply to go through the routine of doing an NIHSS (National Institute of Health Stroke Score). This is not a diagnostic score. It is a measure of the severity of stroke to be used once the stroke has been diagnosed by other means.

Skilled history and examination will also avoid the need in some cases for proceeding to expensive and potentially harmful radiological investigations. We are not in favour of protocols that take patients directly to the CT or MRI scanner without first being seen by a clinician able to exclude mimics through clinical assessment alone. However, that clinical assessment must be very fast so as not to delay the administration of acute treatments. We do not apologise for repeating a table used in this chapter on TIA that summarises key differences between vascular presentations and other causes of brain pathology (Table 10.1).

10.4 Aetiology of Stroke Mimics

A useful review of the literature about stroke mimics by Pohl et al. in 2021 [2] summarises 61 studies including over 62,000 patients [1]. The stroke mimic rate overall was about 25% although this rate will vary considerably depending on when in the patient journey the assessment is made. Figure 10.1 reproduced from the paper shows the frequency of different disorders in percentages.

Table 10.1 Structure for identifying if something is a stroke/TIA

Is it a vascular event or not?
1. Are the neurological symptoms *focal* rather than *non-focal*?
2. Are the focal neurological symptoms *negative* rather than *positive*?
3. Was the *onset* of the focal neurological symptoms *sudden*?
4. Were the focal neurological symptoms *maximal at onset* rather than progressing over a period?
If *YES* to all questions, the symptoms are almost certainly caused by vascular pathology (cerebral ischaemia or haemorrhage)

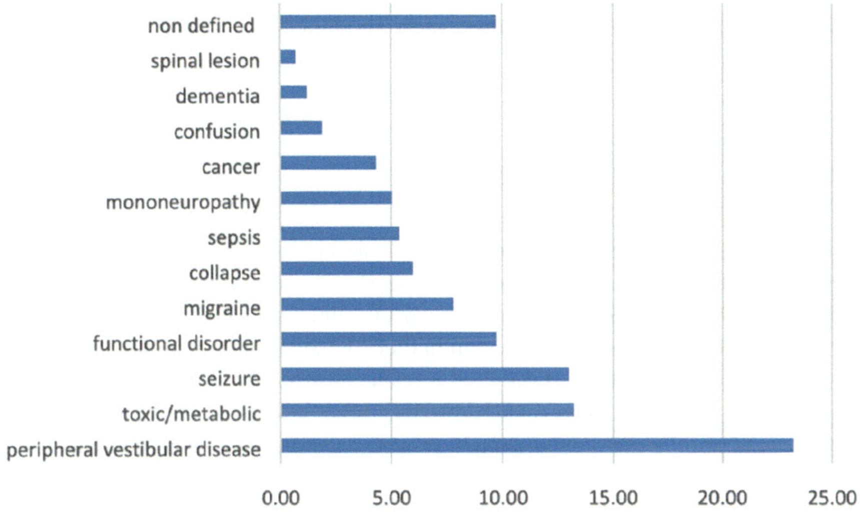

Fig. 10.1 Aetiology of Stroke Mimics

Again, the frequencies will vary according to the setting and particularly will vary according to the population being studied. For example, the incidence of functional disorders is highly dependent on cultural factors.

10.5 Presentation of Mimics

10.5.1 Peripheral Vestibular Disturbance [3]

Peripheral Vestibular disturbance accounts for about 25% of mimics and is often the cause that causes clinicians the most difficulty. Stroke is a rare cause of isolated vertigo or dizziness with less than 3% of strokes presenting with these symptoms. They are more likely to be due to peripheral vestibular disturbance such as paroxysmal positional vertigo, labyrinthitis and vestibulitis. Differentiating between these peripheral causes and a central cause is usually not difficult, particularly with a reasonably compliant patient, but does require the clinician to know how to conduct basic tests of peripheral vestibular function. Association with hearing loss, tinnitus or headache makes a central cause much less likely and often with central causes which are usually brainstem or cerebellar lesions there will be other neurological abnormalities such as ataxia, abnormalities of eye movements and long tract signs. In peripheral lesions symptoms of vertigo may be reduced by visual fixation on a stationary object. The Dix Hallpike manoeuvre can be used to distinguish central from peripheral lesions where there is nystagmus. Vertical or rotatory nystagmus is much less common with peripheral lesions than central ones.

While cerebellar or brainstem lesions can produce vertigo, they are more often associated with additional symptoms such as ataxia and long tract symptoms and signs.

10.5.2 Toxic/Metabolic Causes [4]

These include hypoglycaemia and drug and alcohol poisoning. Hypoglycaemia can produce focal neurological symptoms and signs that exactly mimic stroke. Testing blood sugar should be a routine procedure by the clinicians who first see the patient. Hypoglycaemia is most commonly seen in diabetics on insulin or taking oral hypoglycaemic agents but can also occur as a result of alcohol and rarely insulinoma, when insulin has been given inappropriately to non-diabetic patients and large highly metabolically active malignant tumours. Acute alcohol and recreational drug poisoning is sometimes mistaken for stroke but is less likely to cause focal neurological signs than impaired consciousness. However, the presence of dysarthria and ataxia may result in a misdiagnosis.

10.5.3 Seizure [4, 5]

Where there is a previous history of epilepsy and where there has been witnessed seizure activity the diagnosis of a Todd's paresis should be seriously considered. It can be very difficult to differentiate from stroke and imaging may mislead as the cause of the focal epilepsy may be a previous ischaemic or haemorrhagic stroke. Wherever possible obtain a description of the acute event from a witness and of course if possible, from the patient. Remember that stroke causes negative symptoms and not positive such as Paresthesia, muscle twitching and rarely starts with symptoms in one site spreading to others. Stroke symptoms are also usually maximal at the time of onset. If there is doubt using MRI with diffusion weighted imaging is recommended. Todd's paresis in some series accounts for up to 20% of stroke mimics. It is an important diagnosis to make as giving intravenous thrombolytics to someone with epilepsy could be dangerous. But stroke can present with epilepsy, particularly haemorrhagic stroke so keep an open mind as to the cause.

10.5.4 Functional Disorder [6]

Functional disorders cover a range of different psychiatric pathologies presenting with physical symptoms that cannot be explained by a neurological or other disease. The symptoms are usually real to the patient and cause distress although there are also cases where patients are very deliberately trying to mimic stroke in a type of Munchausen's disease.. There may be evident underlying causes such as anxiety, depression, previous physical illness including stroke, being in an abusive relationship or being the subject of sexual abuse. It is not uncommon for there to be a history of stroke or other neurological disease in close acquaintances.

Reports of the frequency of functional disorders presenting as stroke mimics varies greatly and may reflect cultural variations. In our practice in South London in the UK, it is common with patients being seen on a weekly basis. The key to diagnosis is finding inconsistencies in the history and physical signs. Patients presenting are unlikely to have read anatomy textbooks and unusual combinations of symptoms and signs which would be unlikely to occur due to a single lesion often occur. Furthermore, there are often inconsistencies in the physical signs themselves, varying in presence and intensity. The patient may behave differently when they are in the presence of clinical staff from when they think they are not being observed. One example from my practice was when I was managing a patient using telemedicine on night from home. The clinician on site had performed the neurological examination showing that the patient had complete paresis of her left arm and leg. The nurse left the patient alone in the room for a few minutes, while I still had the telemedicine link, enabling me to observe her lifting her left arm to scratch her nose.

Clinical assessment is more important than brain imaging as a CT scan and occasionally MRI can be normal in the very acute phase of stroke. Hoovers sign is a useful one to elicit. It is positive suggesting a functional cause when pressure is felt in the paretic leg when the non-paretic leg is raised, and no pressure is felt in the non-paretic leg when the paretic leg is being raised. With the patient lying supine, the examiner places a hand under the non-paralysed heel and the patient is asked to raise the paralysed leg. In organic paresis, the examiner feels a downward pressure under the non-paralysed heel. In both the arm and the leg when testing strength, a sign of a non-organic cause is when the strength of the limb suddenly gives way under pressure.

Functional disorders are important to diagnose as soon as possible. It is not uncommon for such patients to be treated unnecessarily with thrombolytics and while tPA is fairly safe in a normal brain, the financial cost is high and treating a patient may reinforce their belief that there is organic brain disease. Likewise, continuing to do multiple investigations may make the patient believe that the doctors believe that there is a structural cause. Early diagnosis and referral to the appropriate psychiatric care may be beneficial.

10.5.5 Migraine [7]

Headache disorders account for about 10% of mimics. Headache is not uncommon in stroke, particularly haemorrhage so do not assume that headache equates to migraine as a cause of stroke. Familial hemiplegic migraine is uncommon. It is an autosomal dominant syndrome with high penetrance and so it is important to ask for a family history. The diagnostic criteria for the International Headache Society requires at least two attacks involving an aura causing fully reversible motor weakness combined with either visual, sensory or language symptoms (usually positive symptoms but maybe negative) and with the aura developing gradually over 5 min or more and lasting not more than 24 h.

10.5.6 Brain Tumour

Symptoms due to brain tumours usually present progressively over days, weeks or months. Occasionally, they do develop suddenly, often as a result of haemorrhage into the tumour or a sudden increase in the surrounding oedema. Patients can also present with a Todd's paresis as a result of a focal seizure caused by the tumour. Brain imaging will usually confirm the diagnosis. Major oedema on a scan done within the first few hours of a stroke should raise the suspicion of an underlying tumour and prompt a contrast enhanced scan. This is particularly the case if the pattern of the oedema is typical of vasogenic oedema rather than the cytotoxic oedema usually associated with vascular disease.

10.5.7 Peripheral Nerve Abnormalities Including Bell's Palsy and Guillain–Barré Syndrome

Isolated peripheral nerve lesions can result in a misdiagnosis of stroke including median, radial, ulnar and common peroneal nerves. Knowledge of neuroanatomy and good clinical skills should make diagnosis straightforward. This should nearly always avoid the need for brain imaging. This is also the case with the common presentation of a lower motor neurone (LMN) facial nerve lesion (Bell's palsy) where the important physical sign is that the facial weakness also involves weakness of the muscles of the upper face impairing eye closure. Where a LMN lesion is suspected look for evidence of herpetic infection around the ear and where present treat with acyclovir or similar. Bell's palsy may resolve more quickly if steroid are given within 72 h after the onset of symptoms.

Guillain–Barre syndrome should not pose a diagnostic problem trying to differentiate it from stroke. Unlike stroke the symptoms usually develop progressively and are bilateral. The one situation where confusion may arise is with Miller Fisher syndrome where the predominant nerves affected are the cranial ones. Again, careful clinical examination should make clinicians question the diagnosis of stroke. The nerve lesions are lower motor neurone rather than upper and onset is gradual.

10.5.8 Sepsis Including Post Stroke Deterioration [7]

Sepsis accounts for about 5% of stroke mimics although it must be remembered that sepsis and stroke can co-exist. Perhaps the most common scenario is of a patient who has had a previous stroke, who then develops infection which results in the old symptoms and signs from the previous stroke becoming more apparent. MRI with DWI is an invaluable tool in differentiating this situation from a new ischaemic lesion. Mycotic aneurysms from infective endocarditis is another situation where stroke and sepsis may occur together.

10.5.9 Transient Global Amnesia [8]

More often presenting as a TIA mimic transient global amnesia is a fairly frequent cause of referral to a neurovascular clinic. The typical case is one where the patient describes losing several hours where he or she has no idea what they have been doing. During this time, they continue to function but independent witnesses will often describe the patient as being confused and asking the same questions repeatedly. It usually occurs in middle aged and older people. Symptoms nearly always resolve within 24 h. The cause is unknown but in the majority, it occurs as a single event and investigations including brain imaging and electroencephalography (EEG) are normal. It appears to be a benign condition and my clinical practice where there is a typical presentation is to reassure the patient and discharge without any further investigations. If attacks recur or are atypical then they should be investigated. The rare transient epileptogenic amnesia should be excluded. With more prolonged amnesia brain imaging to exclude thalamic stroke should be performed and tests to check for possible Wernicke's encephalopathy or other metabolic disorders done and in patients prone to hypoglycaemia of course checking blood glucose.

10.5.10 Spinal Lesions

Stroke affecting the spinal cord is not uncommon and should always be considered when a patient presents with sudden onset paraparesis or quadriparesis. But there are of course many other causes of spinal cord damage that need to be excluded including tumours and trauma. One case example from my practice was where a frail elderly patient fell down some stairs and presented with limb motor weakness. The inexperience doctor who first saw here decided that the lady had sustained a stroke causing the fall. The bruise on her forehead showing where she had hit her head causing a hyperextension injury to the neck and spinal cord damage was the important clinical sign he had missed.

10.6 Summary

Stroke diagnosis is often straightforward when the patient presents a typical history with a clinical examination consistent with a focal brain injury confirmed with brain imaging. But in about half of patients presenting to paramedics and about 30% of patients presenting to the hospital emergency department, the patient will have a stroke mimic. It is important that the correct diagnosis is made promptly not only just to avoid inappropriate stroke treatments but also to ensure that the real pathology is managed effectively. Reading medical textbooks like this one will help but nothing can beat seeing lots of patients and receiving bedside clinical teaching. We all make mistakes, and these are often the most valuable learning experiences.

References

1. Rudd M, Buck D, Ford GA, Price CI. A systematic review of stroke recognition instruments in hospital and prehospital settings. Emerg Med J. 2016;33(11):818–22. https://doi.org/10.1136/emermed-2015-205197. Epub 2015 Nov 16
2. Pohl M, Hesszenberger D, Kapus K, Meszaros J, Feher A, Varadi I, Pusch G, Fejes E, Tibold A, Feher G. Ischemic stroke mimics: a comprehensive review. J Clin Neurosci. 2021;93:174–82.
3. Fetter M. Assessing vestibular function: which tests, when? J Neurol. 2000;247(5):335–42. https://doi.org/10.1007/s004150050599.
4. Brigo F, Lattanzi S. Poststroke seizures as stroke mimics; clinical assessment and management. Epilepsy Behav. 2020;104(Pt B):106297. https://doi.org/10.1016/j.yebeh.2019.04.050. Epub 2019 Jul 11.
5. Bucka BH, Akhtarb N, Alrohimia A, Khana K, Shuaiba A. Stroke mimics: incidence, aetiology, clinical features and treatment. Ann Med. 2021;53:420–36.

6. Popkirov S, Stone J, Buchan AM. Functional neurological disorder: a common and treatable stroke mimic. Stroke. 2020;51(5):1629–35. https://doi.org/10.1161/STROKEAHA.120.029076. Epub 2020 Apr 16
7. Fernandes PM, Whiteley WN, Hart SR, Al-Shahi SR. Strokes: mimics and chameleons. Pract Neurol. 2013;13:21–8.
8. Ropper AH. Transient global amnesia. N Engl J Med. 2023;388(7):635–40. https://doi.org/10.1056/NEJMra2213867.

Chapter 11
Stroke Nursing in Vietnam

Gill Cumberbatch, Thong Van Nguyen, and Ngoc Huy Nguyen

11.1 Introduction

Nurses have a key role in the care of stroke patients and are typically the only health professionals working directly with patients 24 h a day. This provides a unique opportunity and role to monitor and manage patients, to support their daily function and to liaise with other health care professionals. There is evidence that the number of qualified nurses per stroke patient has an impact on mortality after stroke—Fig. 11.1 [1]. Whilst some of this care will involve care around mechanical thrombectomy or thrombolysis treatments this is only for a small proportion of patients and by contrast all stroke patients require effective stroke care in monitoring, preventing complications and supporting rehabilitation. It is therefore important that nurses are suitably skilled in all aspects of stroke care and that sufficient attention is paid to stroke care and rehabilitation.

G. Cumberbatch (✉)
St Georges Hospital, London, UK
e-mail: gillian.cluckie@nhs.net

T. Van Nguyen
Stroke Center, Phutho General Hospital, Phutho, Vietnam

Vietnam Stroke Association, Hanoi, Vietnam

N. H. Nguyen
Phutho Department of Health, Phutho, Vietnam

VNU University of Medicine and Pharmacy, Hanoi, Vietnam

A. Rudd et al. (eds.), *Stroke Management in Vietnam*,
https://doi.org/10.1007/978-981-96-0221-6_11

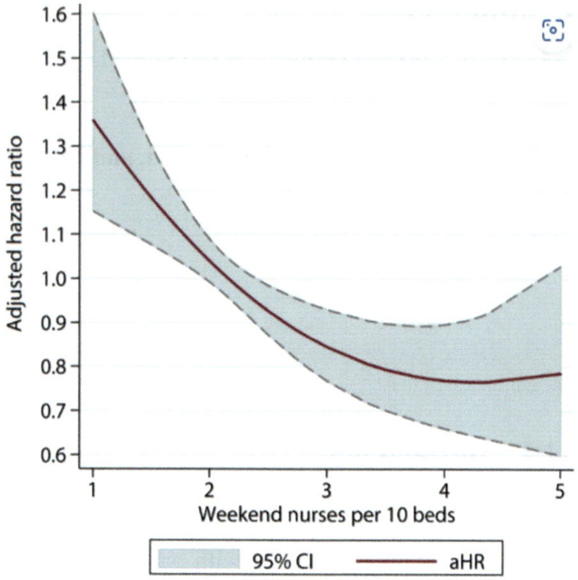

Fig. 11.1 Registered nurse ratio to patient mortality (Bray et al, 2015)

11.2 Hyper-Acute Stroke Care

The role of nurses in the first few hours after a stroke patient's admission is primarily focused upon the monitoring and prevention of complications.

In the emergency department, the nurse may be involved in the assessment and treatment of patients including mechanical thrombectomy, thrombolysis or managing intra-cerebral haemorrhage.

11.2.1 Care in the Emergency Department

Nurses in this setting should be aware of potential complications to be monitored—see Table 11.1.

Patients with suspected stroke in the ED require immediate cardiovascular monitoring including ECG, oxygen saturations, blood pressure monitoring and respiratory monitoring.

Table 11.1 Hyper-acute nursing care

	Condition/complication	Nursing care interventions
Cardiovascular	• Atrial fibrillation (AF) • Cardiac arrhythmias such as ventricular tachycardia • ST segment changes, e.g., indicating myocardial infarction (MI) • Bradycardia or heart block • Hypo or hypertension • Acute heart failure/pulmonary oedema • Critical limb ischaemia	IV rate control, e.g., digoxin/beta blockers IV anti-hypertensives, e.g., labetalol IV anti-arrhythmics IV diuretics IV fluids
Respiratory	• Aspiration pneumonia • Upper airway obstruction • Reduced respiratory effort, e.g., with reduced conscious level • Respiratory failure (type 1 and 2) • Pulmonary embolism	Water swallow screening test prior to oral intake Oxygen therapy Anaphylaxis management Airway adjuncts, e.g., oral or naso-pharyngeal airway Non-invasive ventilation (specialist care required) Anticoagulation
Neurological	• Reduced conscious level, • Seizure (focal or generalized), • Neurological deterioration or fluctuation in symptoms	IV anti-epileptics IV/PR benzodiazepines Seizure monitoring Positioning to manage reduced conscious level
Nutrition and hydration	• Dehydration • Malnutrition • Hyper-glycaemia	Naso-gastric (NG) insertion NG feed provision IV fluids Fluid intake and output monitoring Blood sugar monitoring Administration of insulin and oral glycaemic agents
Pain and infection	• Sepsis and infection • Pain	IV antibiotics IV/oral paracetamol or analgesia IV fluids Obtain bloods/blood cultures, sputum or urine specimens

11.3 Swallow Assessment

It is critical that patients are not provided with any oral intake prior to a water swallow screening test being performed. This is due to the link between dysphagia and aspiration pneumonia and nurses have a key role in screening for dysphagia and ensuring the risk of aspiration is reduced. The paper by Bray et al. 2017 [2] reports the correlation between the time taken to screen for dysphagia and the risk of aspiration showing a clear benefit for early screening.

Using a bedside water screening tool, nurses can identify patients at risk of aspiration on water with good sensitivity and specificity [3]. Patients may then be referred to speech and language therapy or for instrumental assessment of swallow, for example, with videofluoroscopy. In some areas, nurses may perform a more advanced assessment of differing consistencies to check for aspiration risk. Nurses should be trained and skilled to undertake this swallow screening and should complete this within 4 h and prior to the patients being offered any food or drink. Patients should be alert and positioned upright prior to a swallow assessment. Where they remain drowsy or are unconscious or unable to sit upright, the assessment should not be performed and they should be placed nil by mouth with alternative hydration/nutrition until the swallow screen can be completed.

11.4 Patient Assessment, Examination and History Taking

Nurses working in the emergency department (ED) setting may be involved in patient assessment and examination. This may include advanced physical assessment skills such as neurological examination including NIHSS or cardiovascular/respiratory assessment. Completing these tasks should be undertaken with further advanced education, supervision and clinical observations to ensure quality and to provide the nurse with appropriate medico-legal support. In the UK, this is operated via a master level of education in advanced clinical practice.

11.4.1 Mechanical Thrombectomy

Mechanical thrombectomy is an evidence-based intervention to reperfuse ischaemic brain tissue following large vessel arterial occlusion. The evidence base continues to develop with additional time frames or groups of patients included in research trials—see Table 11.2 for current evidence base [4–10].

From a nursing perspective, there is a need to have knowledge of the local mechanical thrombectomy pathway and inclusion criteria. The nurse will be involved in preparing the patient for transfer to the interventional neuroradiology suite which may include securing intravenous access, 12 lead ECG, avoiding hypotension and patient/relative information. Handover to the neuroradiology nurses should include neurological or systems deterioration and medication administered. Urinary catheterization is not usually routinely required unless indicated to manage urinary retention or reduce uncontrolled hypertension.

Table 11.2 Mechanical thrombectomy inclusion criteria

Inclusion criteria	Imaging criteria	Reference
0–6 h from onset, large vessel occlusion (e.g., M1), prior mRS 0–2, NIHSS >5	CTA confirming large vessel occlusion, e.g., carotid/M1 occlusion CT head excluding haemorrhage and less than 1/3 of MCA territory ischaemia	Goyal et al. (2016)
Defuse 6–16 h from onset, large vessel occlusion (e.g. M1), prior mRS 0–2, NIHSS >5 Dawn 6–24 h from onset, large vessel occlusion (e.g. M1), prior mRS 0–2 • Age >80, NIHSS >10, core volume <21 mL • Age <80, NIHSS >10, core volume <31 mL • Age <80, NIHSS >20, core volume 31–50 mL	Advanced imaging—CT perfusion mismatch/MRI mismatch Defuse Core volume <70 mL Mismatch ratio <1.8 Dawn Based on age—core volume <21 mL to <50mL	Albers et al. (2018) Nogueira et al. (2018)
Large core infarct <24 h of onset or last known well time, large vessel occlusion	ANGEL-ASPECT trial—ASPECTS 3–5 or core volume 70–100 mL SELECT 2 trial ASPECTS 3–5, core volume >100 mL on CTP or MRI	Huo et al. (2023) Sarraj et al. (2023)
Basilar artery occlusion BAOCHE trial 18–80 years, 6–24 h from onset, basilar artery occlusion, mRS 0–1, NIHSS >10 ATTENTION trial >18 years, <16 h from onset/last known well time, NIHSS >10 <80 years mRS 0–2 >80 years mRS 0	BAOCHE trial PC-ASPECTS >6, Pons-midbrain index <2 ATTENTION trial PC-ASPECTS >6 (under 80 years) or >8 (over 80 years)	Jovin et al. (2022)

11.5 Post-Thrombectomy Care

Nurses should be skilled in post-thrombectomy care including groin puncture care. There is an increased risk of bleeding from arterial puncture sites at its most severe causing life-threatening retroperitoneal haemorrhage. At completion of thrombectomy, the groin puncture site will be sealed with an angioseal device which is a collagen-based plug to reduce but not fully prevent bleeding. Nurses should therefore monitor the groin puncture site at least hourly for 24 h:

- Direct visualization of the groin puncture site for signs of redness, bruising, swelling or bleeding.
- Vascular check of groin puncture leg including pulses, colour and sensation.
- Avoid leg movement above 30 degrees for 24 h.

If there is bleeding, haematoma development or swelling noted at the groin puncture site, the nurse should apply firm direct pressure with two fingers for 20 min on puncture site. There is no indication for pressure devices as an initial treatment and pressure dressings should be avoided as they prevent direct visualization of the puncture site. Local policy should be followed which is likely to include escalation to the medical staff. Should major bleeding or pseudo-aneurysm be suspected referral to vascular specialists may be required to provide either a thrombin injection for pseudo-aneurysms or emergency surgery for retroperitoneal haemorrhage?

11.5.1 Thrombolysis

Thrombolysis is an intravenous drug administered to breakdown thrombus occluding the intra-cerebral artery. Evidence-based drugs include alteplase and tenectoplase and nurses should be familiar with the differing drug reconstitution and administration methods for each. There are risks of thrombolytic therapy and nurses should be aware of these and ensure suitable monitoring of patients to monitor for these complications—see Table 11.3.

Escalation to medical staff in the case of complications will enable further treatment and escalation to higher care facilities where appropriate.

Table 11.3 Thrombolysis complications

Complication	Observation	Treatment
Intra-cerebral haemorrhage (circa 5–6%)	Regular neurological observation Seizure monitoring Headache, nausea or vomiting Changes in NIHSS Blood pressure surges or persistently raised	Stop thrombolysis infusion Repeat CT imaging Manage blood pressure to prevent hypertension Seizure management Oxygen therapy Analgesia Anti-emetics
Anaphylactoid reaction—typically oro-pharyngeal oedema (circa 1%)	Regular monitoring of airway, respirations and oxygen saturations Observation of tongue and mouth for swelling Blood pressure monitoring	Stop thrombolysis infusion Airway management with adjuncts if needed High flow oxygen IV antihistamine, e.g., chlorphenamine IM adrenaline if systemic effects such as hypotension IV hydrocortisone
Major extra-cranial haemorrhage (circa 1%)	Blood pressure and pulse monitoring Observation of bleeding, e.g., wound site, GI bleeding	Stop thrombolysis infusion IV fluids Compression of bleeding site if compressible

11.5.2 Hyper-Acute Ward Care

Care on the hyper-acute stroke unit primarily involves monitoring and preventing complications and promoting independence for the first 72 h post-stroke. In addition to the cardiovascular, respiratory and neurological observations outlined in Sect. 11.2.1 nurses should be aware of post-stroke changes that can occur.

11.6 Neurological Care

Patients may be at continued risk of neurological deterioration, for example, as a result of further stroke, cerebral oedema such as malignant middle cerebral artery (MCA) syndrome or seizure. The role of the nurse in the hyper-acute stage is to monitor the patients' neurological function to include a score of consciousness such as the Glasgow Coma Scale (GCS), limb assessment such as the NIHSS score and monitoring of cardiovascular and respiratory function to identify any signs of raised intra-cranial pressure. Signs of raised intra-cranial pressure can include:

- Headache.
- Nausea and vomiting.
- Reduced consciousness, e.g., drop in GCS.
- Changes to limb function, e.g., drop in MRS limb grading.
- Late signs—Cushings triad—widened pulse pressure, bradycardia and reduced respirations.

Changes to respiratory patterns such as ataxic, apneustic or Cheyne-Stokes breathing may be central driven and signs of pressure within the brainstem. Nurses should be aware of the early and late signs and should escalate their monitoring when any are suspected and inform medical staff.

Seizures can develop due to cortical ischaemia or pre-existing epilepsy and nurses should be attentive to signs of either focal or generalized seizure activity. Seizures should be monitored to include the nature, affected area and duration. For generalized seizures nurses should additionally provide airway support and oxygenation during the seizure and be able to anxiolytics such as benzodiazepines. These treatments may impact the respiratory function and nurses should be attentive for reduced respiratory function.

11.7 Cardiovascular Care

Nurses should be knowledgeable and skilled in the management of hypertension in acute stroke to prevent haemorrhage or extension of ICH. For patients following thrombolysis or intra-cerebral haemorrhage, this will require active blood pressure reduction using IV agents such as labetalol to prevent complications.

Blood pressure following thrombolysis should be maintained below 185/110 mmHg. For intra-cerebral haemorrhage, there is evidence that reducing systolic blood pressure to below 140 mmHg within 6 h and maintained for 7 days can reduce mortality but should be carefully managed to prevent rapid hypotension based on the patients initial blood pressure [11]. Nurses should be able to follow local policies to manage hypertension and escalate to medical staff where treatments are ineffective.

Nurses should initiate treatment to prevent deep vein thrombosis (DVT). Intermittent pneumatic compression devices are effective in the reduction of DVTs in stroke patients, whereas anti-embolic stocking's are ineffective [12]. The administration of prophylactic anticoagulation can increase the risk of intra-cerebral haemorrhage and therefore is often contraindicated, e.g., in ICH or post-thrombolysis. Nurses should follow local policies for the prevention of DVTs and should monitor the patient's calves every shift for signs of swelling, redness, pain or hardening that may indicate DVT and if identified refer to medical staff.

11.8 Respiratory Care

Nurses should be aware of the ongoing risk of aspiration pneumonia and pulmonary embolism and identify the signs such as hypoxia, increased respiratory secretions, chest pain or hypotension. If suitably trained and clinically appropriate nurses may auscultate the chest to identify additional sounds such as wheeze, crackles or diminished sounds for example indicating consolidation. Nurses should be skilled and familiar with a range of respiratory support in hyper-acute stroke care. This should include the use of oral and naso-pharyngeal suction using adjuncts such as oral and nasal airways, oxygen therapy devices including masks, nasal cannula and humidified circuits and the administration of nebulizers or inhalers.

11.9 Pain and Fever

Stroke patients are at risk of headache and this should be monitored to ensure there are no other concerning features such as neurological deterioration. Otherwise, oral or IV analgesics can support the patients. Nurses should be attentive to the link between pain and hypertension particularly in patients with aphasia or other communication difficulties. Pain due to existing conditions should be noted and monitored.

Fever can be detrimental to stroke mortality and therefore patients' temperature should be monitored regularly and antipyretic medication such as paracetamol administered. Nurses should consider likely sources of infection where pyrexia develops and should obtain appropriate samples such as sputum or urine samples and communicate likely infection source to the medical staff.

11.10 Nutrition and Hydration

Swallow screening may also be required either where not already completed in ED or for clinical changes, e.g., reduced conscious level. Where identified that patients have an unsafe swallow additional fluids and hydration will be required. For some patients, this will require naso-gastric (NG) tube insertion. Nurses should be able to:

- Insert NG tube effectively.
- Check position of NG tube to prevent misplaced tubes, aspiration risk.
- Secure NG tubes securely at nose and onto face.
- Utilize appropriate strategies to maintain NG tube position, e.g., nasal bridle, mittens for agitated or restless patients. Information provision for patient and family on these strategies. Utilize these for shortest possible time.
- Administer NG feed ensuring patient is positioned at least at 30 degrees to prevent reflux and aspiration risk.

Nurses should monitor fluid intake, e.g., via IV fluids identifying dehydration or fluid overload, e.g., increased respiratory effort, pink, frothy sputum. IV cannulae should be removed as soon as possible where they are not required to reduce the potential for infection.

Hyper-glycaemia should be avoided to prevent the risk of further cerebral tissue damage and blood sugar monitoring should be conducted for diabetic patients or those with raised blood sugar levels. Treatment using oral hypoglycaemic agents or insulin should be administered to maintain sugar levels ideally in the range 8–12 mmol/L. Urinary ketones should be checked where the blood sugar level is above 20 mmol/L.

11.11 Positioning and Mobility

In the hyper-acute stage of care, nurses should be assessing the impact of the neurological deficits on the patient's ability to move and re-position themselves. Pressure sore risk assessment should be completed for example using the Waterlow score [13]. Regular repositioning avoiding long periods semi-prone on the back will reduce the risk of sacral pressure sores. There is no evidence that positioning the patient either above 30 degrees or fully flat has an impact on outcomes in stroke therefore patients should be positioned comfortably and in a position that maximizes independence [14].

11.11.1 Acute Stroke Care

In the period of care beyond the first 72 h from stroke onset the nursing focus is based on preventing and managing complication, rehabilitation and encouraging independence.

11.12 Positioning and Mobility

Nurses should continue to be attentive to the risk of pressure sores conducting assessments of skin changes on pressure areas every shift and regularly reviewing the pressure sore risk assessment tool such as the Waterlow score. Where families are supporting the direct care of patients, they should be given both verbal and written information about the risk of pressure sores and the optimal positioning to prevent this. Where additional mattresses are available to minimize the impact of pressure these should be prioritized for the patients at highest risk based on the assessment tool or presence of existing pressure sores.

Nurses should position patients to carefully support the hemiplegic limbs and pay careful attention to the hemiplegic arm due to the risk of shoulder pain and subluxation. The hemiplegic arm should be positioned with support under the elbow such as on a pillow to reduce the drag effect on the shoulder and patients with hemiplegic arms should never be handled or moved by the arm or shoulder. Families should be made aware of this and given training on the optimal handling of their relative to prevent unnecessary shoulder damage and pain.

11.13 Continence

It is common that patients may develop urinary of faecal incontinence after stroke. Urinary continence can develop for a number of reasons and there are differing types and treatments—see Table 11.4.

Patients with communication difficulties such as aphasia should be supported to communicate their toileting needs using written or pictorial support. Signs of agitation should be reviewed to note if it indicates urinary sensation and an awareness of their toileting need. Supporting incontinence with pads should only be utilized where treatment is ongoing and should not be considered long term without interventions to treat incontinence.

Table 11.4 Types and treatment of urinary incontinence

Type	Signs/symptoms	Treatment
Urge incontinence, e.g., detrusor instability	Increased urgency Urine leakage before reaching bathroom	Timed toileting Anticholinergic agents
Stress incontinence	Urine leakage when coughing, laughing or straining	Pelvic floor exercises Regular toileting
Functional incontinence	Urine incontinence Inability to independently mobilize to bathroom Inability to communicate need for toileting	Nursing support for regular timed toileting Nursing support for communication
Overflow incontinence, e.g., urinary retention	Small volume urine output at frequent intervals Palpable bladder	Bladder scan to confirm retention Treat constipation if present Intermittent catheterization for no more than 24 h whilst constipation is treated In-dwelling urinary catheter

Incontinence of faeces can indicate poor sensation, poor mobility, or constipation. Stroke patients are at high risk of constipation due to immobility, altered diet and reduced fluid intake. The use of laxatives should be considered to aim for the patient's usual bowel habit. Where constipation has caused impaction nurses should be aware of overflow loose bowel motions and undertake a rectal examination. Treatment with enemas or suppositories in addition to oral laxatives may be appropriate as a short term treatment.

11.14 Communication

Where patients have an acquired communication impairment such as aphasia nurses have a key role in identifying and supporting optimal routes of communication. This may include using written single words, pictures or gestures to support total communication strategies. Nurses should be aware that in aphasia the patient also will have difficulties with writing, spelling and reading and these may not be suitable support strategies. Asking closed questions can determine the patient's ability to indicate an accurate yes/no response. Using environmental cues such as showing the patient, the activity or space can support understanding. Nurses should liaise with the speech therapist on the optimal strategy for each patient.

11.15 Rehabilitation and Maximizing Independence

Patients in acute stroke care should be supported to optimize their recovery and maximize their independence. Encouraging them to participate in their own personal care and mobility can increase the intensity of any available therapy. Where there is therapy guidance on mobility, positioning or personal care nurses should follow this and encourage family members to promote independence. Encouraging patients to sit out of bed and mobilize to the bathroom where appropriate will support their recovery.

11.16 Psychological Impact of Stroke

Nurses should be aware of the range of psychological impacts of stroke including depression, emotional lability and memory difficulties. Signs of these during nursing care interventions should be noted and the medical or psychology team informed. Nurses should normalize the experience of these conditions for patients and their families.

11.16.1 Community Care

In addition to hospital-based roles, nurses can have a key role in the community care of stroke patients. This may include the optimization of secondary prevention strategies, medication compliance, management of hypertension and identification of further risk factors such as AF. Nurses in this role can also provide ongoing observation and prevention of complications such as spasticity or contractures or urinary incontinence. Nurses can also provide patient and family support for the ongoing impact of stroke such as psychological consequences. Family support and guidance can be crucial in this area.

References

1. Bray BD, Ayis S, Campbell J, Cloud GC, James M, Hoffman A, Tyrrell PJ, Wolfe CD, Rudd AG. Associations between stroke mortality and weekend working by stroke specialist physicians and registered nurses: prospective multicentre cohort study. PLoS Med. 2014;11(8):e1001705.
2. Bray BD, Smith CJ, Cloud GC, Enderby P, James M, Paley L, Tyrrell PJ, Wolfe CD, Rudd AG. The association between delays in screening for and assessing dysphagia after acute stroke, and the risk of stroke-associated pneumonia. J Neurol Neurosurg Psychiatry. 2017;88(1):25–30.
3. Chen PC, Chuang CH, Leong CP, Guo SE, Hsin YJ. Systematic review and meta-analysis of the diagnostic accuracy of the water swallow test for screening aspiration in stroke patients. J Adv Nurs. 2016;72(11):2575–86.
4. Albers GW, Marks MP, Kemp S, et al. Thrombectomy for stroke at 6 to 16 hours with selection by perfusion imaging. N Engl J Med. 2018;378(8):708–18.
5. Goyal M, Menon BK, van Zwam WH, et al. Endovascular thrombectomy after large-vessel ischaemic stroke: a meta-analysis of individual patient data from five randomised trials. Lancet. 2016;387(10029):1723–31.
6. Huo X, Ma G, Tong X, Zhang X, Pan Y, Nguyen TN, Yuan G, Han H, Chen W, Wei M, Zhang J. Trial of endovascular therapy for acute ischemic stroke with large infarct. N Engl J Med. 2023;388(14):1272–83.
7. Jovin TG, Li C, Wu L, Wu C, Chen J, Jiang C, Shi Z, Gao Z, Song C, Chen W, Peng Y. Trial of thrombectomy 6 to 24 hours after stroke due to basilar-artery occlusion. N Engl J Med. 2022;387(15):1373–84.
8. Nogueira RG, Jadhav AP, Haussen DC, et al. Thrombectomy 6 to 24 hours after stroke with a mismatch between deficit and infarct. N Engl J Med. 2018;378(1):11–21.
9. Sarraj A, Hassan AE, Abraham MG, Ortega-Gutierrez S, Kasner SE, Hussain MS, Chen M, Blackburn S, Sitton CW, Churilov L, Sundararajan S. Trial of endovascular thrombectomy for large ischemic strokes. N Engl J Med. 2023;388(14):1259–71.
10. Tao C, Li R, Zhu Y, Qun S, Xu P, Wang L, Zhang C, Liu T, Song J, Sun W, Wang G. Endovascular treatment for acute basilar artery occlusion: a multicenter randomized controlled trial (ATTENTION). Int J Stroke. 2022;17(7):815–9.
11. Moullaali TJ, Wang X, Martin RH, Shipes VB, Robinson TG, Chalmers J, Suarez JI, Qureshi AI, Palesch YY, Anderson CS. Blood pressure control and clinical outcomes in acute intracerebral haemorrhage: a preplanned pooled analysis of individual participant data. Lancet Neurol. 2019;18:857–64. https://doi.org/10.1016/S1474-4422(19)30196-6.
12. Dennis M, Sandercock P, Graham C, Forbes J, Smith J, CLOTS (Clots in Legs Or sTocKing's after Stroke) Trials Collaboration. The Clots in legs or sTocKing's after stroke (CLOTS) 3 trial: a randomised controlled trial to determine whether or not intermittent pneumatic compression reduces the risk of post-stroke deep vein thrombosis and to estimate its cost-effectiveness. Health Technol Assess. 2015;19(76):1.
13. Waterlow J. Pressure sores: a risk assessment card. Nurs Times. 1985;81(48):49–55.
14. Anderson CS, Arima H, Lavados P, Billot L, Hackett ML, Olavarría VV, Muñoz Venturelli P, Brunser A, Peng B, Cui L, Song L, Rogers K, Middleton S, Lim JY, Forshaw D, Lightbody CE, Woodward M, Pontes-Neto O, De Silva HA, Lin RT, Lee TH, Pandian JD, Mead GE, Robinson T, Watkins C. HeadPoST investigators and coordinators. Cluster-randomized, crossover trial of head positioning in acute stroke. N Engl J Med. 2017;376(25):2437–47. https://doi.org/10.1056/NEJMoa1615715.

Chapter 12
Development of Stroke Guidelines and Audit for Vietnam and Department of Health Directives

Tuan Tran Van, Ton Duy Mai, Ngoc Huy Nguyen, and Son Dinh Thanh Le

12.1 Introduction

Development of national standards and guidelines is a key activity that is needed to improve clinical care. While international guidelines such as the European Stroke Guidelines provide an invaluable source for evidence review, each national health system needs to ensure that the evidence is applied in a way that is appropriate for their services and population. We are all starting from different places in terms of how health and social services are organised, how funding is provided and how much funding there is and what the expectations of the population are. That is not to say that the evidence should be reinterpreted or dismissed because it is not convenient for a country, but it does mean that the priorities for a country will inevitably differ. There may be some evidence that while accepted is not a priority, while other treatments, perhaps not subjected to randomised controlled trials may be necessary to implement first.

In 2014, Vietnam published its own quality standards developed by clinical leaders from the country recruited from a range of medical specialties, supported by a

T. T. Van (✉)
Thai Nguyen University of Medicine and Pharmacy, Thai Nguyen, Vietnam
e-mail: tranvantuanyktn@gmail.com

T. D. Mai
Stroke Center, Bach Mai Hospital, Hanoi, Vietnam

VNU University of Medicine and Pharmacy, Hanoi, Vietnam

Hanoi Medical University, Hanoi, Vietnam

N. H. Nguyen
VNU University of Medicine and Pharmacy, Hanoi, Vietnam

Phutho Department of Health, Phutho, Vietnam

S. D. T. Le
Phutho General Hospital, Phutho, Vietnam

A. Rudd et al. (eds.), *Stroke Management in Vietnam*,
https://doi.org/10.1007/978-981-96-0221-6_12

team from an organisation from the United Kingdom called NICE (The National Institute for Clinical Excellence) International who were there to facilitate the meetings and provide technical support, collating the evidence, encouraging an evidence-based approach, and assisting with the drafting of the recommendations. The Quality Standards were developed using the UK National Clinical Guidelines and the NICE Stroke Quality Standards and were subsequently adopted by the Ministry of Health in Hanoi who issued a directive that they should implemented by all hospitals providing stroke care.

This chapter presents those Quality Standards drafted 10 years ago. Clearly some aspects of stroke care have changed since then but the basic principles remain the same and many of the recommendations are still as relevant today as they were then.

Quality Standards and Guidelines are not rules, never to be broken. They are applicable for perhaps 80% of the time for 80% of the population. A skilled clinical team will be aware of the guidelines and their limitations. Most of the time they will provide a clear answer as to how a patient should be treated but often patients will for very justifiable reasons need alternative approaches. Clinical trials tend to exclude very elderly or very young patients, those with multiple comorbidities and there will not be trials covering every aspect of care, even when those aspects are important for the patient.

The Vietnamese Stroke Quality Standards cover most of the important aspects of care (Guidelines on the Implementation of Quality Management of Medical Services in Hospitals (no. 19/2013/TT-BYT; 12 July 2013)). As can be seen from the papers by Mai et al. 2021 [1] and Phan et al. 2022 [2] since their publication, there has been a very rapid development of specialist services across the country. This may not be entirely due to the Ministry of Health directive but we are sure that it helped.

12.2 Vietnamese Stroke Quality Standards

The Ministry of Health of Vietnam made care quality improvement a key priority, as set out in the Circular Guidelines on the Implementation of Quality Management of Medical Services in Hospitals (no. 19/2013/TT-BYT; 12 July 2013).

The document contains the first set of care Quality Standards (QS) [3] developed in Vietnam. The QS were the product of a partnership between the Medical Services Administration (Ministry of Health), the Vietnam Health Economics Association (VHEA), and UK's NICE International, with funding support from the Rockefeller Foundation.

Drawing from local and international evidence-based clinical guidelines based on NICE methodology, the QS contains a set of concise statements and measurable indicators covering the management of acute stroke. The QS is an advisory document aimed at driving improvement in patient care; it is neither legally mandatory nor intended to punish providers and clinicians. It focuses on key areas of variation in current clinical practice and describes what the highest quality care would look like; it does not list all minimum expected standards for a hospital providing care for stroke patients, which are set out in the Hospital Quality Criteria (December 2013) according to the Decision no. 4858/QD-BYT of the Ministry of Health. The QS are expected to apply to the majority of stroke patients; nonetheless every patient is different, and the QS will not apply to all stroke patients all of the time.

The QS requires that stroke services be coordinated across all relevant agencies to encompass the whole stroke care pathway, and this document includes draft suggestions of the potential roles of the Ministry of Health, Provincial Departments of Health, hospitals, clinicians, payers such as Vietnam Social Security (VSS), and patients in ensuring that this QS is implemented. An integrated approach to provision of services, with appropriate training for workforce at all levels, is fundamental to delivering high-quality care to patients with stroke and their carers.

The QS were aspirational, but developed with the vision that in the future all stroke patients in Vietnam will receive high-quality care in specialist stroke units as set out in this document.

The document is summarised here but can be read in full with the following link https://f1000research.com/documents/6-1457/pdf. A budget assessment has also been published which will be discussed in more detail in the chapter on health economics. https://f1000research.com/documents/8-825/pdf [4].

The evidence for each of the standards is given in the relevant chapters in this book and are included in the latest edition of the UK National Clinical Guidelines for Stroke 2023 [5].

12.3 Audit of Stroke Care

Developing Quality Standards is a useless exercise if they are then not implemented and used by all the relevant stakeholders. It is recognised that some of the standards are more difficult to achieve than others and to implement all of them in all hospitals in Vietnam will take many years. One of the most powerful ways of encouraging implementation is to measure performance regularly across all parts of the country and report the measures to the Ministry of Health, Health Authorities, Hospitals, individual clinicians, and the general public. The quality standards are designed to be measurable and any audit could use them to define the specific questions asked. It is preferable that data are collected automatically through electronic health records but often this is not possible and then they need to be collected as a special exercise. Where the clinicians are responsible for collecting the data, it is our view that this is preferable to it being done by people in a back office with little interest in the quality of the data or the messages that are obtained. But this requires valuable clinicians' time which is not always available. However, data is collected, it is essential that the clinicians trust their accuracy and have ownership of the results. In this way, they are much more likely to be used constructively. Our preference is for the data to be put into the public domain. Comparing performance of one's own hospital to others is a powerful driver for improvement. Likewise having the public able to scrutinise the performance of their local hospitals is likely to encourage the health systems to develop. But this system is only possible if audit is seen as being a quality improvement process that is not punitive but rather being used in a constructive and non-judgemental way.

The national stroke audit in England, Wales, and Northern Ireland [6] (Sentinel Stroke National Audit Programme, SSNAP) is one example where the process has been shown to be useful in promoting positive change. Although participation is voluntary 100% of hospitals submit data and about 95% of patients admitted with stroke are included. The audit requires staff centrally to develop and run the audit tool and then to produce reports on a quarterly basis. A summary of some of the ways in which the data have been used is described in the paper by Rudd et al. 2018 [7].

12.4 Quality Standards Committee

The QS Committee was recruited by VHEA, with advice from NICE International, to include policymakers, hospital managers, and clinicians with a broad range of expertise and perspectives of stroke care in the three tiers of hospitals (district, provincial, and central). VHEA convened two workshops in November 2013 and March 2014, during which the QS Committee reached consensus on the priority areas for quality improvement in stroke care and agreed 15 quality standards. NICE International provided technical assistance, in helping the QS Committee identify relevant evidence-based clinical guidelines and develop the quality statements and measures. VHEA and the NICE International team were responsible for overall programme management.

12.4.1 Membership of the Quality Standards Committee

Chair: Prof Le Duc **Hinh**, Neurologist; President of Vietnam Association of Neurology.

Honorary Adviser: Prof Le Quang **Cuong**, Vice Minister, Ministry of Health.

Vice-Chair: Prof Le Van **Thanh**, Chairman of Vietnam Stroke Association.

Vice-Chair: Prof Luong Ngoc **Khue**, Director of Medical Services Administration, Ministry of Health.

Prof Nguyen Trong **Thong**, Neurologist; Vice-President of Vietnam Stroke Prevention Association; Military Hospital 108, Hanoi.

Prof Nguyen Dat Anh, Chief of Emergency Department, Bach Mai Hospital, Hanoi.

Prof Nguyen Trong **Hung**, Neurologist (Director of Neurology Department), National Geriatric Hospital, Hanoi.

Secretary: Dr. Mai Duy **Ton**, Emergency Doctor, Bach Mai Hospital, Hanoi.

Dr. Vu Van **Can,** Vice Director of Department of Health, Ninh Binh Province.

Dr. Nguyen Van **Chi**, Emergency Doctor, Bach Mai Hospital, Hanoi.

Prof Bui My **Hanh**, Doctor (Director, Center for Development of Curriculum and Human Resources in Health), Hanoi Medical University Hospital.

Dr. Nguyen Thanh **Binh**, Neurologist, National Geriatric Hospital, Hanoi.

Dr. Nguyen Huy **Thang**, Neurologist, 115 Hospital, HCMC.

Dr. Pham **Ty,** Neurosurgeon (Director of Neurosurgical Department), Gia Lai Hospital.

Dr. Ngo Van **Dung**, Neurologist, Viet Tiep Hospital, Haiphong.

Dr. Nguyen Hoanh **Sam,** Neurologist (Director of Neurology Department), Thanh Hoa Provincial Hospital.

Dr. Nguyen The **Hao**, Neurosurgeon, Bach Mai Hospital, Hanoi.

Dr. Nguyen Tuan **Hai**, Cardiologist, Bach Mai Hospital, Hanoi.

Dr. Nguyen Dinh **Hien**, Cardiologist, Saint Paul Hospital, Hanoi.

Dr. Pham Thi Phuong **Hanh**, Cardiologist (Director of Emergency Department), Ninh Binh Provincial Hospital.

Dr. Pham Viet **Phuong**, Internal Doctor, Tam Diep District Hospital, Ninh Binh.

Vu Thi Thu **Huong**, Pharmacist, Vice Head of Pharmaceutical Dept., Central Hospital.

Mr. Le Quang **Tri**, Nurse, Bach Mai Hospital.

Dr. Nguyen The **Dung**, Doctor (Former Director of HCMC Health Department); Pham Ngoc Thach Medical University, HCMC.

Dr. Le Truc **Phuong**, HCM People Committee.

12.4.2 Ministry of Health (MoH)

Dr. Nguyen Trong Khoa, Vice Director, Medical Services Administration, Ministry of Health.

Dr. Duong Huy **Luong**, Medical Officer, Medical Services Administration, Ministry of Health.

12.4.3 VHEA

Dr. Dong Huy **Lieu**, Chair of VHEA.

Dr. Vu Van **Chinh**, Director of VHEA.

12.4.4 NICE International Team, United Kingdom

Professor Anthony **Rudd** CBE, Chair of NICE Quality Standard Topic Expert Group for Stroke; Consultant Stroke Physician, Guy's and St Thomas' Hospital, London.

Dr. Françoise **Cluzeau**, Associate Director, NICE International.
Dr. Ryan **Li**, Adviser, NICE International.
Mr. Tommy **Wilkinson**, Adviser (Health Economics), NICE International.

12.5 Summary of Quality Statements

12.5.1 Clinician-Level Quality Standards

1. People with stroke and people with transient ischaemic attack (TIA) receive hospital care from appropriately trained healthcare staff.
2. Patients with suspected stroke receive brain imaging within 1 h of arrival at the hospital if they meet any of the indications for immediate imaging or within 24 h if they do not meet any indication for immediate imaging.
3. People with TIA (whose symptoms have fully resolved) are considered as medical emergencies, assessed and treated by a healthcare professional with expertise in neurovascular disease within 24 h, and started on aspirin treatment immediately.
4. Patients with suspected stroke are assessed and managed in a specialist stroke unit that meets at least Bronze criteria, by a doctor with specialist expertise in stroke and other appropriately trained staff within 24 h of admission to hospital, and by all relevant members of the multidisciplinary rehabilitation team within 72 h, with documented multidisciplinary goals agreed within 5 days.
5. Patients with stroke are treated with dignity, including their hygiene maintained, provided care to prevent and manage pressure ulcers, and given privacy.
6. Patients with suspected stroke arriving at a hospital with facilities to provide thrombolysis are admitted directly to a specialist stroke unit and assessed for thrombolysis, receiving it within 4.5 h of stroke onset if clinically indicated.
7. Patients with acute stroke (ischemic and haemorrhagic) are mobilised and helped to sit up as soon as they are awake, unless medically unstable; and supported to stand and walk as soon as possible.
8. Patients with acute stroke have their swallowing screened by specially trained healthcare staff within 4 h of admission to the hospital, before being given any oral food, fluid or medication; and have an ongoing management plan for the provision of adequate nutrition.
9. People at high risk of stroke, including those who have already had a TIA or stroke, are assessed for and given information about lifestyle risk factors (exercise, smoking, diet, weight, and alcohol); these people, and their carers where

possible, given accessible information, advice, and support in possible strategies to modify lifestyle and risk factors.

10. Patients after stroke are offered appropriate medication to reduce risk of future strokes.

12.5.2 Service-Level Quality Standards

1. A telemedicine service in a specialist stroke unit that does not have a specialist stroke physician on site has: a video link that enables a specialist stroke physician to observe a clinical examination, discuss the case with the examining clinician on site, and see and talk to the patient and carer directly; a link that enables a specialist stroke physician to review radiological investigations remotely.
2. Central hospitals with expert training facilities in stroke care lead in disseminating expertise to provincial hospitals and organise regular joint meetings; and provincial hospitals lead in disseminating expertise to other hospitals within the province and organise regular joint meetings.
3. Emergency care staff can screen for stroke and TIA using a validated tool and respond to these as emergencies.
4. Members of the public can identify the main symptoms of stroke and TIA and respond to these as emergencies.
5. Patients with stroke have their quality of care monitored, and systems are in place to address problems that are identified.

12.5.3 Where Will the QS Be Implemented?

The QS should be implemented in all hospitals in Vietnam where acute stroke is managed, from district level hospitals to specialist central hospitals, and including private hospital facilities. However, differences in the administrative and technical classes of hospitals means that some hospitals will be able to implement the QS more rapidly and without major reorganisation or costs, while others may need substantial changes to clinical practice, organisational environment, and existing payment and activity regulation policies.

The maximum potential for implementing each QS in hospitals by administrative type and class, under current Ministry of Health policies, is given in Table 12.1.

Table 12.1 Potential for implementing each QS within different hospital categories

Quality standard	Central hospital		Provincial hospital	District hospital			Private
	Specialised	Class I	Class I	Class II	Class III	Class IV	
QS1: Trained staff	✓	✓	✓	✓	✓	✓	✓
QS2: Imaging	✓	✓	✓	✓	✗	✗	Hospital decision
QS3: Stroke units	Gold	Gold	Gold	Silver	Bronze	Bronze	Bronze at minimum
QS4: Dignity	✓	✓	✓	✓	✓	✓	✓
QS5: Thrombolysis	✓	✓	✓	✗	✗	✗	Competency dependent
QS6: TIA	✓	✓	✓	✓	Referral	Referral	Competency dependent
QS7: Early mobilisation	✓	✓	✓	✓	✓	✓	✓
QS8: Swallowing and nutrition	✓	✓	✓	✓	✓	✓	✓
QS9: Prevention (lifestyle advice)	✓	✓	✓	✓	✓	✓	✓
QS10: Secondary prevention (medication)	✓	✓	✓	✓	✓	✓	✓
QS11: Telemedicine	Hub	Hub	✓	✓	✓	✓	✓
QS12: Disseminating expertise	Hub	Hub	Hub / recipient	Hub / recipient	Recipient	Recipient	Hospital decision
QS13: Screening (emergency response)	✓	✓	✓	✓	✓	✓	✓
QS14: Public awareness	✓	✓	✓	✓	✓	✓	✓
QS15: Monitoring quality of care	✓	✓	✓	✓	✓	✓	✓

12.6 Clinical-Level Quality Standards

12.6.1 People with Stroke and People with Transient Ischaemic Attack (TIA) Receive Hospital Care from Appropriately Trained Healthcare Staff

12.6.1.1 Quality Measure—Structure

- Evidence of locally agreed protocols to ensure that staff in the relevant hospital departments (such as emergency department, stroke unit, ICU, neurology) are appropriately trained to deliver care for people with a suspected or confirmed diagnosis of stroke or TIA.

12.6.1.2 Quality Measure—Process

Numerator: The number of people who have received care from appropriately trained staff.

Denominator: The number of people with stroke or TIA admitted to the hospital.

12.6.1.3 What Quality Statement Means for Each Audience

Ministry of Health: Ensure that training programmes and standards for healthcare professionals are regularly reviewed in line with international best practice.

Provincial health departments: Ensure that hospitals adhere to training standards.

Hospitals: Ensure appropriate training for healthcare staff in the relevant hospital departments.

Healthcare staff: Adhere to training and local protocols in the management of acute stroke.

Payers (VSS, other health insurers, patients who pay for a service): Can use adherence to QS to inform payment.

Patients: Can expect to receive care from hospital staff.

12.6.2 Patients with Suspected Stroke Receive Brain Imaging Within 1 H of Arrival at the Hospital If They Meet Any of the Indications for Immediate Imaging, or within 24 H If they Do Not Meet any Indication for Immediate Imaging

12.6.2.1 Quality Measure—Structure

- Evidence of equipment for brain imaging, e.g., a cranial tomography (CT) scanner.
- Evidence of locally agreed protocols to prioritise any patients with acute stroke to receive imaging within 1 h of arrival at the hospital if they meet indications for immediate imaging, or within 24 h if they do not meet such indications.
- Availability of appropriately trained staff to perform imaging within the specified times 24 h a day and 7 days a week.
- Availability of appropriately trained staff, either locally or via an electronic link, to interpret the findings of brain imaging within the specified times 24 h a day and 7 days a week.
- Evidence of locally agreed protocols to identify patients with acute stroke and to refer them to another hospital with facilities for timely brain imaging, where these are not locally available.

12.6.2.2 Quality Measure—Process

(a) **Numerator:** The number of patients who have had brain imaging within 1 h of arrival at the hospital.

Denominator: The number of patients with acute stroke who meet any indication for immediate imaging admitted to the hospital.

(b) **Numerator:** The number of patients who have had brain imaging within 24 h of arrival at the hospital.

Denominator: The number of patients with acute stroke who do not meet any indication for immediate imaging admitted to the hospital.

12.6.2.3 What Quality Statement Means for each Audience

Ministry of Health: Consider revising hospital classifications so that all public hospitals could have brain imaging facilities.

Provincial health departments: Ensure resources for hospitals to provide brain imaging facilities.

Hospitals: Ensure adequate equipment, human resources and protocols to provide brain imaging within the specified times 24 h a day, 7 days a week.

Healthcare staff: Adhere to training and local protocols to provide imaging within the specified times 24 h a day, 7 days a week.

Payers (VSS, other health insurers, patients who pay for a service): Can use adherence to QS to inform payment.

Patients: Can expect to receive brain imaging within the specified times 24 h a day, 7 days a week.

12.6.3 People with TIA (Whose Symptoms Have Fully Resolved) Are Considered as Medical Emergencies, Assessed and Treated by a Healthcare Professional with Expertise in Neurovascular Disease within 24 H, and Started on Aspirin Treatment Immediately

12.6.3.1 Quality Measure—Structure

- Evidence of locally agreed protocols for the assessment and treatment of TIA as medical emergencies within 24 h, and not necessarily as inpatients.
- Availability of staff with expertise in neurovascular disease.
- Availability of aspirin.

12.6.3.2 Quality Measure—Process

(a) Numerator: The number of patients treated as medical emergencies, and assessed and treated by a healthcare professional with expertise in neurovascular disease within 24 h of arrival at the hospital.

Denominator: The number of patients with TIA admitted to the hospital.

(b) Numerator: The number of patients started on aspirin treatment immediately.

Denominator: The number of patients with TIA admitted to the hospital who do not have contraindications to aspirin.

12.6.3.3 What Quality Statement Means for Each Audience

Ministry of Health: Ensure that training programmes and standards for healthcare professionals include recognition of stroke risk following TIA (for example, using the ABCD2 tool), and treating TIAs as emergencies.

Provincial health departments: Ensure the resources for hospitals to assess and treat TIA as medical emergencies.

Hospitals: Ensure the appropriate skillset and resources to assess and treat TIA as medical emergencies, and not necessarily as inpatients.

Healthcare staff: Ensure adherence to training and protocols to assess and treat TIA as medical emergencies, and not necessarily as inpatients.

Payers (VSS, other health insurers, patients who pay for a service): Can use adherence to QS to inform payment.

Patients with TIA: Can expect to be assessed and managed as an outpatient medical emergency, and started on aspirin immediately.

12.6.4 *Patients with Suspected Stroke Are Assessed and Managed in a Specialist Stroke Unit that Meets at Least Bronze Criteria, by a Doctor with Specialist Expertise in Stroke and Other Appropriately Trained Staff within 24 H of Admission to Hospital, and by all Relevant Members of the Multidisciplinary Rehabilitation Team within 72 H, with Documented Multidisciplinary Goals Agreed within 5 Days*

12.6.4.1 Quality Measure—Structure

- Evidence of a designated ward, part of a ward, or geographically identified unit for stroke patients.
- Evidence of locally agreed protocols to assess and manage stroke patients in a specialist stroke unit within 24 h of arrival at the hospital.
- Availability of a multidisciplinary team with appropriately trained staff to perform the specified assessment and management.
- Evidence that patient rehabilitation plans are discussed at a multidisciplinary meeting including a doctor, a nurse and a therapist, within 5 days of arrival at the hospital.

12.6.4.2 Quality Measure—Process

(a) Numerator: The number of patients assessed and managed in a specialist stroke unit that meets at least Bronze criteria by a doctor with specialist expertise in stroke and other appropriately trained staff within 24 h of admission to the hospital.

Denominator: The number of patients with suspected stroke admitted to the hospital.

(b) Numerator: The number of patients assessed and managed by all relevant members of the multidisciplinary rehabilitation team within 72 h of admission to the hospital.

Denominator: The number of patients with stroke admitted to the hospital.

(c) Numerator: The number of patients with documented multidisciplinary goals agreed within 5 days of admission to the hospital.
Denominator: The number of patients with stroke admitted to the hospital.

12.6.4.3 What Quality Statement Means for each Audience

Ministry of Health: Establish and maintain an accreditation or regulatory system for specialist stroke units, within current hospital classification and auditing frameworks; and ensure that training programmes and standards for healthcare professionals include necessary competencies and multidisciplinary working in the context of a stroke unit.

Provincial health departments: Ensure the resources for hospitals to establish specialist stroke units.

Hospitals: Ensure the appropriate facilities and skillset are available in the specialist stroke unit.

Healthcare staff: Assess and manage all patients with stroke at a stroke unit that meets Level 1 (Bronze) criteria with relevant appropriately trained staff and document multidisciplinary goals, within the specified times.

Payers (VSS, other health insurers, patients who pay for a service): Can use adherence to QS to inform payment.

Patients: Can expect to be assessed and managed in a stroke unit that meets at least Level 1 criteria by relevant appropriately train staff and have documented multidisciplinary goals, within the specified times.

Specialist stroke units are an evidence-based and internationally recognised method of providing timely and effective care to stroke patients in the acute phase. As of 2014, there are 21 stroke units across Vietnam, almost entirely in Hanoi and Ho Chi Minh City (Prof Le Van Thanh presentation to QS Committee, 2014). Establishing stroke units do not necessarily require new specialist staff to be recruited, but does require existing resources to be reorganised.

12.6.4.4 Specialist Stroke Units Are Classified Using the Following Criteria

Bronze

- A designated ward or part of a ward set aside for stroke patients.
- At least one nurse with stroke management experience and training will be on duty at all times.
- Access to a doctor with expertise in stroke/neurology at least during normal working hours.
- Agreed management protocols for common problems, based on available evidence.

Silver

- As for Bronze, plus:
- Access to brain imaging during normal working hours.
- Access to a physiotherapist with neurological/stroke training during normal working hours.
- Access to a speech therapist with neurological training during normal working hours.
- Has a coordinated multidisciplinary team that meets at least once a week for the interchange of information about individual patients.
- Educational programmes and information are provided for staff, patients, and carers.

Gold

- As for Silver, plus:
- A geographically identified unit.
- Staff has specialist expertise in stroke and rehabilitation.
- Provision of imaging and laboratory services.
- Access to rehabilitation specialist staff.
- All nurses caring for the stroke patients are experienced and competent in the management of acute stroke covering neurological, general medical, and rehabilitation aspects.
- Medical staff are specially trained in the delivery of acute medical care to stroke patients, including the diagnostic and administrative procedures needed for safe, effective delivery of thrombolysis available 24 h, 7 days a week.
- Organised as a single team of staff with specialist knowledge and experience of stroke and neurological rehabilitation including:
- consultant physician(s),
- nurses,
- physiotherapists,
- occupational therapists,
- speech and language therapists,
- dietitians,
- psychologists,
- social workers
- Easy access to services providing: pharmacy; orthotics; orthoptists; specialist seating; patient information, advice and support; and assistive devices.
- Have an education programme for all staff providing the stroke service and offer training for junior professionals in the specialty of stroke.

12.6.5 *Patients with Stroke Are Treated with Dignity and Respect, Including Their Hygiene Maintained, Provided Care to Prevent and Manage Pressure Ulcers, and Given Privacy*

12.6.5.1 Quality Measure—Structure

- Evidence of locally agreed protocols to ensure that patients' hygiene is maintained and provided care to pressure area provided;
- Evidence of curtains around each patient's bed, and locally agreed protocols to ensure curtains are closed when medical or personal care is being provided.

12.6.5.2 Quality Measure—Process

(a) Numerator: The number of patients with their hygiene maintained.
  Denominator: The number of patients with stroke admitted to the hospital.
(b) Numerator: The number of patients provided care to prevent and manage pressure ulcers.
  Denominator: The number of patients with stroke admitted to the hospital.
(c) Numerator: The number of patients with a curtain around their bed.
  Denominator: The number of patients with stroke admitted to the hospital.

12.6.5.3 What Quality Statement Means for Each Audience

Ministry of Health: Include indicators in the MoH hospital auditing programme on hygiene maintenance, care to prevent and manage pressure ulcers, and privacy.

Provincial health departments: Ensure resources and protocols for hospitals to maintain hygiene, provide care to prevent and manage pressure ulcers, and giving privacy.

Hospitals: Ensure resources, training and protocols to maintain hygiene, provide care to prevent and manage pressure ulcers, and giving privacy.

Healthcare staff: Adhere to training and local protocols to maintain hygiene, provide care to prevent and manage pressure ulcers, and give privacy.

Payers (VSS, other health insurers, patients who pay for a service): Can use adherence to QS to inform payment.

Patients: Can expect to have hygiene maintained, provided care to prevent and manage pressure ulcers and be given privacy.

12.6.6 Patients with Suspected Stroke Arriving at a Hospital with Facilities to Provide Thrombolysis Are Admitted Directly to a Specialist Stroke Unit and Assessed for Thrombolysis, Receiving it within 4.5 H of Stroke Onset if Clinically Indicated

12.6.6.1 Quality Measure—Structure

- Evidence of a stroke unit meeting Gold criteria.
- Evidence of equipment for brain imaging, e.g., a cranial tomography (CT) scanner.
- Evidence of locally agreed protocols to prioritise any patients with acute stroke to receive imaging within 1 h of arrival at the hospital and for the results to be interpreted as soon as possible.
- Availability of appropriately trained staff to perform imaging within 1 h of arrival at the hospital and to interpret the results as soon as possible, 24 h a day and 7 days a week.
- Evidence of locally agreed protocols to ensure that patients with suspected stroke are assessed for and given thrombolysis if clinically indicated.
- Availability of thrombolytic medications.
- Availability of appropriately trained and experienced staff to perform thrombolysis, including knowledge of contraindications, and specialist monitoring.

12.6.6.2 Quality Measure—Process

(a) Numerator: The number of patients admitted directly to a specialist stroke unit and assessed for thrombolysis.

Denominator: The number of patients with suspected stroke arriving at a hospital with facilities to provide thrombolysis.

(b) Numerator: The number of patients who receive thrombolysis within 4.5 h of stroke onset.

Denominator: The number of patients with suspected stroke assessed to require thrombolysis.

12.6.6.3 What Quality Statement Means for Each Audience

Ministry of Health: Ensure specialist training standards for stroke clinicians to deliver thrombolysis.

Provincial health departments: Ensure resources for hospitals to provide thrombolysis as soon as possible 24 h a day, 7 days a week.

Hospitals: Ensure adequate facilities and human resources to provide thrombolysis as soon as possible 24 h a day, 7 days a week.

Healthcare staff: Adhere to training and local protocols to provide thrombolysis as soon as possible 24 h a day, 7 days a week.

Payers (VSS, other health insurers, patients who pay for a service): Can use adherence to QS to inform payment.

Patients: Can expect to receive thrombolysis as soon as possible 24 h a day, 7 days a week.

12.6.7 *Patients with Acute Stroke (Ischemic and Haemorrhagic) Are Mobilised and Helped to Sit up As Soon as they Are Awake, unless Medically Unstable; and Supported to Stand and Walk As Soon as Possible*

12.6.7.1 Quality Measure—Structure

- Evidence of locally agreed protocols for early mobilisation.
- Availability of appropriately trained staff to support early mobilisation.
- Availability of sufficient floor space around each patient.
- Availability of a chair beside each bed in order to practice sitting.
- Availability of other appropriate equipment for early mobilisation, including walking sticks and frames.
- Evidence of locally agreed protocols to provide basic practical training for family carers to assist in early mobilisation.

12.6.7.2 Quality Measure—Process

(a) Numerator: The number of patients who are mobilised and practice sitting.
Denominator: The number of patients with acute stroke admitted to hospital who are awake and not medically unstable.

(b) Numerator: The number of patients who are supported to stand and walk .
Denominator: The number of patients with acute stroke admitted to hospital are who are able to stand and walk, and not medically unstable.

12.6.7.3 What Quality Statement Means for Each Audience

Ministry of Health: Ensure that training programmes and standards for healthcare professionals include early mobilisation.

Provincial health departments: Ensure resources for hospitals to provide appropriate skillsets and facilities (including sufficient floor space, chairs, and other equipment) for early mobilisation.

Hospitals: Ensure the appropriate skillset and facilities (including sufficient floor space, chairs, and other equipment) to allow for early mobilisation.

Healthcare staff: Adhere to training and protocols to mobilise stroke patients appropriately and as soon as possible.

Payers (VSS, other health insurers, patients who pay for a service): Can use adherence to QS to inform payment.

Patients: Can expect to be mobilised within 24 h.

Family carers: Can ask for practical training and assist the patient in early mobilisation.

12.6.8 Patients with Acute Stroke Have their Swallowing Screened by Specially Trained Healthcare Staff within 4 H of Admission to the Hospital, Before Being Given any Oral Food, Fluid or Medication; and Have an Ongoing Management Plan for the Provision of Adequate Nutrition

12.6.8.1 Quality Measure—Structure

- Evidence of locally agreed protocols for swallowing screening and nutritional management.
- Availability of specially trained staff to perform swallowing checks.
- Availability of specially trained staff to administer nutrition management plans.

12.6.8.2 Quality Measure—Process

(a) Numerator: The number of patients who have their swallowing screened by a specially trained healthcare professional within 4 h of admission to hospital, before being given any oral food, fluid or medication.

Denominator: The number of patients with acute stroke admitted to hospital.

(b) Numerator: The number of patients with an ongoing management plan for the provision of adequate nutrition.

Denominator: The number of patients with acute stroke admitted to hospital.

12.6.8.3 What Quality Statement Means for Each Audience

Ministry of Health: Ensure that training programmes and standards for healthcare professionals include swallowing screening and nutrition management.

Provincial health departments: Ensure the resources for hospitals to provide perform swallowing screening within 4 h of admission, and to administer ongoing management plans for the provision of adequate nutrition.

Hospitals: Ensure appropriate training for staff to perform swallowing screening within 4 h of admission, and to administer ongoing management plans for the provision of adequate nutrition.

Healthcare staff: Adhere to training and protocols to perform swallowing screening within 4 h of admission, and to administer ongoing management plans for the provision of adequate nutrition.

Payers (VSS, other health insurers, patients who pay for a service): Can use adherence to QS to inform payment.

Patients: Can expect to receive swallowing screening within 4 h of admission, and have an ongoing management plan for the provision of adequate nutrition.

12.6.9 People at High Risk of Stroke, Including Those Who Have Already Had a TIA or Stroke, Are Assessed for and Given Information about Lifestyle Risk Factors (Exercise, Smoking, Diet, Weight, and Alcohol); These People, and Their Carers Where Possible, Given Accessible Information, Advice and Support in Possible Strategies to Modify Lifestyle and Risk Factors

12.6.9.1 Quality Measure—Structure

- Evidence of locally agreed protocols for the provision of information, advice and support to reduce lifestyle risk factors for stroke.
- Evidence of accessible written information, such as leaflets, for the general public.

12.6.9.2 Quality Measure—Process

(a) Numerator: The number of people whom are assessed for lifestyle risk factors (exercise, smoking, diet, weight, and alcohol).

Denominator: The number of people at high risk of stroke.

(b) Numerator: The number of people whom or whose carers are given accessible information, advice and support in possible strategies to modify their lifestyle risk factors (exercise, smoking diet, weight, and alcohol).

Denominator: The number of people at high risk of stroke.

12.6.9.3 What Quality Statement Means for each Audience

Ministry of Health: Ensure that training programmes and standards for healthcare professionals include identifying people at high risk of stroke and offering appropriate referral or support for reducing lifestyle risk factors; and ensure resources for central hospitals to provide these.

Provincial health departments: Ensure the resources for hospitals to identify people at high risk of stroke and to offer appropriate referral or support for reducing lifestyle risk factors.

Hospitals: Ensure appropriate training and protocols for staff in all hospital departments to identify people at high risk of stroke and to offer appropriate referral or support for reducing lifestyle risk factors.

Healthcare staff: Adhere to training and protocols to assess people at high risk of stroke for lifestyle risk factors and offer appropriate referral or support.

Payers (VSS, other health insurers, patients who pay for a service): Can use adherence to QS to inform payment.

People at increased risk of stroke: Can (alongside their carers) expect to receive information and advice on reducing lifestyle risk factors and offered medications for secondary prevention (if they have already had stroke).

12.6.10 Patients After Stroke Are Offered Appropriate Medication to Reduce Risk of Future Strokes

12.6.10.1 Quality Measure—Structure

- Evidence of locally agreed protocols to offer appropriate medication for secondary prevention of stroke, in line with international guidance.
- Availability of appropriate medication.

12.6.10.2 Quality Measure—Process

Numerator: The number of patients given appropriate medication to reduce risk of future strokes.

Denominator: The number of patients who have had stroke.

12.6.10.3 What Quality Statement Means for Each Audience

Ministry of Health: Ensure that training programmes and standards for healthcare professionals include offering appropriate medication for secondary prevention of stroke.

Provincial health departments: Ensure the resources for hospitals to offer appropriate medication for secondary prevention of stroke.

Hospitals: Ensure protocols and resources to offer appropriate medication for secondary prevention of stroke.

Healthcare staff: Adhere to protocols to offer appropriate medication for secondary prevention of stroke.

Payers (VSS, other health insurers, patients who pay for a service): Can use adherence to QS to inform payment.

Patients: Can expect to be offered medications for secondary prevention.

12.7 Service-Level Quality Standards

12.7.1 A Telemedicine Service in a Specialist Stroke Unit that Does Not Have a Specialist Stroke Physician on Site Has: A Video Link that Enables a Specialist Stroke Physician to Observe a Clinical Examination, Discuss the Case with the Examining Clinician on Site, and See and Talk to the Patient and Carer Directly; and a Link that Enables a Specialist Stroke Physician to Review Radiological Investigations Remotely

12.7.1.1 Quality Measure—Structure

- Evidence of joint working agreements and protocols with specialist stroke unit in another hospital that does have a local specialist stroke physician.
- Availability of video-conferencing facilities at the location of clinical examination, including adequate broadband Internet connection and equipment.
- Availability of facilities to capture and transmit radiological images electronically (e.g., via email) for timely remote reviews.

12.7.1.2 Quality Measure—Process

Numerator: Hospital has a telemedicine service with a video link to a specialist stroke physician for observing clinical examinations, discussing cases with a trained assessing clinician, and seeing and talking to patients and carers directly; and a link for reviewing radiological investigations remotely.

Denominator: Hospital with a specialist stroke unit meeting all Bronze criteria except having a specialist stroke physician on site.

12.7.1.3 What Quality Statement Means for Each Audience

Ministry of Health: Include standards for telemedicine services as part of an accreditation or regulatory system for specialist stroke units.

Provincial health departments: Ensure the resources for hospitals to provide a telemedicine service, and facilitate joint working between hospitals.

Hospitals: Ensure joint working agreements and protocols with another hospital that does have a local specialist stroke physician, and adequate facilities for providing a telemedicine service.

Healthcare staff: Adhere to protocols to implement a telemedicine service in order to facilitate early diagnosis and treatment of patients with stroke.

Payers (VSS, other health insurers, patients who pay for a service): Can use adherence to QS to inform payment.

Patients: Can expect to be assessed and managed appropriately within the stroke unit, whether or not the hospital has a specialist stroke physician on site.

12.7.2 Central Hospitals with Expert Training Facilities in Stroke Care Lead in Disseminating Expertise to Provincial Hospitals and Organise Regular Joint Meetings; and Provincial Hospitals Lead in Disseminating Expertise to Other Hospitals within the Province and Organise Regular Joint Meetings

12.7.2.1 Quality Measure—Structure

- Evidence of joint working agreements and protocols between central hospitals with expert training facilities and provincial hospitals, and between provincial hospitals and other hospitals within the province, to disseminate expertise via regular meetings, e.g. weekly or monthly case reviews, training workshops, clinical placements, etc.
- Evidence of regular joint meetings, e.g., meeting agendas, attendance lists, summaries and reports, workshop training materials.

12.7.2.2 Quality Measure—Process

(a) Numerator: Hospital has a programme of regular joint meetings to disseminate expertise to provincial hospitals.

Denominator: Central hospital with expert training facilities in stroke care.

(b) Numerator: Hospital has a programme of regular joint meetings to disseminates expertise to other hospitals within the province.

Denominator: Provincial hospital.

(c) Number of joint meetings per month.
(d) Numerator: Number of staff that have taken part in training events.
    Denominator: Number of staff in the hospital who are involved in the assessment and management of stroke patients.

12.7.2.3 What Quality Statement Means for Each Audience

Ministry of Health: Ensure that central hospitals with expert training facilities are responsible for disseminating expertise.

Provincial health departments: Ensure that leading provincial hospitals are responsible for disseminating expertise, and facilitate joint working between hospitals within the province.

Hospitals: Establish regular joint meetings with other hospitals to facilitate exchange of expertise.

Healthcare staff: Engage in regular joint meetings to exchange expertise with staff in other hospitals.

Payers (VSS, other health insurers, patients who pay for a service): Can use adherence to QS to inform payment.

Patients: Can expect to be assessed and managed appropriately within a local hospital that receives regular dissemination of expertise from a more specialised hospital.

12.7.3 Emergency Care Staff Can Screen for Stroke and TIA Using a Validated Tool, and Respond to These as Emergencies

12.7.3.1 Quality Measure—Structure

- Evidence of a professional education campaign for emergency contact healthcare professionals outside of the hospital setting.
- Evidence of a professional education campaign for emergency and outpatient healthcare professionals in the hospital.

12.7.3.2 Quality Measure—Process

(a) Numerator: Hospital has in place a professional education campaign for emergency contact healthcare professionals to screen for stroke and TIA using a validated tool, and responding to these as emergencies.
    Denominator: Any hospital.

(b) Government has established professional training standards for emergency contact healthcare professionals to screen for stroke and TIA using a validated tool, and responding to these as emergencies.

12.7.3.3 What Quality Statement Means for Each Audience

Ministry of Health: Ensure that training programmes and standards for emergency contact healthcare professionals including screening for stroke and TIA using a validated tool, and responding to these as emergencies.

Provincial health departments: Ensure training for emergency contact healthcare professionals to screen for stroke and TIA using validated tools, and treat them appropriately as emergencies.

Hospitals: Initiate professional education campaigns within the hospital.

Emergency healthcare contact professionals: Adhere to training to screen for stroke and TIA using validated tools, and treat them appropriately as emergencies.

Patients: Can expect to be assessed by emergency healthcare professionals using a validated tool and be treated appropriately as emergencies.

12.7.4 Members of the Public Can Identify the Main Symptoms of Stroke and TIA, and Respond to These as Emergencies

12.7.4.1 Quality Measure—Structure

- Evidence of posters displayed and accessible written material made available in public areas of the hospital, e.g., emergency and outpatient departments.
- The presence of mass-media public education campaigns, conducted within the framework of a formal evaluation.

12.7.4.2 Quality Measure—Process

(a) Numerator: Hospital has a public education campaign in place.
    Denominator: Any hospital.
(b) Government has established mass-media public education campaigns within the framework of a formal evaluation.

12.7.4.3 What Quality Statement Means for Each Audience

Ministry of Health: Initiate mass-media public education campaigns within the framework of a formal evaluation.

Provincial health departments: Initiate public education campaigns within the province.

Hospitals: Initiate public education campaigns within the hospital.

Healthcare staff: Educate patients and carers to the main symptoms of stroke and TIA, and how to respond to these as emergencies.

General public: Be aware of the main symptoms of stroke and TIA, and how to respond to these as emergencies.

12.7.5 Patients with Stroke Have Their Quality of Care Monitored, and Systems Are in Place to Address Problems that Are Identified

12.7.5.1 Quality Measure—Structure

- Evidence of locally agreed protocols to monitor quality, and to identify and address problems (e.g., regular review meetings).
- Evidence of audit standards (including specific measures and indicators) based on the Quality Standards for Stroke.
- Evidence of data collection tools for audit standards.

12.7.5.2 Quality Measure—Process

Numerator: The number of patients with stroke who have their quality of care monitored.

Denominator: The number of patients with stroke admitted to the hospital.

12.7.5.3 What Quality Statement Means for Each Audience

Ministry of Health: Include indicators specific to stroke quality improvement in the MoH hospital auditing programme.

Provincial health departments: Establish Provincial Stroke Quality Improvement Groups to monitor the quality of care.

Service providers: Ensure regular auditing system in place to monitor quality of care and address any identified problems.

Healthcare staff: Adhere to quality monitoring systems and address any problems that are identified.

Payers (VSS, other health insurers, patients who pay for a service): Can use adherence to QS to inform payment.

People at high risk of stroke: Can expect to have their quality of monitored, and systems in place to address any identified problems.

References

1. Mai DT, Phan H, Hoang VM, et al. Treatment of stroke patients in the context of the COVID-19 pandemic: lessons learnt from a major stroke center in Vietnam. J Glob Health. 2021;11:03092. https://doi.org/10.7189/jogh.11.03092.
2. Phan HT, Nguyen TH, Watkins C, et al. Organisational survey for acute stroke care in Vietnam: regional collaboration Programme. J Stroke Cerebrovasc Dis. 2022;31(11):106792.
3. Vietnamese Stroke Quality Standards. 2013. https://f1000research.com/documents/6-1457/pdf.
4. Vietnamese Quality Standards. Budget Assessment. https://f1000research.com/documents/8-825/pdf.
5. National Clinical Guidelines for Stroke for the United Kingdom and Ireland 2023. https://www.strokeguideline.org.
6. Sentinel Stroke National Audit Programme. https://www.strokeaudit.org/.
7. Rudd AG, Hoffman A, Paley L, Bray B. 20 years of researching stroke through audit. Clin Rehabil. 2018;32(8):997–1006.

Chapter 13
Health Economics of Stroke

Ngoc Huy Nguyen and Thanh Ngoc Le

13.1 Introduction

With stroke as the second commonest cause of death worldwide and one of the most important causes of acquired disability, it is evident that stroke is a significant drain on economic resources both in terms of the costs of providing acute care but also the cost to the individual, family and society of long-term disability.

There are limited published data on the health economics of stroke in Vietnam but this chapter reviews some of the data available internationally and specifically for low-and middle-income countries.

13.2 Global, Regional and National Consequences of Stroke

The Global Burden of Disease Study [1] published in 2021 based on 2019 data provides the basis for several estimates of stroke costs. This includes Gerstl et al. in 2023 [2] who published a useful summary of the economic consequences of stroke using data from the Global Burden of Disease (GBD) database from 2019. Disability adjusted life year (DALY) data for overall stroke and its subtypes (ischemic stroke, intracerebral haemorrhage and subarachnoid haemorrhage) were collected. Gross

N. H. Nguyen (✉)
Phutho Department of Health, Phutho, Vietnam

VNU University of Medicine and Pharmacy, Hanoi, Vietnam
e-mail: ngochuynguyen8888@gmail.com

T. N. Le
VNU University of Medicine and Pharmacy, Hanoi, Vietnam

A. Rudd et al. (eds.), *Stroke Management in Vietnam*,
https://doi.org/10.1007/978-981-96-0221-6_13

domestic product (GDP, adjusted for purchasing power parity [PPP]) data were collected from the World Bank; GDP and disability adjusted life year data were combined to estimate the macroeconomic losses using a value of lost welfare (VLW) approach (Fig. 13.1). This takes account of the age at which a patient has their stroke and therefore the likely longer term costs. The results were presented in 2017 international US dollars adjusted for PPP. Globally, in 2019, VLW due to stroke was $2059.67 billion or 1.66% of the global GDP. The data for Vietnam suggest that the consequences of stroke as a proportion of their GDP are significantly higher than the mean global figure. The overall VLW was $23.5 billion which is 3.03% of the GDP. The figures for primary intracerebral haemorrhage alone were $14.19 billion and 1.83% of GDP, for ischaemic stroke $7.92 billion and 1.02% and for subarachnoid haemorrhage $1.40 billion and 0.18% of GDP.

Stroke is therefore a major economic burden in Vietnam with the major factors being the high incidence rate, the low average age of the patients and specifically the high incidence of primary intracerebral haemorrhage. The relative costs are much greater than in the high-income countries of Europe and North America. It also follows that there is great potential to reduce costs particularly by investing in stroke prevention through the management of risk factors and by providing better acute care and rehabilitation to reduce the rates of long term dependency.

As Gerstl et al [2] comment the 2016 GBD study on stroke, revealed that 87.9% of ischemic stroke DALYs and 89.5% of haemorrhagic stroke DALYs were due to potentially modifiable risk factors. It follows that there is a vast potential to decrease stroke disease burden by reducing risk factor exposure; for example, for every $1 spent on stroke and cardiovascular disease prevention, there is a $10.9 return on investment. The most important risk factors to address are diabetes and hypertension which are both becoming more prevalent as LMIC adopt western patterns of behaviour and diet and reducing tobacco use. The World Health Organization estimates that population wide interventions to modify risk factors would amount to only, 4% of health spending in low-income countries, 2% in lower middle-income countries and less than 1% in upper middle-income countries. Vietnam is classified as a lower middle-income country by the World Bank. These data need to be interpreted with caution as they are largely based on modelling rather than real life data due to the lack of good population based epidemiological information.

13.3 Stroke Cost Studies

A systematic review of the cost of stroke in LMIC published in 2014 [3] found ten articles suitable to include. It looked specifically at the costs associated with acute care which varied hugely between countries with the highest being Nigeria at $8424 and the lowest reported in Senegal at $214. No papers reporting Vietnamese costs were included in the review. The main driver to costs that the authors found was length of hospital stay. The main message is probably that if you provide very little or no care for acute stroke the acute costs will be low. However, the consequences

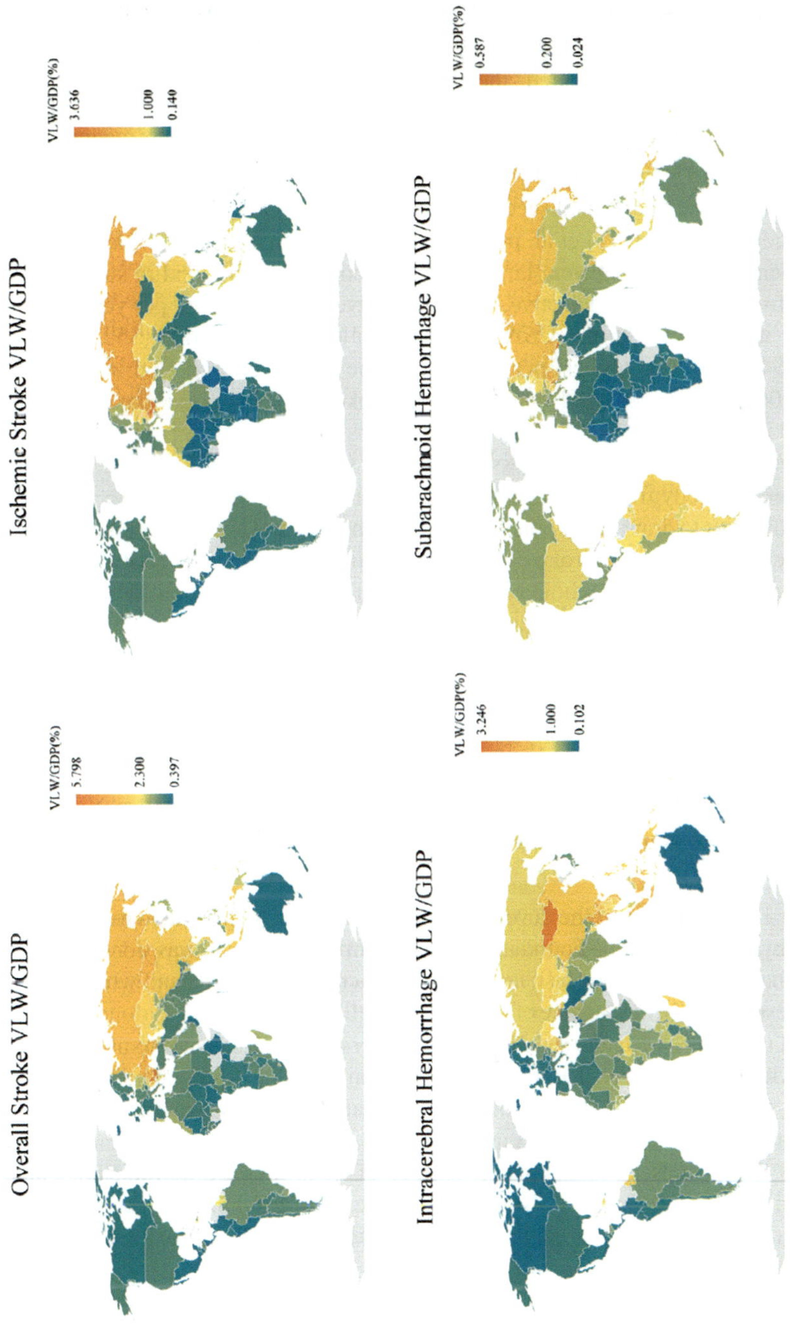

Fig. 13.1 World heat maps of value of lost welfare (VLW)/gross domestic product (GDP) in 2019 by country for stroke overall, ischemic stroke, intracerebral haemorrhage and subarachnoid haemorrhage

are likely to be high mortality rates and high levels of long-term disability and dependency. A more up-to-date publication from 2023 [4] looked at stroke care costs in high-income countries as well as LMIC and included 25 studies. They varied as to whether they included just the acute care or also longer term patient, carer and societal costs. As expected, there are huge variations in reported costs. For example, costs for primary prevention (management of atrial fibrillation and hypertension varied between €4750 and €23,064/patient/year. Costs for acute care ranged between €5798.15 and €140,048 and with similar large variations for provision of rehabilitation, social care and secondary prevention.

A study by Strilciuc [5] et al. published in 2021 found 46 cost of illness studies. Per patient per year costs were larger in high-income countries and in studies conducted from the payer perspective. The highest average per patient per year cost by country was reported in the USA ($59,900), followed by Sweden ($52,725) and Spain ($41,950). The highest per patient lifetime costs were reported in Australia ($232,100) for all identified definitions of stroke. Some of these data are summarised in Fig. 13.2.

How these are distributed across the globe is illustrated in Fig. 13.3 taken from the paper. No study from Vietnam was included in this report.

It is difficult to draw many conclusions from the data in any of these studies apart from the evident fact that stroke is an expensive disease and that we badly need high quality data covering the whole of the stroke pathway to understand where investment is best made and what returns such investment might have. The paper also makes the case for a more standardised approach to cost studies so that data from different health systems can be usefully compared.

13.4 Costs and Benefits of Implementing the Vietnamese Stroke Quality Standards

Chapter 13 gave details of the development of the Stroke Quality Standards. Funded in part by the Rockefeller Foundation a budget impact analysis was done to determine what resources would be needed to implement the standards and what savings might result from better quality of care [6]. Modelling of the data was done for three hospital types. Type 1 facilities are large centrally or provincially administered hospitals which admit many patients with stroke (more than 1000 patients annually) such as Bach Mai hospital in Hanoi admitting about 5500 stroke patients a year. There are about 30 such hospitals in Vietnam.

Type 2 hospitals have a smaller number of beds and are administered at a Provincial or District level. These hospitals have a lower number of admissions at approximately 100–200 annually. It is estimated that there are approximately 250 of these hospitals in Vietnam.

Type 3 hospitals are typically smaller, usually administered at the district level. They refer a significant number of their patients to type 1 and 2 hospitals for their

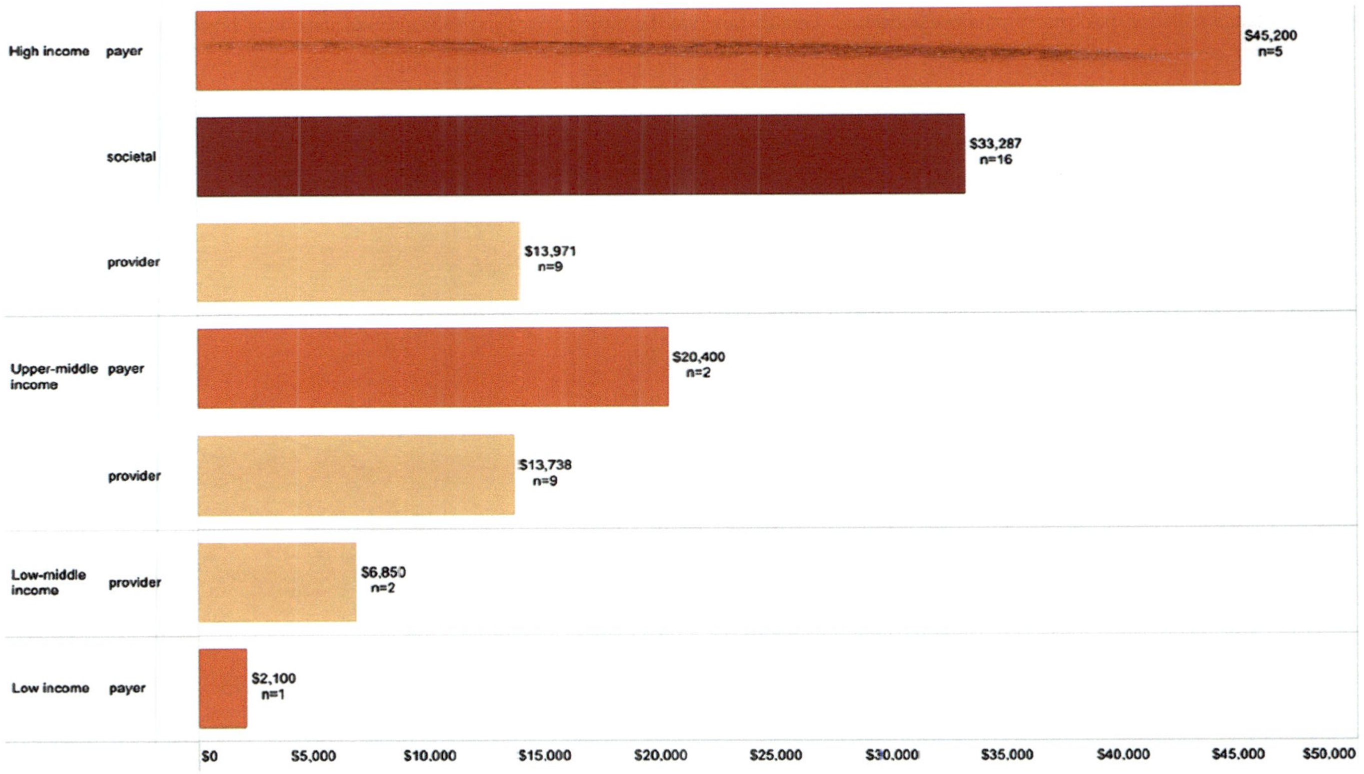

Fig. 13.2 Average per patient per year costs in US dollars by country classification and study perspective. Light orange provider perspective, orange payer perspective, dark orange societal perspective. n = number of studies

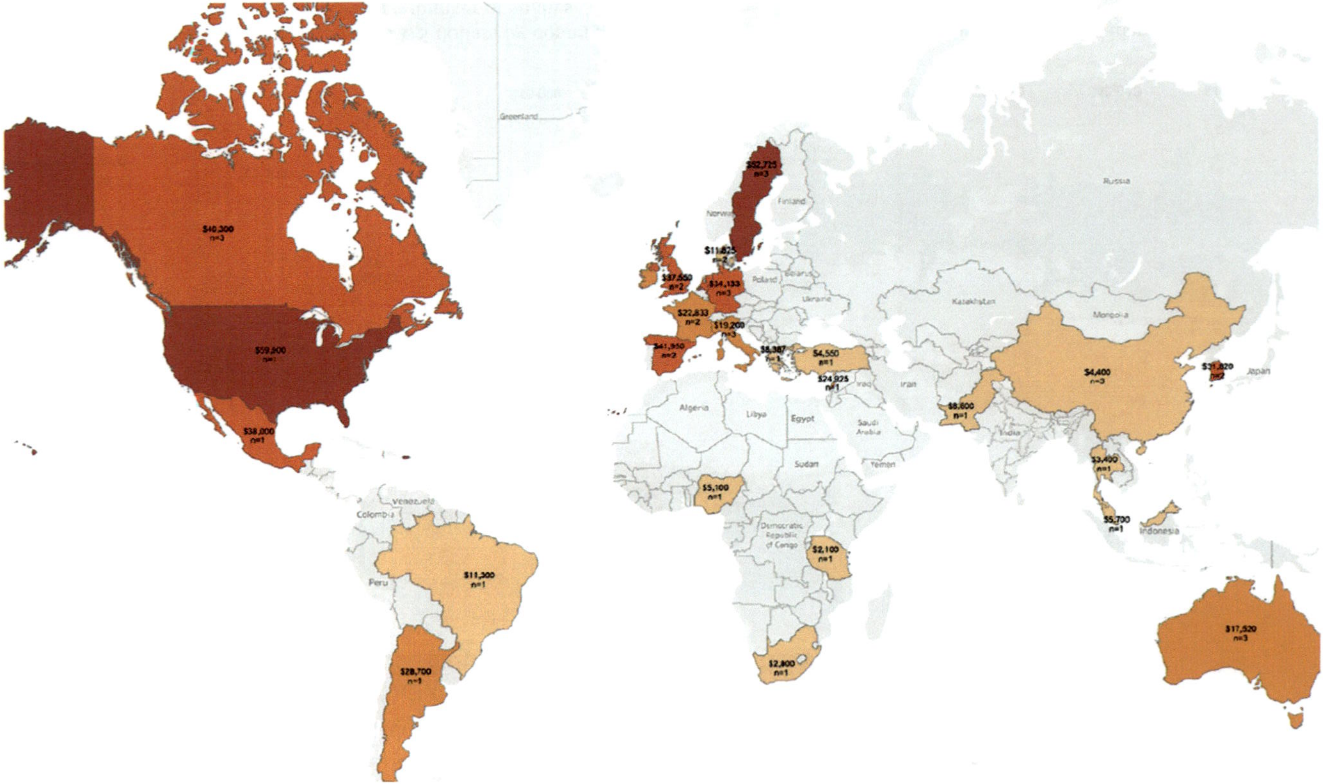

Fig. 13.3 World map reflecting per patient per year costs (USD 2020). Map figures show country averages across studies analysed (colour gradient light = lower values, dark = higher values. *N* = number of studies. OpenStreetMap®

acute care and receive back some patients for further care after the acute phase. The patient case-mix in such facilities is of a lower complexity and in some instances represents referral from Type 1 or 2 hospitals after acute stroke care has been provided. It is estimated that there are approximately 780 Type 3 hospitals in Vietnam.

The data on which the modelling for this paper was based is summarised in Fig. 13.2 and is based on 2010 Global Burden of Disease data.

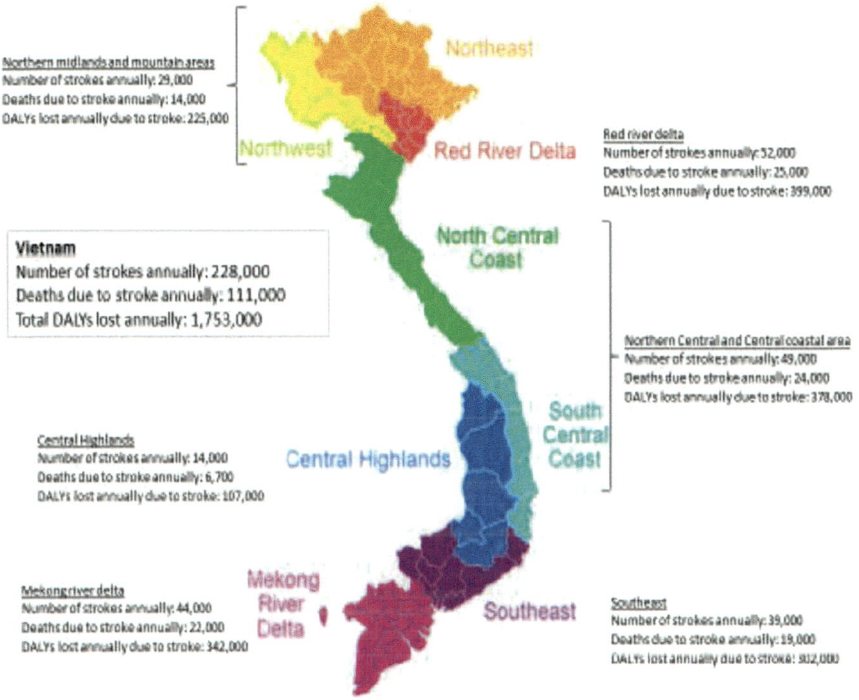

It is estimated that the management of acute stroke in Vietnamese health facilities costs VND 1026 billion (US$48 million). It is assumed that most of the Quality Standards should be implemented in all three hospital levels, apart from the stroke unit standard where level 1 hospitals would be expected to deliver the Gold level standards, level 2, Silver and level 3 Bronze. There are five cost main cost groupings (cost drivers) that result from implementing the QS as a package of care and which are included in this analysis: training, protocol development, administrative support, equipment and medications.

Training costs which are central to the implementation of all the QS are shown in Table 13.1 using Level 1 hospitals as the example.

Table 13.2 summarises the cost drivers to implement all of the five domains and also includes potential cost savings obtained predominantly from reducing the length of hospital stay.

Table 13.1 Training costs in Level 1 Hospitals in Vietnam Type 1 Hospitals n = 30

Training subject area	To whom (staff type)	To meet which QS	Frequency of training/year	Number of staff requiring training/ facility	Annual cost per facility (Dong)	Total cost (all facilities Type 1) (Dong)
Appropriate management of stroke including routine care, maintaining dignity, early mobilisation, swallowing and nutrition, stroke unit	Clinicians, nurses, allied health professionals	QS1; QS4 (gold SU); QS5; QS7; QS8	2	25	11 million	330 million
Diagnostic imaging	Clinicians, radiographers	QS2	2	10	5 million	150 million
Management of TIA	Clinicians, nurses, allied health professionals	QS1; QS3	2	25	11 million	330 million
Thrombolysis	Specialist clinicians	QS6	Specialist training programmes			
Multifacility working and expertise dissemination	Clinicians, nurses, allied health professionals	QS11; QS12	1	25	6 million	180 million
Screening for stroke	Emergency healthcare staff	QS13	2	10	5 million	150 million
Clinical audit (monitoring care)	Clinicians, nurses, allied health professionals, administrative staff	QS15	1	30	7 million	210 million
Protocol implementation	Clinicians, nurses, allied health professionals, administrative staff	All	1	30	7 million	210 million
			Total	40	52 million	1560 million
				Total cost (US$)	2433	72,992

In summary, the implementation of Quality Standards for the hospital management of stroke will require an investment of VND 82.2 billion (US$ 3.8 million) per year at full capacity. It is expected to result in gross savings of VND 117 billion (US$5.five million) (VND 35 billion net) each year across all acute care hospitals in

Table 13.2 Cost drivers for the five groups of Quality Standards

Hospital type	Type 1	Type 2	Type 3	Total
Cost drivers	**In VND (millions) and US$ (millions)**			
Training	1560	6750	11,700	20.010
Us$	*0.07*	*0.32*	*0.55*	*0.94*
Equipment	40	299	461	1163
Us$	*0.02*	*0.01*	*0.02*	*0.05*
Drugs	44,096	4079	1989	50,163
Us$	*2.06*	*0.19*	*0.09*	*2.35*
Protocol development	570	3500	3900	7970
Us$	*0.03*	*0.16*	*0.18*	*0.37*
Administrative support	1185	988	770	2943
Us$	*0.06*	*0.05*	*0.04*	*0.14*
Total costs	**47,814**	**15,615**	**18,820**	**82,249**
Us$	*2.24*	*0.73*	*0.88*	*3.85*
Savings				
LOS reduction	71,339	38,688	7228	117,256
Us$	*3.34*	*1.81*	*0.34*	*5.49*
Estimated annual net impact	**23,524**	**23,073**	**−11,591**	**35,006**
Us$	*1.10*	*1.08*	*−0.54*	*1.64*

Vietnam through a reduction in hospital length of stay. The largest net savings (VND23.5 billion, US$1.1 million) are expected in high-concentration hospitals (high number of stroke admissions per facility) which account for an estimated 48% of admissions. Implementing the Quality Standards in low-concentration hospitals is estimated to result in a net cost of VND11.6 billion (US$0.54million) as expected reductions in length of stay at these facilities may not offset implementation costs, however, savings from improved care and referral processes at low-concentration hospitals may be realised in better outcomes and further savings in high-concentration hospitals.

A significant proportion of expenditure associated with the implementation of the Quality Standards is increased use of medications for thrombolysis (alteplase). Meeting the thrombolysis quality standard is expected to increase the access of this drug to 3300 additional patients annually at a cost of VND 38.5 billion (US$1.8 million). The modelling does not take into account longer term costs such as the need for longer term rehabilitation and loss of earning and contribution of taxes from both the patient and potentially carers. Overall savings may well therefore be quite substantial by improving the quality of care.

This study reported before the evidence emerged for the benefits of endovascular thrombectomy (EVT). While a fairly small proportion of patients, less than 10%, will receive EVT even when it is made available to all appropriate patients in Vietnam and maybe 3–5% of patients benefitting from it the overall impact is likely to be important for those patients but relatively small at a population level.

13.5 Summary

There are limited data globally on the true costs of stroke from primary prevention through to longer term social costs and there are even fewer data from low- and middle-income countries including Vietnam. Using what data are available, mainly from modelling studies it does seem likely that costs are extremely high and that significant savings could be made by nations willing to invest in population based prevention programmes and high quality acute and rehabilitation care. It is very encouraging that Vietnam has made such good progress implementing their Quality Standards. This should result not just in benefits for the patients but also the state from a reduction in health care expenditure.

References

1. Gerstl JVE, Blitz SE, Qu QR, Yearley AG, Lassarén P, Lindberg R, Gupta S, Kappel AD, Vicenty-Padilla JC, Gaude E, Atchaneeyasakul KC, Desai SM, Yavagal DR, Peruzzotti-Jametti L, Patel NJ, Aziz-Sultan MA, Du R, Smith TR, Bernstock JD. Global, regional, and National Economic Consequences of Stroke. Stroke. 2023;54(9):2380–9. https://doi.org/10.1161/STROKEAHA.123.043131. Epub 2023 Jul 27. PMID: 37497672; PMCID: PMC7614992.
2. GBD 2019 Stroke Collaborators. Global, regional, and national burden of stroke and its risk factors, 1990–2019: a systematic analysis for the Global Burden of Disease Study 2019. Lancet Neurol. 2021;20(10):795–820. https://doi.org/10.1016/S1474-4422(21)00252-0. Epub 2021 Sep 3. PMID: 34487721; PMCID: PMC8443449.
3. Kaur P, Kwatra G, Kaur R, Pandian JD. Cost of stroke in low and middle income countries: a systematic review. Int J Stroke. 2014;9(6):678–82. https://doi.org/10.1111/ijs.12322. Epub 2014 Jul 7.
4. Lucas-Noll J, Clua-Espuny JL, Lleixà-Fortuño M, Gavaldà-Espelta E, Queralt-Tomas L, Panisello-Tafalla A, Carles-Lavila M. The costs associated with stroke care continuum: a systematic review. Health Econ Rev. 2023;13(1):32. https://doi.org/10.1186/s13561-023-00439-6. PMID: 37193926; PMCID: PMC10190015.
5. Strilciuc S, Grad DA, Radu C, Chira D, Stan A, Ungureanu M, Gheorghe A, Muresanu FD. The economic burden of stroke: a systematic review of cost of illness studies. J Med Life. 2021;14(5):606–19. https://doi.org/10.25122/jml-2021-0361. PMID: 35027963; PMCID: PMC8742896.
6. Wilkinson T. Quality standards for the Hospital Management of Stroke in Vietnam: budget impact analysis [version 1; not peer reviewed]. F1000 Res. 2019;8:825. https://doi.org/10.7490/f1000research.1116853.1.

Chapter 14
Training in Stroke for Doctors, Nurses and Therapists

Ngoc Huy Nguyen, Thanh Ngoc Le, and Thong Van Nguyen

14.1 Introduction

This chapter describes the skills required for clinicians involved in stroke care. Some of the documents have been prepared specifically for use in Vietnam and other material has been used from international sources. But there should not be much difference. Care given to stroke patients at all points along their pathway should be based on good general principles taught to doctors, nurses and therapists throughout their training augmented by a good understanding of the specific needs of the patient with stroke. Stroke however, rarely occurs in patients without any other medical, psychological or social problems. It is a disease that becomes much more prevalent with increasing age and is usually associated with multiple comorbidities. Once a patient has had a stroke, they are then at increased risk of many other medical problems including chest and urinary infections, venous thromboembolism, pressure sores, depression, dementia, malnutrition, dehydration and many more. Therefore, the clinicians caring for patients with stroke need to be excellent generalists as well as specialists.

What matters is whether the clinician has the knowledge and skills to do the job. It is not simply a question of how long a doctor, nurse or therapist has worked with stroke patients or how long they have studied. Nor is it appropriate to be rigid in terms

N. H. Nguyen (✉)
Phutho Department of Health, Phutho, Vietnam

VNU University of Medicine and Pharmacy, Hanoi, Vietnam
e-mail: ngochuynguyen8888@gmail.com

T. N. Le
VNU University of Medicine and Pharmacy, Hanoi, Vietnam

T. Van Nguyen
Vietnam Stroke Association, Hanoi, Vietnam

Stroke Center, Phutho General Hospital, Phutho, Vietnam

A. Rudd et al. (eds.), *Stroke Management in Vietnam*,
https://doi.org/10.1007/978-981-96-0221-6_14

of which profession takes responsibility for any particular clinical activity or leadership role. There are several examples in the UK, for example, of a nurse leading the whole stroke team. There are also examples where nurses have been trained to prescribe a defined list of drugs and to manage post-stroke issues and to therefore be able to run stroke follow-up clinics. In some hospitals, the stroke specialist nurse runs the intravenous thrombolysis pathway in the hospital emergency department. There are therapists who run rehabilitation units. The traditional model where a senior doctor oversees the whole team is not the only way to deliver effective clinical care.

So, the curriculum needs to be flexible to adapt to the needs of the person training and performance needs to be assessed for both theoretical knowledge as well as practical and social skills.

Training in stroke is not a once and for all exercise. All clinicians need to continue to learn throughout their career through continuing professional education. The quantity and quality of this training needs to be monitored and systems in place to regularly re-evaluate a person's fitness to practice. Many countries have now developed systems for revalidation of clinicians. In the UK, doctors need to go through a process of revalidation every 5 years and this is now being extended to other professional groups as well. For people who practice extremely complex practical procedures such as endovascular thrombectomy for stroke, there is also a requirement to demonstrate that they are performing at least a minimum number of treatments each year.

Conducting continuous audit for a clinical team is an essential way of ensuring that the skills of the team are being maintained and provides early warning of problems. This must always be augmented by having in place robust systems that enable patients and their relatives as well as clinical colleagues to highlight clinical failings, to investigate them and then to take appropriate action. This should be done in a way that does not, in any way, penalise the person making the complaint.

14.2 Medical Training

There are big variations between countries in the systems in place to train in stroke medicine. In Vietnam most if not all physicians managing stroke patients will have initially trained in neurology and this is also the case in many other countries including some European countries and the USA. In the UK doctors wanting to train in stroke can first train in geriatric medicine, rehabilitation medicine, general medicine or neurology. They then need to do a further year of specialist training in an accredited stroke service. Whatever the route a country chooses it is important to recognise that stroke medicine covers a wide range of issues. A doctor aiming to manage patients across the pathway needs to understand stroke prevention, acute stroke diagnosis and management, general medicine as related to stroke, rehabilitation and some elements of psychiatry and end of life care. Some countries divide up the patient pathway and have different specialties managing the acute, rehabilitation and prevention. That is acceptable but, in our view, does result in some loss of continuity of care as well as failing to recognise that each of these stages of care overlap considerably. Rehabilitation needs to start at the moment of admission. Acute stroke

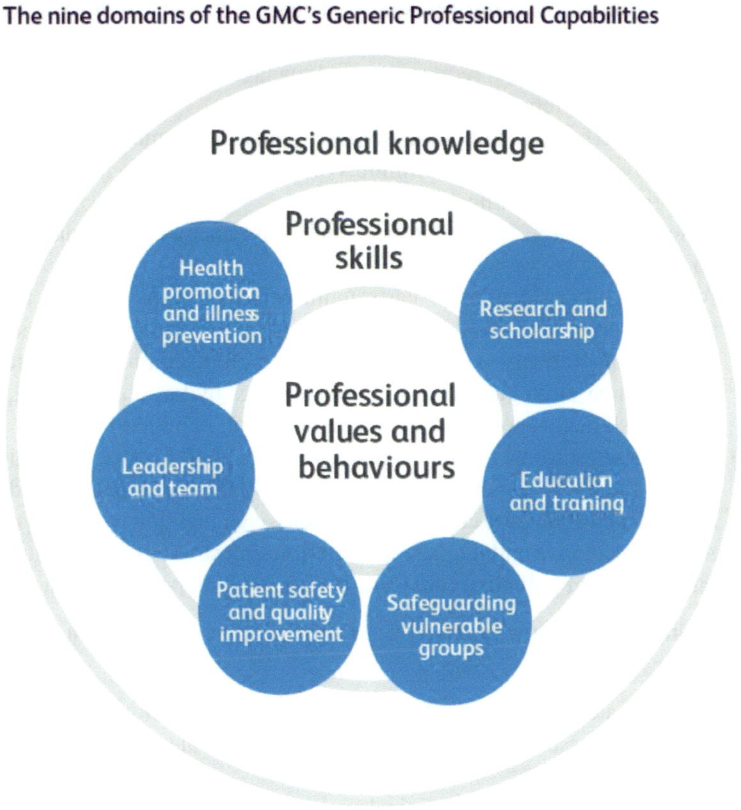

Fig. 14.1 UK Stroke training Curriculum

issues can occur weeks or months after the first acute event at a time when the patient is supposed to be in the rehabilitation phase and prevention of course is a lifelong issue for the patient. The curriculum below (Fig. 14.1) is one developed by the training authorities in the UK for stroke physicians. It is comprehensive but will need adapting to fit the Vietnamese health system [1].

14.3 Core Skills that all Doctors Should Have

14.3.1 Specialist Stroke Skills

1. **Managing the care of acute stroke patients, including hyperacute care and cerebral reperfusion strategies.**
   (a) Able to conduct an up-to-date hyperacute stroke clinical assessment efficiently (including face to face and virtually [e.g., telemedicine]) with appro-

priate use of imaging to safely deliver treatment including cerebral reperfusion strategies where indicated.
(b) Able to demonstrate a recognition and management of complications relating to cerebral reperfusion strategies.
(c) Able to perform a comprehensive, specialist assessment, investigate and treat patients with stroke or mimic syndromes relevant to the patient's age, comorbidities and clinical presentation.
(d) Able to manage comorbidities and risk factors relevant to stroke appropriately.
(e) Able to apply principles of early multi-professional assessment to understand the physical, psychological and social impact of stroke on patients and work collaboratively with the stroke unit multidisciplinary team to guide management strategies including positioning, hydration, nutrition, continence, risk factor modification and participation in rehabilitation.
(f) Able to use up-to-date knowledge of evidence, guidelines, appropriate monitoring and measurement scales (including NIHSS and mRS) to guide management and anticipate early complications, e.g., malignant MCA syndrome.
(g) Able to recognise and manage the deteriorating stroke patient including the introduction of palliative care (e.g., communicating prognostic uncertainty).

2. **Managing the primary and secondary prevention of stroke and Transient Ischaemic Attack.**

   (a) Demonstrates knowledge of the different pathophysiological mechanisms, disease processes and causes that underlie the clinical syndrome of stroke (and its subtypes).
   (b) Able to conduct an urgent clinical evaluation and prioritise safely: initiating appropriate investigations in a timely manner, interpreting the results and communicating the management plan effectively (including face to face and virtually [e.g., telemedicine]).
   (c) Able to provide an accurate diagnosis and appropriate comprehensive management of patients with suspected TIA or stroke including identification of vascular risk factors and lifestyle modification.
   (d) Able to identify conditions that mimic TIA and stroke and manage these effectively or make an appropriate referral.
   (e) Able to manage comorbidities and risk factors relevant to TIA and stroke in an outpatient clinic (including tolerating uncertainty where investigation or intervention may not have high utility or benefit).
   (f) Awareness of up-to-date primary and secondary prevention treatment strategies for TIA and stroke (including knowledge and application of national guidance).

(g) Able to prioritise referrals received through different mechanisms (e.g., electronic, telephone, in person) and by all healthcare professionals.
(h) Able to provide appropriate driving, vocational and social advice for patients with TIA or stroke working in partnership where necessary with the stroke multidisciplinary team.

3. **Managing early and late stroke rehabilitation in hospital and community settings.**

(a) Understands the anatomy and pathophysiology of stroke with regard to patterns of recovery relevant to stroke subtypes and other factors to guide planning and expectations for an individual's recovery.
(b) Demonstrates an understanding of the diverse factors that can influence outcome including problems often associated with non- dominant hemisphere stroke (e.g., higher mental function), neuropsychiatric consequences, post-stroke pain and spasticity.
(c) Appropriately manages common post-stroke complications (seizures, thromboembolism, dysphagia, dehydration, shoulder girdle dysfunction, spasticity) and takes into account how these may affect participation in rehabilitation.
(d) Ensures rehabilitation is individualised, patient focused and recognises how the consequences of stroke disability can impact on participation in rehabilitation.
(e) Co-ordinates the multidisciplinary team to optimise post-stroke recovery, participation in goal setting, measurement of rehabilitation outcome and participation in national audit.
(f) Demonstrates good communication and understanding with patients and families and identifies carer's long-term needs and participation in goal planning.
(g) Demonstrates an understanding of medico-legal issues relating to clinically assisted nutrition and hydration in patients both with and without capacity.
(h) Contributes to and leads effective discharge planning to support transition to the community and facilitate life after stroke, including engaging with social services that may help optimise on-going recovery and/or provide support including impact on function, vocation and driving.
(i) Understands the impact of ethnicity and socioeconomic patient backgrounds on stroke severity, prognosis and rehabilitation outcomes.

Able to recognise and manage the deteriorating stroke patient including the introduction of palliative care (e.g. communicating prognostic uncertainty).

14.4 Summary of the Range of Presentations and Conditions that a Stroke Physician Should Have Experience and Expertise

Clinical area	Presentations	Conditions/issues
Acute stroke or mimic	Weakness, unilateral or bilateral Inattention Dysarthria Dysphasia Dysphagia Vertigo Unsteadiness Monocular visual loss Visual field impairment Altered sensation Sudden loss consciousness	Acute cerebral infarction Acute intracerebral haemorrhage TIA Cerebral amyloidosis Transient amnesias Acute seizure Cerebral venous thrombosis Migraine Syncope Subdural haemorrhage Subarachnoid haemorrhage Amaurosis fugax Space occupying lesion Bell's palsy Functional neurological disorder Facial mononeuropathy Peripheral neuropathy Vestibular disorders Systemic/metabolic disorders
Primary or secondary prevention of stroke, transient Ischaemic attack or mimic	Weakness, unilateral or bilateral Inattention Dysarthria Dysphasia Dysphagia Vertigo Unsteadiness Visual loss Altered sensation Cognitive decline	Acute cerebral infarction Acute intracerebral haemorrhage TIA Cerebral amyloidosis Transient amnesias Acute seizure Cerebral venous thrombosis Migraine Syncope Subdural haemorrhage Subarachnoid haemorrhage Amaurosis fugax Space occupying lesion Bell's palsy Atrial fibrillation Cervical arterial disease Cardiac disease Vascular cognitive impairment

Clinical area	Presentations	Conditions/issues
Medical care and rehabilitation following stroke	Incontinence of urine Incontinence of Faeces Oral feeding failure Immobility, including problems with standing and transfers Communication problems Disorders of conduct and behaviour Spasticity Pain Seizures Disorders of mood Musculoskeletal complications of neurological disease Visual loss Disorders of perception and visuospatial neglect Abnormal sensation Disorders of cognition Fatigue Complications of immobility	Cerebral infarction Intracerebral haemorrhage Pneumonia Incontinence Post-stroke pain Post-stroke depression Post-stroke epilepsy Vascular cognitive impairment Venous thromboembolic disease Upper motor neurone syndrome
	Disorders of perception and visuospatial neglect abnormal sensation disorders of cognition fatigue Complications of Immobility	

14.4.1 Recommended Training

- Training in acute reperfusion therapy.
- Use of scales and other tools for the assessment of stroke patients.
  - National Institutes of Health Stroke Scale NIHSS.
  - ASPECTS.
  - BARTHEL.
  - Modified Rankin Scale mRS.
  - Course in Stroke reperfusion therapy.
- Training in neurovascular brain imaging, e.g., CT, MRI and angiography techniques.
- Spasticity and Botulinum toxin injection treatment.

14.4.2 Palliative and End of Life Care

Palliative and end of life care is a core component of the Internal Medicine (IM) curriculum and trainees will continue to develop their knowledge and skills throughout specialty training. Palliative and end of life care is one of the eight clinical capabilities in practice.

Palliative care is very pertinent to stroke and experience of end of life care can be achieved during attachments to the stroke service.

14.5 Training to Perform Endovascular Thrombectomy (EVT) for Ischaemic Stroke

EVT as a proven therapy for stroke emerged suddenly on the scene in 2015. It is a technique that requires highly specialist skills previously confined to interventional neuroradiologists whose main workload was management of aneurysms after subarachnoid haemorrhage and arteriovenous malformations. The numbers of these cases is relatively small and the work mainly done as cold cases during usual working hours. Suddenly the need for these skills increased dramatically and needed to be done very rapidly regardless of day of week or time of day. Because the benefits of EVT are so dramatic, there was an imperative to provide the service as quickly as possible and this led, in some places, to clinicians without the training and skills to start performing the procedure, potentially doing more harm than good. An international group published a consensus statement on the training needs for anyone who is providing EVT. It recognises that countries will differ in their training systems and requirements but our view is that the general principle that anyone treating patients should be properly trained in what they are doing is irrefutable. The following information is extracted from the consensus statement [2].

14.6 Baseline Training and Qualifications

1. **Residency training in radiology, neurology or neurosurgery** which should include documented training in the diagnosis and management of acute stroke, the interpretation of cerebral arteriography and neuroimaging. The residency programme and supervising physicians should be accredited according to national standards as they pertain to the countries involved. Those physicians who did not have adequate such training during their residencies must spend an additional period (typically one year) by training in clinical neurosciences and neuroimaging.
2. **Dedicated training in Interventional Neuroradiology** under the direction of a neuro-interventionist, at a high-volume centre. A training programme accredited by a national accrediting body is strongly preferred but not required. Within these programmes, specific training for intraarterial therapy for acute ischemic stroke should

be performed, including obtaining appropriate access even in challenging anatomy, microcatheter navigation in the cerebral circulation, knowledge, and training of the use of stroke specific devices and complication avoidance and management.
3. **Maintenance of physician qualifications:** It is vital that the physician has ongoing stroke-specific continuing medical education. A minimum of 16 h of stroke specific education every 2 years is suggested. Individual physician outcomes should conform to national standards and institutional requirements. In addition, the physician should participate in an ongoing quality assurance and improvement programme. The quality assurance programme must review all emergency interventional stroke therapy patients. While threshold levels for recanalization, complication rates, etc. have yet to be established, we suggest the following as a minimum: 1. Successful recanalization (modified TICI 2b or 3) in at least 60% of cases. 2. Embolization to new territory of less than 15%. 3. Symptomatic intracranial haemorrhage (i.e., parenchymal hematoma on imaging with clinical deterioration) rate less than 10%.

This statement is not specific as to the number of procedures an individual clinician should undertake each year to maintain their skills. In the UK this has been set at 40 procedures per year which do not necessarily need to be EVT for stroke but could include catheterisation of intracranial vessels for any reason [3].

What none of the articles that we have seen mention, but we consider to be important is that the personality of the person doing the procedure is right for extremely high pressure and high risk situations. It needs to be someone who can remain calm when things go wrong.

14.7 Nurse Training

Based on the UK Stroke Nurse training programme [4], the following list of stroke nurse competencies was developed for used by nurses in Vietnam. They cover both the knowledge required as well as the clinical skills. They were designed to be taught to qualified general nurses while they are working in a stroke service and to be evaluated in several stages over a period of months or even years. They do not include the very specific skills needed by a nurse in the vascular suite for patients who are undergoing endovascular thrombectomy.

14.7.1 Vietnam Stroke Nursing Competencies

1. Neurological care	
Able to describe the anatomy of brain including the function of lobes of the brain	Able to name lobes and areas of the brain Able to describe areas responsible for motor, sensory, language, coordination, vision and higher cognitive functions

1. Neurological care	
Able to describe the blood supply to and within the brain	Able to name the blood vessels supplying the brain Able to name the blood vessels within the brain
Able to describe the different types of stroke and the risk factors for each	Able to name the two main types of stroke and the risk factors for each
Able to describe the causes and signs of neurological deterioration in stroke patients	Able to name likely causes for and signs of deterioration including neurological, cardiovascular, infective and respiratory causes
Able to complete a neurological assessment in a stroke patient	Able to assess tone, motor and sensory function and coordination of a patient Able to identify stroke related deficits and relate these to function
Able to identify changes in a patients' neurological function	Able to specify alterations in function based on previous assessments
Able to assess and plan nursing care for a patient who is: – unconscious – having seizures	Able to plan nursing care to ensure the following areas are attended to: Complication prevention, safety, medical treatment, privacy and dignity
2. Thrombolysis	
Able to describe the indications for thrombolysis in stroke	Able to describe the indications for thrombolysis including type of stroke, previous medical history, time from onset and medication history
Able to describe the action and drugs used for thrombolysis in stroke	Able to describe how thrombolysis drugs work in stroke Able to name commonly used thrombolysis drugs
Able to describe the possible complications of thrombolysis	Able to name common thrombolysis complications Able to describe the signs of thrombolysis complications
Able to safely administer thrombolysis treatment	Able to describe the preparation and dose calculation of thrombolysis treatment
Able to monitor the patient following thrombolysis	Able to describe the patient monitoring required after thrombolysis including blood pressure monitoring, neurological monitoring and monitoring for signs of complications
Able to identify changes in patient's neurological function as a result of thrombolysis and inform doctors	Able to specify alterations in function based on previous assessments
3. Respiratory	
Able to describe common respiratory complications of stroke	Able to name common respiratory complications including neurological, infective and cardiovascular causes
Able to describe the importance of positioning on the respiratory system	Able to describe the benefits of changing position, upright positioning and mobilisation
Able to describe the indications for oxygen therapy for stroke patients	Able to describe the rationale for providing oxygen therapy
Able to assess respiratory function	Able to complete assessment of airway, respiratory rate, depth, regularity and comment on any additional features such as wheeze

1. Neurological care	
Able to demonstrate optimal upright positioning to aid lung expansion	Able to appropriately position stroke patient in an upright position
4. Cardiovascular	
Able to describe common cardiac conditions in stroke	Able to name common cardiac conditions including the effects of these on the patient's blood pressure, pulse and respiratory rate
Able to describe the relevance of atrial fibrillation in stroke	Able to describe mechanism of atrial fibrillation as a risk factor for stroke
Able to describe the importance of blood pressure management in stroke	Able to describe the rationale for active blood pressure lowering in stroke Able to list commonly used anti-hypertensive agents
Able to assess cardiac function	Able to complete assessment of cardiac function including BP, pulse and ECG
5. Post-stroke complications	
Able to name common post-stroke complications	Able to name common complications including: Cardiovascular, peripheral, renal, infective, metabollic
Able to describe nursing care to prevent post-stroke complications including: Blood sugar control, hydration, prevention and management of infection, positioning	Able to describe the nursing care involved to prevent post-stroke complications
Able to describe why urinary catheters should be avoided in stroke patients	Able to rationalise the potential complications from urinary catheters in stroke patients including effects on continence, infection risk and positioning
Able to describe the causes of pressure areas in stroke patients	Able to list reasons why stroke patients are at risk of pressure area breakdown
Able to describe the importance of early mobilisation and independence post-stroke	Able to list the reasons why early mobilisation and independence is important after stroke Able to explain potential complications of immobility
Able to complete a pressure area risk assessment tool	Able to complete assessment of pressure sore risk for a stroke patient
Able to implement nursing care to reduce the risk of pressure are breakdown	Able to use available equipment and positioning to minimise the risk of pressure area breakdown
Able to demonstrate good positioning of a stroke patient: In bed and in a chair	Able to provide appropriate support for the patient to achieve good positioning including care of the hemiplegic arm and leg
Able to initiate nursing care and treatment to prevent dehydration and poor nutrition	Able to initiate fluid monitoring taking account of patient's conscious level and swallowing ability Able to demonstrate maintenance of accurate fluid and food intake monitoring to prevent dehydration and poor nutrition
6. Swallow and nutrition	
Able to describe why swallowing problems occur after stroke	Able to describe the four stages of a normal swallow and the potential impact of stroke on each of these stages

1. Neurological care	
Able to describe the potential impact of poor swallowing after stroke	Able to describe the impact of poor swallow on the respiratory system
Able to describe the rationale and stages of a formal swallowing assessment	Able to describe the use of a swallow screening tool Able to describe situations where a swallow screen is not indicated
Able to describe the reasons that stroke patients can become malnourished	Able to describe common causes of malnutrition post-stroke
Able to complete a swallow screening tool for a stroke patient	Able to assess a patient's ability to safely swallow according to the tool Able to identify reasons to stop the assessment
Able to initiate alternative feeding strategies including modified food and nasogastric tube feeding as indicated by the swallow screening tool	Able to rationalise the indications for: Modified food and fluids Nasogastric feeding Able to monitor the safety of modified food and fluids
7. Communication	
Able to describe common communication problems post-stroke	Able to name common communication difficulties including receptive dysphasia, expressive dysphasia and dysarthria
Able to describe the areas of the brain responsible for communication	Able to describe the areas of the brain responsible for the understanding and expression of language
Able to describe strategies which can help communication with patients who have receptive and expressive dysphasia	Able to describe the use of verbal and non-verbal strategies to improve communication
Able to assess a patient's communication abilities using verbal and non-verbal strategies	Able to assess a patient's ability to follow verbal and non-verbal instructions Able to assess a patient's ability to verbalise including naming objects or speaking in sentences
8. Secondary prevention	
Able to describe modifiable and non-modifiable risk factors for stroke	Able to describe modifiable and non-modifiable risk factors including: Medical history, medication, lifestyle
Able to describe common medications used for secondary prevention of stroke	Able to name medication used for: Antiplatelet treatment, anticoagulation, cholesterol reduction, blood pressure management
Able to describe lifestyle changes which may reduce the risk of stroke	Able to describe suggested lifestyle changes for patients including smoking, diet, exercise, alcohol
Clinical skills	
Able to discuss lifestyle changes and medication for secondary prevention of stroke with a patient or carer	Able to provide lifestyle and medication advice and recommendations to patients and their carers
9. Basic rehabilitation	

1. Neurological care	
Able to describe the importance of rehabilitation in stroke care	Able to describe the benefits of rehabilitation on stroke recovery Able to describe the complications of lack of rehabilitation on stroke recovery
Able to describe the basic principles of neuroplasticity	Able to describe the creation of new neural pathways in the brain
Able to discuss the impact of encouraging patient independence on rehabilitation	Able to describe the importance of encouraging patients to regain independent function on their stroke recovery Able to discuss the role of the family in encouraging independence
10. Team working	
Able to describe the role of different team members including doctor, nurse, physiotherapist, rehabilitation assistant	Able to describe the role and function of different team members to patients and carers Able to describe how the role of each team member impacts stroke recovery
Able to identify appropriate short term goals for a stroke patient	Able to appropriately identify 3 short term goals for a stroke patient. These goals will be specific, measurable, achievable, realistic and have a specified time for achievement
Able to discuss the impact of a multidisciplinary team meeting on ensuring effective stroke care	Able to describe the role of a multidisciplinary meeting on a stroke unit Able to present a patient to a multidisciplinary team and discuss their goals

This is a very long list of knowledge and skills but then stroke nursing is a particularly complex specialty within nursing. As with medical training, the nurse needs to be expert at both the management of intensive care situations with an extremely sick physiologically unstable patient as well as being able to manage the frequent psychological and physical problems that occur after stroke and be able to understand and advise patients on stroke prevention. Surely on the most challenging roles in nursing!

14.8 Therapist Training

A programme run by Professor Morgan Head of the Department of Physiotherapy from Monash University and Lê Thanh Vân, Head of the physiotherapy course at Ho Chi Minh University and vice president of the Vietnam Physical Therapy Association (VNPTA) have been running a 5 year programme to achieve the following objectives [5]:

- Development of a new **national physiotherapy curriculum** that is evidence-based and outcomes-focused, and aligned with international expectations of physiotherapy practice.

- Provision of **continuous professional development** to physiotherapy academics and clinicians to upskill in clinical reasoning and clinical decision-making skills.
- Development of a **national standard in physiotherapy** for endorsement by the professional body and government.
- Facilitation of a **national physiotherapy association in Vietnam** to develop physical therapy standards and provide support to achieve greater recognition of the scope of practice of the physical therapy profession.

A systematic assessment of rehabilitation in Viet Nam released by the Vietnam Ministry of health in 2020 [6] found that most health facilities were equipped to provide rehabilitation services: the proportion ranged from 75% at the district level to 100% at the central level However, only 7200 individuals had a pre-service training qualification in rehabilitation; the majority were physiotherapists with 2-year diploma certificates. Other qualified professionals included prosthetists, orthotists, speech language therapists and occupational therapists. In addition, a range of other health workers had undertaken short orientation courses in rehabilitation of 3–12 months' duration. For a population of about 100 million people, this is clearly insufficient to be able to provide comprehensive stroke rehabilitation services across the country in addition to all the other conditions that also require the skills provided by rehabilitation staff.

A 2017 report from the World Health Organization, entitled Rehabilitation 2030 [7]was a call for action to build an adequate, well-trained and multi-occupation rehabilitation workforce worldwide, so as to strengthen rehabilitation in health systems. Figure 14.2 summarises the key elements within the document.

The final version of the Vietnamese curriculum is as far as we know not yet available but will be an important document that will hopefully guide the way towards developing a workforce that is able to provide comprehensive specialist rehabilitation for all stroke patients that require it in the country.

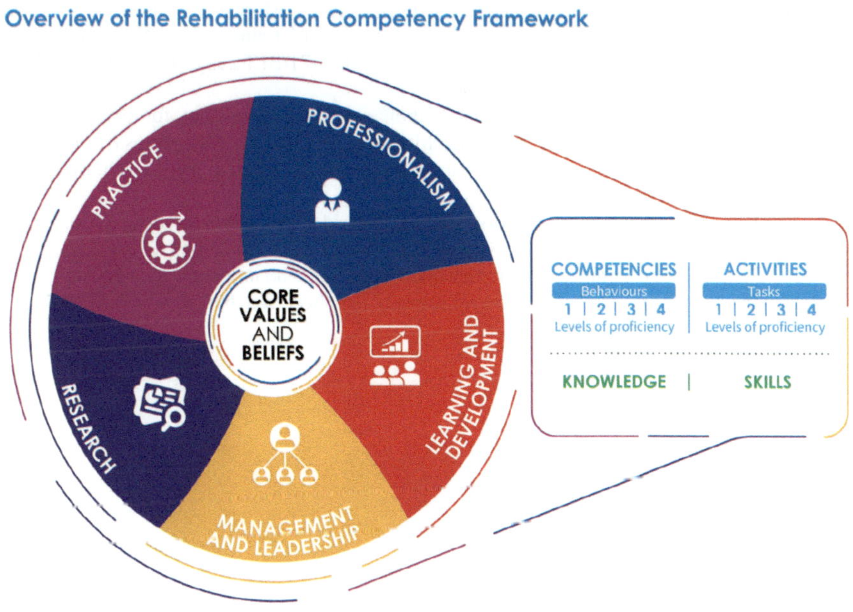

Fig. 14.2 WHO Rehabilitation Competency Framework [8]

14.9 Summary

Effective stroke treatment both in the acute phase as well as in longer term management and rehabilitation requires effective teamwork with the team comprised of well-trained specialists in a range of different fields able to combine their knowledge to provide high quality personalised care for their patients. This chapter summarises some of those skills but it does not cover important issues such as how teams work effectively, team leadership and it also has not addressed the need for a range of important professional groups. These include speech and language therapy, occupational therapy, psychology, dietetics, social work, orthoptists, orthotics, foot health and pharmacists as well as several others.

References

1. UK Joint Colleges Training Board Stroke Curriculum. https://www.gmc-uk.org/-/media/documents/stroke-medicine-2022-subspecialty-curriculum-final_pdf-92054187.pdf.
2. Lavine SD, Cockroft K, Hoh B, et al. Training guidelines for endovascular stroke intervention: an international multi-society consensus document. Neuroradiology. 2016;58(6):537–41.
3. EVT Credential. Royal College of Radiologists UK. https://www.gmc-uk.org/-/media/documents/credential-in-mt-for-acute-ischaemic-stroke%2D%2D-curriculum-final-(1).pdf.
4. London Stroke Nurse Competency Workbook. https://www.england.nhs.uk/london/wp-content/uploads/sites/8/2019/09/london-stroke-nurse-competency-workbook.pdf.

5. Demey D, Dieye SO, Feipel V, Holey LA, Kruger J, Le VT, Morgan P, Skinner MA, Willems P. International collaboration to improve physiotherapists' training, Viet Nam. Bull World Health Organ. 2022;100(11):733–8. https://doi.org/10.2471/BLT.22.288100. Epub 2022 Sep 2. PMID: 36324559; PMCID: PMC9589383.
6. Approving the national plan for rehabilitation service development for the 2014–2020 period. 4039/QD-BYT. Hanoi: Vietnam Ministry of Health; 2014. https://vanbanphap-luat.co/decision–4039-qd-byt–2014-approving-the-national-plan-for-rehabilitation-service -development.
7. Rehabilitation competency framework. Geneva: World Health Organization; 2020. https://www.who.int/publications/i/item/ 9789240008281 [cited 2022 Jan 25].
8. WHO Rehabilitation Competency Framework. https://cdn.who.int/media/docs/default-source/documents/health-topics/rehabilitation/rcf-information-sheet_web.pdf?sfvrsn=6e4528b9_5.

Chapter 15
Stroke Units in Vietnam. The Evidence Base and Key Components

Ton Duy Mai, Tuan Tran Van, and Son Dinh Thanh Le

15.1 Introduction

Until about 35 years ago, the prevailing view among the public and clinicians was that stroke was a condition for which very little could be done. Some patients would spontaneously improve but that was nature healing rather than anything that the medical profession was able to offer. Hippocrates wrote around 400 years BC that '*Persons are most subject to apoplexy between the ages of forty and sixty and it is impossible to remove a strong attack of apoplexy, and not easy to remove a weak attack*'. Apoplexy was the term used up until about 100 years ago for what we now call stroke.

The famous British neurologist, William Osler, wrote at the end of the nineteenth century '*it is the duty of the physician to explain to the patient, or to his friends, that the condition is past relief, that medicines and electricity will do no good, and that there is no possible hope of cure*'. And that view prevailed right up until fairly recently and certainly within the professional lifetime of one of the authors of this chapter.

The single piece of research that transformed these views was the meta-analysis of the trials of stroke unit care published in 1993 by Langhorne et al. [1]. The first small

T. D. Mai (✉)
VNU University of Medicine and Pharmacy, Hanoi, Vietnam

Stroke Center, Bach Mai Hospital, Hanoi, Vietnam

Hanoi Medical University, Hanoi, Vietnam
e-mail: tonresident@gmail.com

T. T. Van
Thai Nguyen University of Medicine and Pharmacy, Thai Nguyen, Vietnam

S. D. T. Le
Phutho General Hospital, Phutho, Vietnam

A. Rudd et al. (eds.), *Stroke Management in Vietnam*,
https://doi.org/10.1007/978-981-96-0221-6_15

trials of stroke units were published in the 1960s but each trial was small and failed to produce results that were persuasive that stroke unit care was better than conventional care. The first large trial with over 300 patients included came from Norway and was published in 1991 showing benefit for the specialist care [2]. Conventional care varied hugely between hospitals and between countries. In many places, stroke patients were managed by general physicians or physicians specialising in the care of older people. In others, the care was provided by general neurologists. In all cases, very little other than basic medical and nursing care was provided in the acute phase. Sometimes people were transferred after the first few weeks to the care of rehabilitation specialists or geriatricians where there was the tradition of multidisciplinary care, but such care was far from universal and the evidence to support it was scanty.

The stroke unit meta-analysis showed that stroke unit care saved lives [3]. There were insufficient trials reporting disability for the authors to be able draw any conclusions about whether stroke care had any impact on function. Most of the trials included in the meta-analysis compared were trials of stroke units in the rehabilitation phase of the patients' illness. Few had admitted patients acutely or provided intensive care. The definition of stroke units did vary between the trials with some providing care in a geographically defined area of the hospital by a specialist medical, nursing, and rehabilitation team and some providing care by a multidisciplinary team moving around the hospital giving advice on patients on multiple general wards. It should be remembered that the results showing the benefits of stroke units came before the evidence was published about the effectiveness of intravenous thrombolysis and long before the positive trials of clot retrieval. A good summary of how the evidence has accumulated over the years was published by Langhorne in a 30th anniversary review in 2021 [4].

15.2 What Types of Stroke Unit Are There?

Over the years since the first publication of the meta-analysis more trials have been added and it has become clearer what constitutes an effective stroke unit [5]. Also, as the evidence for acute interventions has accumulated so has the definition of what is needed for high quality stroke care. There is now strong evidence to show that specialist stroke care from a multidisciplinary team is important at all stages after the stroke from the:

- Prehospital. The evidence supports mobile stroke units (MSUs) where there is specialist care delivered at the roadside in an ambulance equipped with a CT scanner and staff able to deliver intravenous thrombolysis. At the time of writing, there are no MSU in Vietnam.
- Hyperacute phase (usually defined as from arrival at the hospital to about 48 h). The 'intensive care' type setting Hyperacute Stroke Unit (HASU) in the hospital able to provide specialist monitoring, control of homeostasis, delivery of revascularisation treatments, and early rehabilitation. This model of care is now developing rapidly in Vietnam with many hospitals now opening hyperacute units.

- Acute phase usually taken as covering the period after the intensive care unit, so about 48 h until the patient is physiologically stable. This may be just a few days or as long as a few weeks depending on the severity of the stroke and the co-morbidities. Again, there are an increasing number of such units in Vietnam.
- Hospital rehabilitation phase. This again depends on the patient. For someone who recovers rapidly it may not be required at all. For others with severe stroke, perhaps on a background of frailty it may require weeks or even months of inpatient care. In Vietnam, these units are still needed as most of the rehabilitation takes place on generic or neurological rehabilitation wards which evidence suggests is less effective than focussing just on stroke rehabilitation.
- Early treatment at home. Trials of early supported discharge (ESD), where some of the multidisciplinary care in hospital is substituted with a team providing care in the patients own home, have shown this model to be effective and should be included in our definitions of stroke unit care. The model of ESD has not yet been developed in Vietnam where there is still a lack of organised rehabilitation after discharge from hospital but is perhaps something that might emerge in future years.

15.3 Mobile Stroke Units

The biggest trial published so far by Grotta et al. 2021 [6] showed significantly better outcomes as measured by the modified Rankin Score for patients in the MSU group compared to conventional care. The chances of a good outcome (modified Rankin score of 0 or 1) was 55.2% compared to 47% for those patients treated conventionally by emergency medical services.

These data are confirmed when analysed in the meta-analysis by Turc et al. [7]

The summary of the review states that compared with usual care, MSU use was associated with an approximately 65% increase in the odds of excellent outcome and a 30-min reduction in onset-to-IVT times, without safety concerns. The number needed to treat (NNT) to get one good outcome is 11. Reviews also show that MSUs are cost effective. However, they have only so far been tested using controlled trials in urban settings and in high-income countries. In many parts of the world where there are not even basic ambulance services, the idea that funding should go to MSUs is hardly feasible or realistic.

15.4 Inpatient Stroke Units

The most recent Cochrane review of the Stroke Unit Triallists' Collaboration [5] included 29 trials (5902 participants) that compared organised inpatient (stroke unit) care with an alternative service: 20 trials (4127participants) compared organised (stroke unit) care with a general ward, six trials (982 participants) compared different forms of organised (stroke unit) care, and three trials (793 participants) incorporated more than one comparison.

At an average of 12 months after their stroke, people who received organised inpatient (stroke unit) care were more likely to be alive with an extra two people surviving for every 100 receiving stroke unit care and living at home with an extra six patients for every 100 receiving stroke unit care. They also were more likely to be independent in daily activities (an extra six patients for every 100 receiving stroke unit care). The apparent benefits were seen in men and women, older and younger patients, and people with different types of stroke and different stroke severity. Benefits were most obvious when the stroke unit was based in a discrete stroke ward rather than stroke care being delivered by mobile teams. There was no indication that organised stroke unit care resulted in a longer hospital stay. Mixed rehabilitation wards also did not appear to be as effective as geographically defined wards specialising only in stroke care.

The following figures taken from the Cochrane review summarise some of the key findings, although the full review contains many more analyses that are worth reading.

Figure 15.1 compares the outcomes for patients treated on medical wards and stroke units. Fig. 15.2 gives the data that shows that mobile stroke units are not as effective as geographically based units. Fig. 15.3 shows that the benefits of stroke unit care seem to apply to patients of all ages, gender and stroke type and severity.

Analysis 2.1. Comparison 2: Stroke ward versus general medical ward, Outcome 1: Poor outcome by the end of scheduled follow-up

Study or Subgroup	Treatment Events	Treatment Total	Control Events	Control Total	Weight	Peto Odds Ratio Peto, Fixed, 95% CI
2.1.1 Comprehensive stroke ward vs general medical ward						
Athens 1995	138	302	145	302	21.6%	0.91 [0.66 , 1.25]
Beijing 2004	113	195	118	197	13.6%	0.92 [0.62 , 1.38]
Edinburgh 1980	93	155	94	156	10.7%	0.99 [0.63 , 1.56]
Goteborg-Ostra 1988	49	215	43	202	10.3%	1.09 [0.69 , 1.73]
Goteborg-Sahlgren 1994	108	166	54	83	7.2%	1.00 [0.58 , 1.74]
Huaihua 2004	83	324	39	73	7.3%	0.27 [0.16 , 0.47]
Joinville 2003	18	35	23	39	2.6%	0.74 [0.30 , 1.84]
Perth 1997	10	29	15	30	2.1%	0.54 [0.19 , 1.49]
Svendborg 1995	18	31	20	34	2.3%	0.97 [0.36 , 2.58]
Trondheim 1991	54	110	81	110	7.5%	0.36 [0.21 , 0.61]
Subtotal (95% CI)		**1562**		**1226**	**85.2%**	**0.78 [0.66 , 0.91]**
Total events:	684		632			
Heterogeneity: Chi² = 28.31, df = 9 (P = 0.0008); I² = 68%						
Test for overall effect: Z = 3.11 (P = 0.002)						
2.1.2 Rehabilitation stroke ward vs general medical ward						
Dover 1984 (GMW)	54	98	50	89	6.6%	0.96 [0.54 , 1.70]
Nottingham 1996 (GMW)	63	98	52	76	5.5%	0.83 [0.44 , 1.56]
Orpington 1993 (GMW)	38	53	39	48	2.6%	0.59 [0.24 , 1.48]
Orpington 1995	34	34	37	37		Not estimable
Subtotal (95% CI)		**283**		**250**	**14.8%**	**0.83 [0.57 , 1.23]**
Total events:	189		178			
Heterogeneity: Chi² = 0.76, df = 2 (P = 0.69); I² = 0%						
Test for overall effect: Z = 0.92 (P = 0.36)						
Total (95% CI)		**1845**		**1476**	**100.0%**	**0.78 [0.68 , 0.91]**
Total events:	873		810			
Heterogeneity: Chi² = 29.19, df = 12 (P = 0.004); I² = 59%						
Test for overall effect: Z = 3.22 (P = 0.001)						
Test for subgroup differences: Chi² = 0.12, df = 1 (P = 0.73), I² = 0%						

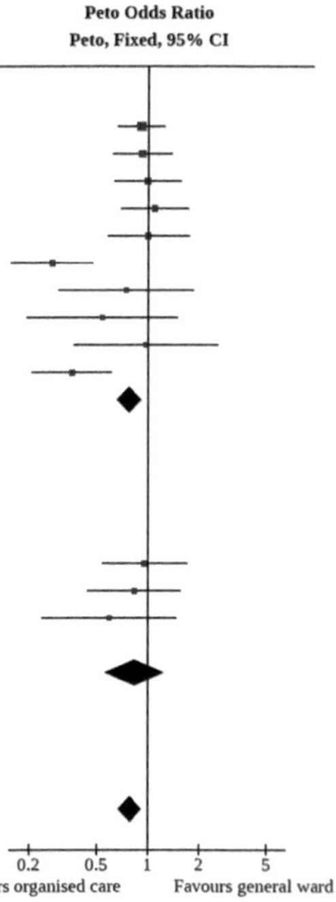

Fig. 15.1 Stroke unit care vs general medical ward comparing poor outcome (Modified Rankin Score 3–6 or Institutional Care)

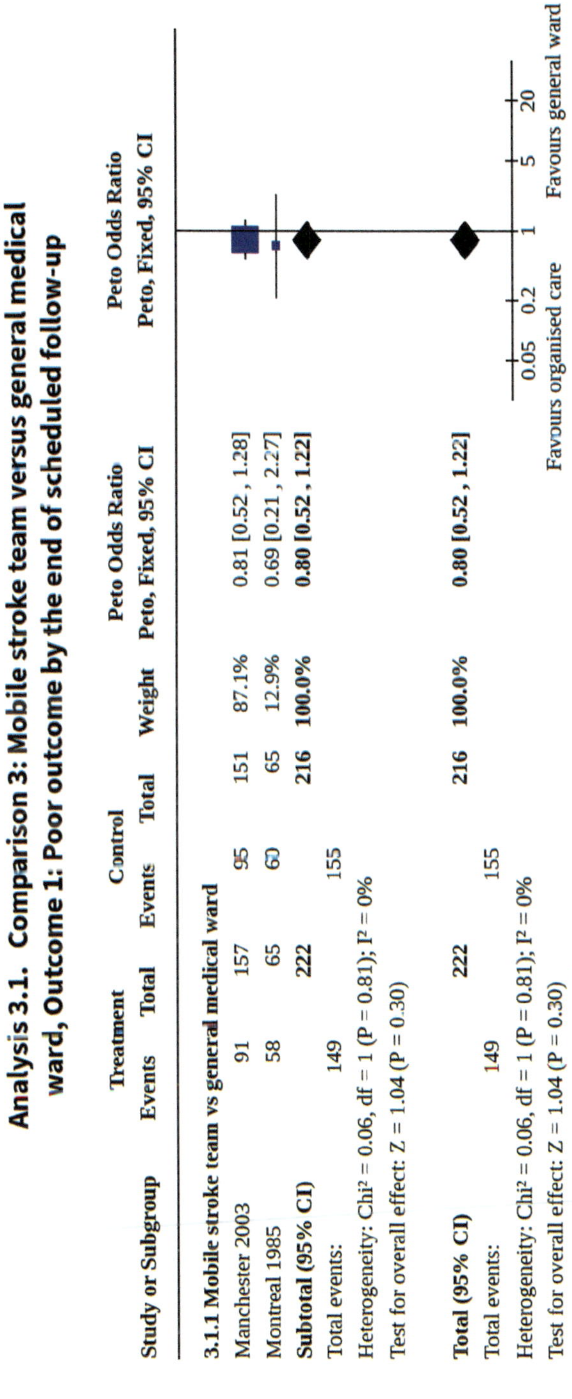

Fig. 15.2 showing that Mobile Stroke Teams do not perform as well as Geographically-based Stroke Wards

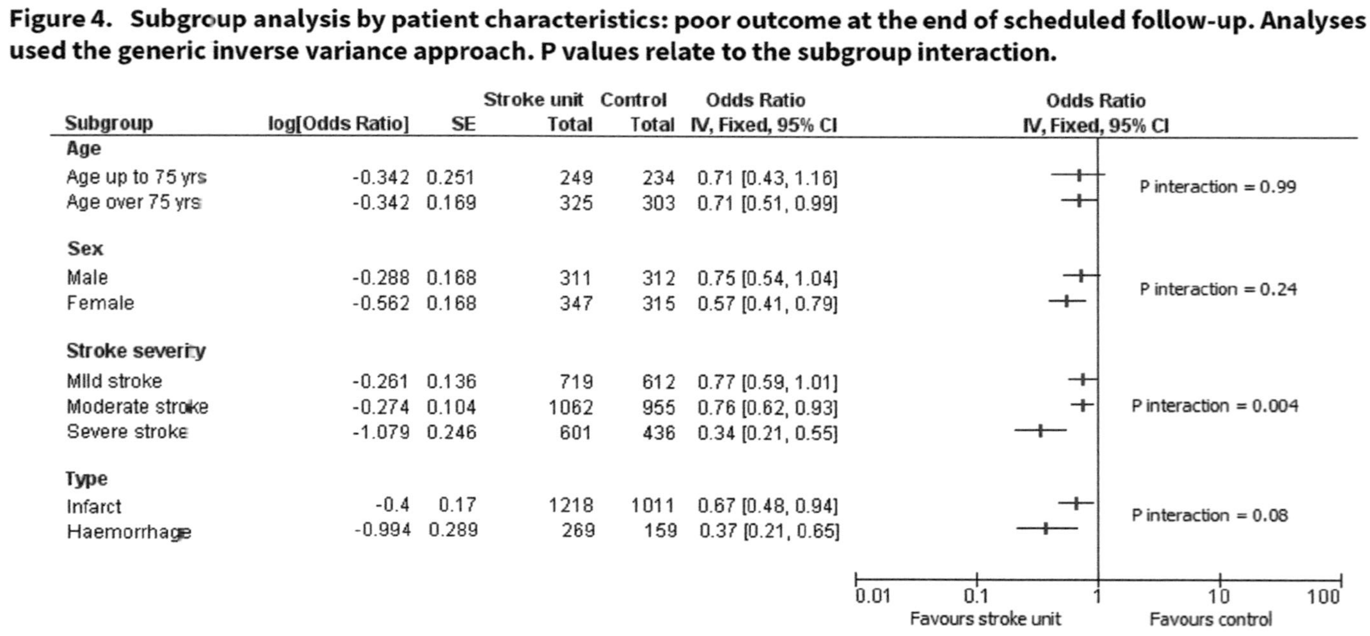

Fig. 15.3 showing that specialist Stroke Unit care benefits patients of all ages, gender, stroke type and stroke severity

15.5 What Is It About Stroke Units that Improves Outcomes?

The stroke unit is a complex system and we still cannot be certain about what components are the ones that make a difference. However, there are some clues from large audit datasets that have looked at differences in outcomes between units that are delivering some aspects of care compared to those that do not. Bray et al. 2013 [8] present very striking data shows that early assessment by a stroke consultant, early nurse and therapist assessment, early swallow assessment and nutrition management, and early intravenous fluids combined with giving aspirin within 24 h of admission all significantly reduce the risk of 30-day mortality (Fig. 15.4).

The number of staff on the stroke unit is also correlated with mortality. In a paper primarily looking at the differences in outcomes between patients admitted at weekends and during the week, Bray et al. [9] showed that having fewer than three nurses on duty at any one time for every 10 beds on the stroke unit significantly increases the risk of patient death within 30 days (Fig. 15.5).

A further paper also using data from the UK national stroke audit dataset showed that providing rapid assessment of the patients ability to swallow safely reduces the chances of the patient developing pneumonia even after adjustment for possible confounder [10].

The key factors then are likely to be the presence of sufficient numbers of staff with expertise in stroke, delivery of timely interventions such as dysphagia screening, maintenance of homeostasis, particularly avoidance of dehydration, early prevention by giving aspirin to the patients with ischaemic stroke and prevention of complications. It is our view that the nurses are the most important members of the stroke team in the early days after a stroke. This is the professional group that is present 24 h a day and if there are sufficient numbers and with the right expertise will recognise early deterioration, will be able to implement the predefined protocols of care and call for medical help when needed. The other key element of stroke

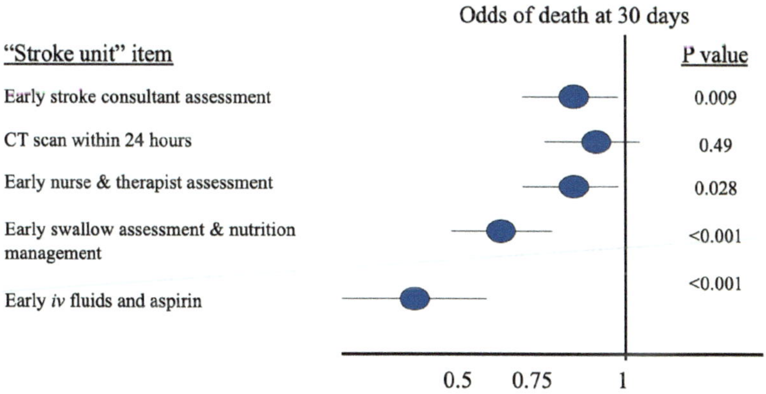

Fig. 15.4 Association between processes of care on stroke units and the odds of death at 30 days

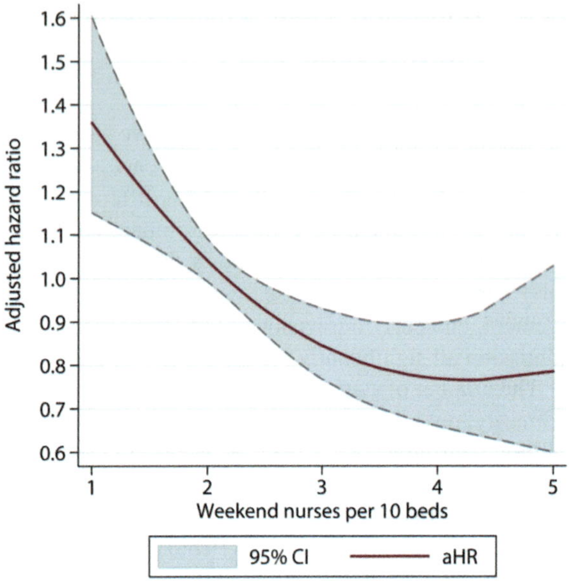

Fig. 15.5 Association between nurse staff levels and 30-day mortality

unit care is the provision of an effectively led multidisciplinary team where each team member are providing their own expertise but working in collaboration with their colleagues to deliver the right interventions for each specific patient. Putting the patient at the centre of the decision making and providing the patient and their carers with education and support are also likely to be important components in getting good long term outcomes.

15.6 Hyperacute Stroke Units (HASU)

Data from London published by Morris et al. [11] where stroke care was reorganised from a service providing stroke care in 32 stroke units to one where all care is provided in eight HASUs has shown major improvements in both processes, with higher rates of intravenous thrombolysis and improved elements of essential basic care as well as improved outcomes in terms of mortality. Similar findings have been demonstrated from other services undergoing similar reorganisation. The features of a HASU are that they admit patients directly from the emergency department with minimal delay, they are staffed by specialist nurses, doctors, and therapists at a higher level than general wards (Fig. 15.6) and there is effective multidisciplinary care. The wording of the UK national Stroke Guidelines [12] is:

- A hyperacute stroke unit should have immediate access to: specialist medical staff trained in the hyperacute and acute management of people with stroke, including the diagnostic and administrative procedures needed for the safe and timely delivery of emergency stroke treatments;

Physiotherapy	Occupational therapy	Speech and language therapy	Clinical psychology / neuropsychology	Dietetics	Nursing	Consultant stroke physician	Consultant-level practitioner-led ward rounds
Whole-time equivalents (WTE) per 5 beds*					WTE per bed	24/7 availability; minimum 6.0 thrombolysis trained physicians on rota	Twice daily ward round
1.02	0.95	0.48	0.28	0.21	2.9 (80:20 registered: unregistered)		

Fig. 15.6 Recommended staffing levels for the hyperacute stroke unit

- specialist nursing staff trained in the hyperacute and acute management of people with stroke, covering neurological, general medical and rehabilitation aspects;
- Stroke specialist rehabilitation staff.
- diagnostic, imaging, and cardiology services;
- tertiary services for endovascular therapy, neurosurgery, and vascular surgery.
- There should be continuous access to a consultant physician with expertise in stroke medicine, with consultant review 7 days per week.

Further recommendations are that there should be management protocols for common problems and regular monitoring of processes and outcomes. Examples of protocols are given in Chap. 16.

15.7 Acute Stroke Units and Rehabilitation Stroke Units

Acute stroke units will usually take patients from the HASU once the patient has received revascularisation treatment or no longer require intensive monitoring to maintain homeostasis. They may be in the same hospital as the HASU or in a lower level hospital. The UK National Clinical Guidelines recommend the following staffing levels (Fig. 15.7).

The recommendations as to how they should operate are:

- An acute stroke unit should provide.
  - Specialist medical staff trained in the acute management of people with stroke.
  - specialist nursing staff trained in the acute management of people with stroke, covering neurological, general medical and rehabilitation aspects;
  - stroke specialist rehabilitation staff,
  - access to diagnostic imaging and cardiology services,
  - access to tertiary services for neurosurgery and vascular surgery.

	Physio-therapy	Occupational therapy	Speech and language therapy	Clinical psychology / neuro-psychology	Dietetics	Nursing	Consultant stroke physician	Consultant-level practitioner-led ward rounds
Acute stroke unit & stroke rehab-ilitation unit	1.18	1.13	0.56	0.28	0.21	1.35 (65:35 registered: unregis-tered)	Acute stroke unit: 7 day cover with adequate out of hours arrange-ments**	Acute stroke unit: daily ward round** Stroke rehabilit-ation unit: twice-weekly ward round**

Fig. 15.7 Recommended staffing levels in acute stroke and rehabilitation stroke units

- continuous access to a consultant physician with expertise in stroke medicine, with consultant review 5 days per week,

- An inpatient stroke unit should be:
  - a geographically defined unit;
  - have a co-ordinated multidisciplinary team that meets at least once a week for the exchange of information about inpatients with stroke;
  - information advice and support for people with stroke and their family and carers,
  - management protocols for common problems, based upon the best available evidence;
  - close links and protocols for the transfer of care with other inpatient stroke services, early supported discharge teams and community services;
  - training for healthcare professionals in the specialty of stroke,
- A stroke rehabilitation unit should have a single multidisciplinary tea including specialists in.
  - Medicine.
  - Nursing.
  - Physiotherapy.
  - Occupational therapy.
  - Speech and language therapy.
  - Dietetics.
  - Clinical psychology.
  - Social work.
  - Orthoptics.

And with

- with timely access to rehabilitation medicine, specialist pharmacy, orthotics, specialist seating, assistive technology and information, advice and support (including life after stroke services) for people with stroke and their family/carers.

15.8 Clinical Protocols for Hospitalised Stroke Patients

Each unit should develop their own protocols for the management of stroke associated issues. Examples of some protocols for the most common issues are given in Chap. 17. These were developed for use in some Vietnamese hospitals in the Red River Region. But recommendations will vary according to local factors such as availability of drugs and local hospital policies and facilities.

15.8.1 Early Supported Discharge

Rudd et al. published the first large trial of early supported discharge in 1996 [13]. The rationale was that once the patient was medically stable and could survive at home with whatever care was available to him or her, rehabilitation might be more relevant to patients than continuing to practice in hospital. For example, teaching someone to get on and off a hospital toilet may not be relevant to the transfer they will need to do in their own bathroom. Furthermore, it was hypothesised that patients might be more motivated to practice when they could see the direct relevance to them coping in their own home. Patients, particularly those with significant post stroke disability can also become very dependent on the help that they get in hospital and may not realise that they are becoming institutionalised. It was also hypothesised that care might be more cost effective given that hospital care can be very expensive. Most of the trials have included patients who are able to transfer independently if they live along or with the help of a willing partner with whom they live. They had to be physiologically stable and not require constant nursing care for such things as intravenous drugs or fluids. They also had to have accommodation suitable to deliver rehabilitation. The range of health professionals available to provide home-based rehabilitation aimed to mirror that available in hospital. All teams offered physiotherapy, occupational therapy, and speech and language therapy and some also provided nursing care, medical care and psychology. Intensity also varied with the initial trials offering daily therapy of each of the therapies that the individual patient required. But all had the common feature, essential to all stroke unit type care that there was co-ordinated multidisciplinary working with regular meetings of the teams to discuss progress and set objectives. The latest Cochrane review [14] analysed 17 trials, with 2422 participants.

The ESD group showed reductions in the length of hospital stay equivalent to approximately 6 days. The odds ratios (OR) for the outcome of death or dependency at the end of scheduled follow-up (median 6 months; range 3–12) was OR 0.80 (95% (Confidence Interval) CI 0.67 to 0.95, $P = 0.01$, which equates to five fewer adverse outcomes per 100 patients receiving ESD. The results for death and death or requiring institutional care were OR 1.04 (95% CI 0.77 to 1.40, $P = 0.81$. Small improvements were also seen in participants' extended activities of daily living scores and satisfaction with services (OR 1.60, 95% CI 1.08 to 2.38, $P = 0.02$, low-grade evidence). The greatest reductions in death or dependency were seen in the trials evaluating a co-ordinated ESD team.

It is surprising that mortality was lower in the ESD group. The explanation is not obvious but conceivably could be due to less exposure at home to infectious diseases and perhaps earlier mobilisation.

15.8.2 Equipping a Stroke Unit

15.8.2.1 For Acute Stroke Unit Beds

- Multi-functional beds with as a minimum high-low function and backrest option. These should be available for all stroke patients while they remain severely disabled (needing assistance with bed mobility and transfers). The number should be determined by an audit of the severity of stroke patients being managed currently in the hospital
- Pressure area care mattresses for every bed—foam at least 2 ½ inch thick
- Air mattress for patients at high risk of pressure sores—1 per 10 beds
- Armchair for every bed—with as a minimum high back support and armrests
- Bedside height adjustable table for each bed
- ECG machine per 20 beds
- One full assistance manual handling hoist per 10 beds
- Rotastand or standing hoist per 10 beds
- One sliding sheet per 5 beds
- Feeding pump for nasogastric feeding—1 per 5 beds
- One wheelchair for every 5 beds
- Adapted toilet and shower facilities with wheelchair access and handrails
- One commode per 5 beds for bedside toileting

15.8.2.2 In Addition, the Hyperacute Stroke Beds Would Require

- 1 cardiac monitor per bed with non-invasive blood pressure, oxygen saturations and 3 lead ECG facilities
- Bedside oxygen and suction for every bed

15.8.2.3 Rehabilitation Equipment for the Acute Stroke Unit or Rehabilitation Stroke Unit

- One plinth for every 10 beds with as minimum high-low facility
- Gait aids—walking sticks, quad sticks, elbow crutches, Zimmer frames
- Full length mirror
- One set of parallel bars
- Wall bars around therapy space
- Standing hoist or rotastand
- Orthotics available for shoulder support, splints, ankle-foot orthoses
- Pillows and foam rolls for positioning
- Practice steps

15.8.3 Stroke Units in Low-and Middle-Income Countries (LMIC)

An important review of this topic was published by Langhorne et al. in 2013 [15]. The paper remains very relevant in 2024. Little appears to have changed. Most of the stroke unit trials have been conducted in high income countries and as revascularisation treatments have achieved such success, albeit for a very small percentage of stroke patients, it may have been forgotten that the success of stroke units, particularly of the early trials, occurred before 'high tech' medicine came to dominate stroke clinicians thinking. The burden of stroke is increasing in LMICs at a relatively higher rate than in high-income countries but specialist stroke care is not developing at a similar pace. Reperfusion treatment depends on access to highly skilled interventionists, especially for endovascular thrombectomy who are a scarce resource in high-income countries and often non-existent in LMIC and expensive equipment ranging from the scanners to the intravascular devices. Intravenous thrombolysis requires an efficient prehospital service by paramedics, immediate access to brain imaging, clinicians experienced at using a potentially dangerous drug and a alteplase or tenecteplase both of which are likely to be out of reach of low-income populations, especially those without access to free at point of access health service. But many of the interventions that are likely to be delivering benefit in a stroke unit are low technology and cheap. Maintaining hydration and nutrition, preventing pressure sores, identifying dysphagia and therefore reducing the likelihood of aspiration pneumonia, controlling blood sugar and early mobilisation are all things that do not require expensive equipment but do require a well-trained nursing and medical workforce. For secondary prevention, there is no need to use any expensive drugs. Generic antihypertensives and antiplatelet drugs should be available for very little money. Figure 15.8 shows the potential benefit for stroke interventions for a population of one million with an estimated number of 2500 strokes per year.

There have been some stroke unit trials performed in LMIC and these show similar results to those obtained in the high-income countries. Again, taken from the Langhorne et al. paper 2013 [15] Fig. 15.9 summarises these.

The theory is then that stroke units should be feasible in LMIC and would produce major population benefits. But of course, it is a lot easier to write that than actually implement it. Even though they do not require major expenditure on expensive equipment and drugs they do require a lot of other things that do not come without expenditure and commitment. They require the political leadership at local, regional, or national level. They require clinical leadership and drive to persuade hospitals to provide the space for the unit and they require the willingness to employ and train the workforce of doctors, nurses, and therapists. They also need to overcome the problem of competition between hospitals. For stroke units to be feasible and effective, they need to be of a reasonable size, perhaps a minimum of 10 patients at any one time. Not all hospitals will therefore be required to provide a stroke unit, so there needs to be cooperation between hospitals to deliver high quality care. This

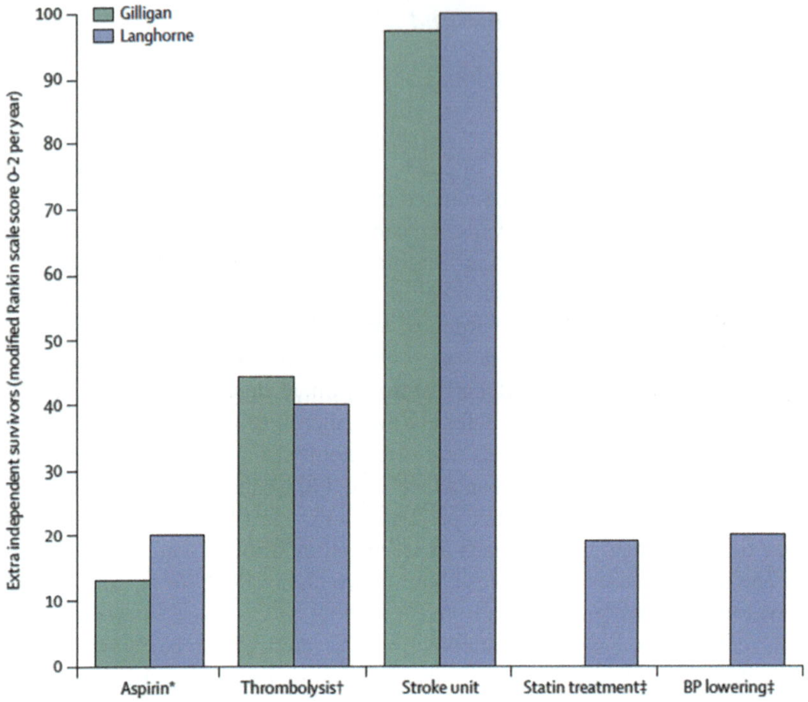

Fig. 15.8 Taken from Langhorne et al. 2013 [15]. Potential population effect of stroke interventions in a district of one million population with 2500 strokes per year. Estimates are shown for the number of extra independent survivors (modified Rankin scale score 0–2 points) resulting from an intervention during 1 year. The assumptions and calculations are detailed by Gilligan and colleagues [16] and Langhorne et al. [17]. *BP* blood pressure. *Acute aspirin treatment. †0–6 h of thrombolysis. ‡Prevention

is easier in a centralised funded service and may be more difficult where hospitals are competing for patients to maintain financial viability.

This chapter has set out details of staffing levels, equipment and elsewhere in the book we discuss training needs. The question is whether to wait to open a stroke unit until all these requirements are fulfilled or whether to start a unit even if all the resources are not yet available. Our view is that it is better to start and then gradually evolve rather than wait for a time that may never come. Even an under-resourced unit is likely to be better than nothing and bringing all the stroke patients together will demonstrate the size of the problem and why investment is needed. The chapter on health economics also may provide some evidence to show that effective acute stroke care can save money in both the short and long term.

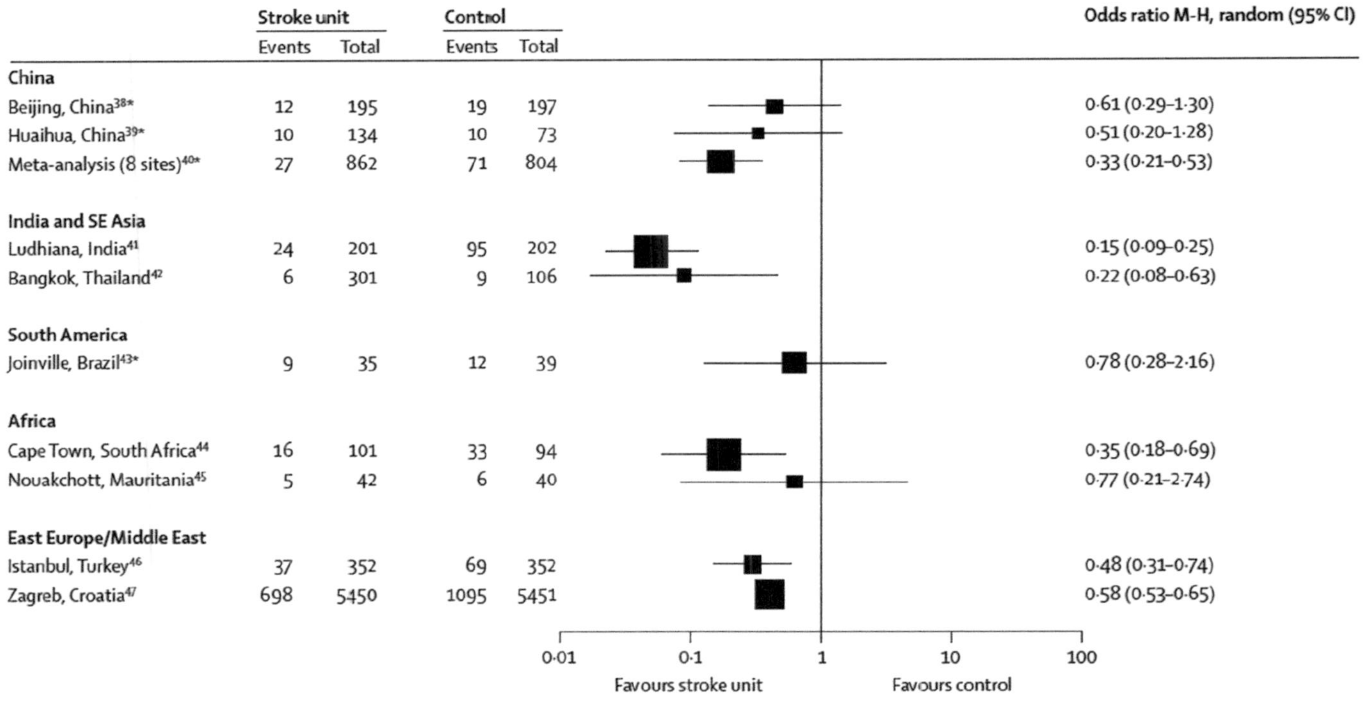

Fig. 15.9 Stroke unit trials in middle-and low-income countries Case fatality at the end of scheduled follow-up. Figure shows the study, deaths (events), study group population (total), and the odds ratio for death in a stroke unit vs. a general ward

Table 15.1 Change in the number of specialist stroke services between 2016 and 2021 [18]

	2016	2021	
	Number	Number	Percentage
Comprehensive stroke Centre	1	6	7.4
Stroke department	2	8	9.9
Stroke units	9	67	82.7
Total	12	81	100

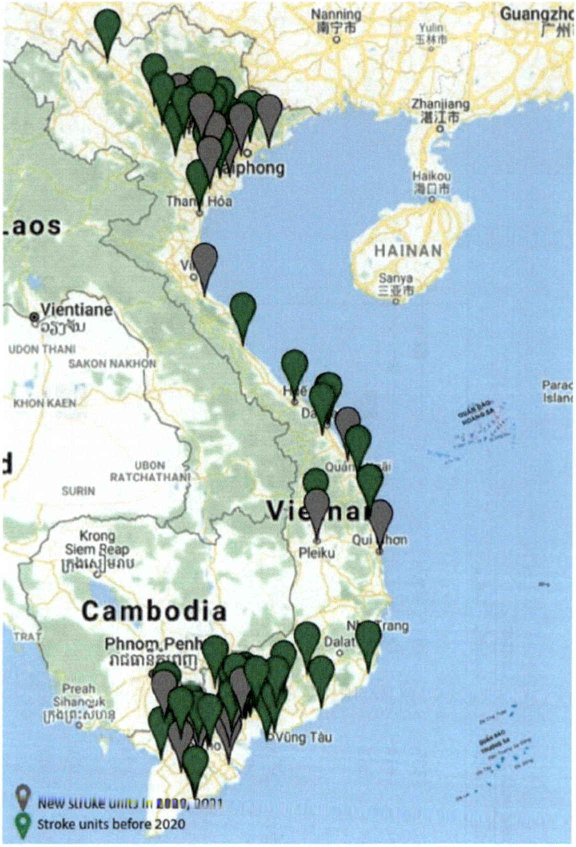

Fig. 15.10 Location of Stroke Units in Vietnam. Green markers are those in existence before 2020 and in grey opened between 2020 and 2021 [18]

15.8.4 *Stroke Units in Vietnam*

Mai DT et al. published an article in 2022 [18] summarising progress with the development of stroke units in Vietnam. Great progress has been made since 2016 as can be given in Table 15.1.

Figure 15.10 shows the geographical distribution of the stroke centres in Vietnam with most being in the large urban areas but with clear evidence that the model of care has become widely accepted in the country.

15.9 Conclusions

The evidence for the benefits of stroke unit care, from the intensive care phase at the beginning through the acute stroke unit and inpatient rehabilitation is extremely strong. There is also evidence to extend stroke unit care both into the prehospital phase by using mobile stroke units and after discharge from hospital by the provision of early supported discharge. Vietnam is making good progress with the development of inpatient stroke units. More are needed particularly outside of the main cities and more may need to be done to provide specialist care for the whole of the stroke pathway and not just for the early days.

References

1. Langhorne P, Williams BO, Gilchrist W, Howie K. Do stroke units save lives? Lancet. 1993;342:395–8.
2. Indredavik B, Bakke F, Solberg R, Rokseth R, Haahein LL, Home I. Benefit of stroke unit: a randomised controlled trial. Stroke. 1991;22:1026–31.
3. Stroke Unit Trialists' Collaboration. Collaborative systematic review of the randomised trials of organised inpatient (stroke unit) care after stroke. BMJ. 1997;314:1151–9.
4. Langhorne P. The stroke unit story: where have we been and where are we going? Cerebrovasc Dis. 2021;50(6):636–43. https://doi.org/10.1159/000518934. Epub 2021 Sep 21. PMID: 34547746.
5. Langhorne P, Ramachandra S. Stroke Unit Trialists' Collaboration. Organised inpatient (stroke unit) care for stroke: network meta-analysis. Cochrane Database Syst Rev. 2020;4(4):CD000197. https://doi.org/10.1002/14651858.CD000197.pub4. PMID: 32324916; PMCID: PMC7197653.
6. Grotta JC, Yamal JM, Parker SA, et al. Prospective, multicenter, controlled trial of Mobile stroke units. N Engl J Med. 2021;385(11):971–81. Erratum in: N Engl J Med 2023 Jun 29;388(26):2495–2496.
7. Turc G, Hadziahmetovic M, Walter S, et al. Comparison of Mobile stroke unit with usual care for acute ischemic stroke management: a systematic review and meta-analysis. JAMA Neurol. 2022;79(3):281–90.
8. Bray BD, Ayis S, Campbell J, et al. Associations between the organisation of stroke services, process of care, and mortality in England: prospective cohort study. BMJ. 2013;346:f2827.
9. Bray BD, Ayis S, Campbell J, et al. Associations between stroke mortality and weekend working by stroke specialist physicians and registered nurses: prospective multicentre cohort study. PLoS Med. 2014;11(8):e1001705.
10. Bray BD, Smith CJ, Cloud GC, SSNAP Collaboration. The association between delays in screening for and assessing dysphagia after acute stroke, and the risk of stroke-associated pneumonia. J Neurol Neurosurg Psychiatry. 2016;88:25–30.
11. Morris S, Ramsay AIG, Boaden RJ, Hunter RM, McKevitt C, Paley L, Perry C, Rudd AG, Turner SJ, Tyrrell PJ, Wolfe CDA, Fulop NJ. Impact and sustainability of centralising acute stroke services in English metropolitan areas: retrospective analysis of hospital episode statistics and stroke national audit data. BMJ. 2019;364:11.
12. UK National Clinical Guidelines for Stroke 2023. https://www.strokeguideline.org/.
13. Rudd AG, Wolfe CDA, Tilling K, Beech R. The effectiveness of an early discharge policy and a package of community care on one year outcome of stroke patients. BMJ. 1997;315:1039–44.

14. Anon. Early supported discharge services for people with acute stroke. Cochrane Database Syst Rev. 2017;7:CD000443. https://doi.org/10.1002/14651858.CD000443.pub4. Accessed 28 Jan 2024.
15. Langhorne P, de Villiers L, Pandian JD. Applicability of stroke-unit care to low-income and middle-income countries. Lancet Neurol. 2012;11(4):341–8. https://doi.org/10.1016/S1474-4422(12)70024-8. Epub 2012 Mar 19. PMID: 22441195.
16. Gilligan AK, Thrift AG, Sturm JW, Dewey HM, Macdonell RA, Donnan GA. Stroke units, tissue plasminogen activator, aspirin and neuroprotection: which stroke intervention could provide the greatest community benefit? Cerebrovasc Dis. 2005;20:239–44.
17. Langhorne P, Sandercock P, Prasad K. Evidence-based practice for stroke. Lancet Neurol. 2009;8:308–9.
18. Mai DT, Dao XC, Luong NK, et al. Current state of stroke Care in Vietnam. Stroke. 2022;2(2):e000331. https://doi.org/10.1161/SVIN.121.000331.

Chapter 16
Protocols for the Management of Common Issues in Acute Stroke

Thong Van Nguyen, Quan Hong Nguyen, Ngoc Huy Nguyen, and Anthony Rudd

16.1 Introduction

As presented in this chapter on Stroke Units, one of the important components for effective specialist stroke care is that units should have clear protocols for the management of common problems affecting acute stroke patients. While it is important that there are always staff on duty with expertise in stroke, there will inevitably be many situations, particularly outside normal working hours, where there will be doctors and nurses who are not familiar with stroke issues and may be tempted to treat or not treat inappropriately.

Each hospital should develop their own protocols as part of the process of setting up their own specialist unit. Particularly when it comes to drug treatments, there are often several equally good options but also some that are less good. The examples in this chapter are ones that the authors developed for use in Vietnam and the UK. Many of the recommendations are discussed in other chapters in this book where references are given. We have not included them in this section to keep it shorter and clearer. To find the evidence for some of the statements, we would

T. Van Nguyen (✉)
Vietnam Stroke Association, Hanoi, Vietnam

Stroke Center, Phutho General Hospital, Phutho, Vietnam
e-mail: nguyenvanthongbv108@gmail.com

Q. H. Nguyen
Department of Neurology, 108 Military Central Hospital, Hanoi, Vietnam

N. H. Nguyen
Phutho Department of Health, Phutho, Vietnam

VNU University of Medicine and Pharmacy, Hanoi, Vietnam

A. Rudd
King's College, London, UK

A. Rudd et al. (eds.), *Stroke Management in Vietnam*,
https://doi.org/10.1007/978-981-96-0221-6_16

recommend referring to the UK National Clinical Guidelines for Stroke 2023 https://www.strokeguideline.org/.

The scores mentioned in these protocols are reproduced at the end of this chapter.

16.2 Protocol for Neurological Observations After Acute Stroke

Regular neurological observations can identify deterioration in acute stroke. The neurological observations should follow a standardised system such as the Glasgow Coma Scale [1] (Fig. 16.1) and/or the NIHSS[2] (National Institute of Health Stroke Severity Score) (Fig. 16.2).

16.2.1 Recommendations

1. Healthcare staff should be trained in the use of the standardised neurological assessment tools to ensure reliability and consistency.
2. Neurological observations should be performed at least 1–2 hourly for all patients with acute stroke for at least 24 h. Where there is alteration in the patient's neurological status, the frequency of observations should be increased to 15–30 minutely as appropriate. Neurological observations should not be performed any less frequently than 2 hourly in order to identify sudden changes. If no longer required after 24 h from admission, neurological observations should be stopped by the medical staff.
3. An alteration in patients' neurological status should be reported to the medical staff as soon as possible. As a general guide:
   (a) A reduction of more than two points on the Glasgow Coma Scale.
   (b) A reduction of more than four points on the NIHSS.
   (c) A sudden or gradual deterioration of limb function or language ability.
4. The patient should be fully assessed by medical staff to identify new neurological deficits and consider whether further brain imaging is indicated for example to identify malignant MCA syndrome or an expanding haematoma.
5. Patients with a Glasgow Coma Scale below 8 should be assessed by an anaesthetist to consider if intubation may be indicated.
6. Neurological observations for patients having received thrombolysis should follow the thrombolysis protocol.

Glasgow Coma Scale*

Area Assessed	Response	Points
Eye opening	Open spontaneously	4
	Open to verbal command	3
	Open in response to pain applied to the limbs or sternum	2
	None	1
Verbal	Oriented	5
	Disoriented, but able to answer questions	4
	Inappropriate answers to questions; words discernible	3
	Incomprehensible speech	2
	None	1
Motor	Obeys commands	6
	Responds to pain with purposeful movement	5
	Withdraws from pain stimuli	4
	Responds to pain with abnormal flexion (decorticate posture)	3
	Responds to pain with abnormal (rigid) extension (decerebrate posture)	2
	None	1

* Combined scores < 8 are typically regarded as coma.

Fig. 16.1 Glasgow Coma Score [1]

National Institutes of Health Stroke Scale (NIHSS)		Score		
Instructions	**Scale Definition** **Date/Time**	**Baseline**	**24 Hrs Post TPA**	**Discharge**
Date/Time				
1a. LOC	0 = **Alert** keenly responsive 1 = **Not Alert** but arousable by minor stimulation to obey, answer, respond 2 = **Not Alert**; requires repeat stimulation, obtunded, requires strong stimuli 3 = **Reflex motor** or autonomic effects response, totally unresponsive, flaccid			
1b. LOC Questions. Ask the patient the month & age	0 = **Answers both** questions correctly 1 = **Answers one** question correctly 2 = **Answers neither** questions correctly			
1c. LOC Commands. Ask to open & close eyes, then grip & release with non-paretic hand.	0 = **Performs both** tasks correctly 1 = **Performs one** task correctly 2 = **Performs neither** task correctly			
2. Best Gaze. Asked to follow with eyes thru horizontal plane (or oculocephalic maneuver).	0 = **Normal** 1 = **Partial Gaze Palsy**; gaze is abnormal in 1 or both eyes, but forced deviation or total gaze paresis is not present. 2 = **Forced deviation**; total gaze paresis not overcome by oculocephalic man.			
3. Visual fields (quadrants) tested with finger counting or visual threat.(done by confrontation)	0 = **No visual loss** 1 = **Partial** hemianopia 2 = **Complete** hemianopia 3 = **Bilateral** hemianopia (including cortical blindness).			
4. Facial Palsy. Asked to show teeth & raise eyebrows	0 = **Normal** symmetrical movement 1 = **Minor paralysis** (flattened nasolabial fold, asymmetry on smiling) 2 = **Partial paralysis** (total or near total paralysis of lower face) 3 = **Complete paralysis** of one or both sides (no upper/lower face mvmt).			
5. Motor Arm. Asked to extend arms (palm down) 90° (if sitting) or 45° (if supine) & hold for 10 seconds. Begin with non-paretic limb.	0 = **No drift**; limb holds 90°(or 45°) for full 10 seconds 1 = **Drift**, limb holds 90°(or 45°) but drifts down before full 10 seconds but does not hit bed or other support 2 = **Some effort against gravity**, limb cannot get to or maintain (if cued 90°or 45°) drifts down to bed, but has some effort against gravity. 3 = **No effort against gravity**, limb falls 4 = **No movement** *UN = Amputation, joint fusion: Explain________	**Left:** **Right:**	**Left:** **Right:**	**Left:** **Right:**
6. Motor Leg. While supine, asked to hold leg at 30° for 5 seconds.	0 = **No drift**; leg holds 30° for full 5 seconds 1 = **Drift**, leg falls but does not hit bed 2 = **Some effort against gravity**, falls to bed w/in 5 sec 3 = **No effort against gravity**; leg falls to bed immediately 4 = **No movement** *UN = Amputation, joint fusion: Explain________	**Left:** **Right:**	**Left:** **Right:**	**Left:** **Right:**
7.Limb Ataxia. Finger – nose & heel – shin test on both sides	0 = **Absent** 1 = **Present in one** limb 2 = **Present in two** limbs *UN = Amputation, joint fusion: Explain________			
8. Sensory. Sensation or grimace to pin prick or withdrawal from noxious stimuli to limbs in obtunded or aphasic patient.	0 = **Normal**, no sensory loss 1 = **Mild/moderate** sensory loss; may be dulled/"Not as sharp" 2 = **Severe/total** sensory loss; not aware of face/arm/leg being touched.			
9.Best Language. Describe what is happening in picture, name items of figures, read list of sentences on attached figures.	0 = **No aphasia**, normal 1 = **Mild / moderate aphasia**; some loss of fluency / comprehension, without limitation of expression of ideas. (can identify what is happening in picture) 2 = **Severe aphasia**; (cannot identify pictures) 3 = **Mute**; global aphasia; no usable speech; or auditory comprehension			
10.Dysarthria. Read or repeat words from list.	0 = **Normal** articulation 1 = **Mild / Moderate**; slurs some words; understood w/some difficulty. 2 = **Severe**, so slurred as to be unintelligible; mute/anarthric *UN = Intubated or other physical barrier. Explain________			
11.Extinction & Inattention. Look at visual (from #3) and double simultaneous tactile. Do both arms & legs.	0 = No abnormality 1 = **Visual, tactile, auditory, spatial or personal inattention** or extinction to bilateral stimulation in one sensory modalities. 2 = **Profound hemi-inattention** or inattention to more than one modality; does not recognize own hand; orients to only one side of space.			
*UN = untestable	**TOTAL SCORE**			
Initials				
Physician or Nurse Signature				

Fig. 16.2 National Institute of Health Stroke Score (NIHSS) [2]

16.3 Protocol for the Management of Hypertension After Acute Stroke

Approximately, 50% of patients admitted with stroke will be known to have hypertension and will be on anti-hypertensive medication. Many of the patients, whether hypertensive or not will have raised blood pressure in the immediate aftermath of the stroke. Some of these will have undiagnosed hypertension; others will only have transient hypertension, probably as a physiological response to the cerebral ischaemia. Lowering blood pressure acutely may result in a reduction in cerebral blood flow to critically ischaemic areas and increase the size of the infarct. It is clear from evidence that hypotension results in increased infarct size and poorer outcomes. Hypotension should be avoided, treated if present, and investigated.

16.3.1 Recommendations

1. Examine the patient for evidence of end organ hypertensive damage, e.g., retinopathy, left ventricular hypertrophy (including ECG).
2. Patients with acute ischaemic stroke should only receive blood pressure lowering treatment if there is an indication for emergency treatment, such as:
   (a) systolic blood pressure above 185 mmHg or diastolic blood pressure above 110 mmHg,
   (b) when the patient is otherwise eligible for treatment with alteplase hypertensive encephalopathy;
   (c) hypertensive nephropathy,
   (d) hypertensive cardiac failure or myocardial infarction;
   (e) aortic dissection;
   (f) pre-eclampsia or eclampsia.
3. Patients with primary intracerebral haemorrhage who present within 6 h of onset with a systolic blood pressure above 150 mmHg should be treated urgently using a locally agreed protocol for blood pressure lowering to a systolic blood pressure below 140 mmHg for at least 7 days, unless:
   (a) the Glasgow Coma Scale score is 5 or below;
   (b) the haematoma is very large and death is expected;
   (c) a structural cause for the haematoma is identified;
   (d) immediate surgery to evacuate the haematoma is planned.
4. Monitor blood pressure, at least twice daily during the first week after admission and ensure a recording of blood pressure from each arm at least once within the first week.
5. Continue preadmission anti-hypertensive drugs where the patient is able to take oral medication. Where the patient is 'nil by mouth' withhold drug treatment until the decision is made to insert an NG or PEG tube.
6. The cerebral perfusion pressure should be maintained above 60 mmHg at least—calculated by the formula—CPP = MAP—CVP/ICP(whichever is thought to be highest). Generally, this means maintaining the MAP above 70 mmHg with the provision of adequate hydration and treating causes of hypotension, i.e., sepsis.

7. When initiating anti-hypertensive medication do so cautiously using a thiazide diuretic and subsequently a long acting ACE inhibitor, if the blood pressure remains above 140 mm systolic or 90 mm diastolic.
8. Investigate the underlying cause for the hypertension where appropriate.
9. For longer term secondary prevention aim for as low a blood pressure as the patient can tolerate without symptoms of hypotension. Use of a long acting ACE inhibitor and thiazide diuretic is supported by well conducted randomised controlled trials.

16.4 Protocol for the Management of Pyrexia After Acute Stroke

Evidence from animal studies suggests pyrexia is harmful to ischaemic brain and evidence from humans shows poorer outcomes inpatients who have fever after stroke. No trial has yet been conducted which shows that treating or preventing fever improves outcome. Until such evidence is available the following protocol should be observed.

16.4.1 Recommendations

1. Monitor temperature at least 4 hourly for the first 48 hours after stroke and then according to clinical situation.
2. When the temperature rises above 37 °C examine the patient for signs of infection, check for neutrophilia and obtain urine, sputum (where available), throat swabs, and blood for culture. Check needle sites for evidence of inflammation. Consider drug reaction as a cause of fever. Stroke itself can cause fever.
3. Treat infection with appropriate antibiotics.
4. Administer paracetamol 1 g 4 hourly until temperature returns to normal.
5. Consider the use of fans and tepid sponging for high fever.

16.5 Protocol for Fluid Management After Acute Stroke

Many patients become dehydrated following stroke because of swallowing difficulties, problems gaining access to fluids, anxiety about being incontinent of urine, disturbed homeostasis, and the hot dry atmosphere of the hospital ward. Patients who become dry have poorer outcomes in terms of mortality and morbidity than those who remain adequately hydrated.

16.5.1 Recommendations

1. Assess hydration clinically on a daily basis and measure urea and electrolytes daily for the first 72 h after stroke. Calculate osmolality using the formula [Na) x 2 + [K] x 2 + Glucose + Urea, aiming for levels of 280–295 mmol/l. Keep hydrated with isotonic fluids (initially 3 L daily for someone who is not taking any fluids by mouth but adjust according to the individual requirements of the patient).
2. Fluids can be administered by intravenous infusion or subcutaneously. If using the subcutaneous route, use only normal saline and change the infusion site daily. Dextrose should be avoided to prevent the precipitation of transient hyperglycaemia or unstable blood sugar levels as well as local inflammation and sepsis.
3. When an enteral tube is in place give fluids through the tube rather than using a separate IV or SC route.
4. Encourage oral hydration whenever possible.

16.6 Protocol for the Management of Hyperglycaemia After Acute Stroke

As with ischaemic heart disease, hyperglycaemia is probably harmful to ischaemic brain. Approximately, 25% of stroke patients occur in known diabetics and many others develop transient hyperglycaemia in the acute phase of stroke. Recent research evidence suggests lower blood sugar levels are important for longer term outcomes—at least maintained below 10 mmol/l but other studies are investigating maintaining levels less than 7 mmol/l. Recent evidence also suggests that transient hyperglycaemia can have an onset of 12–36 h and may not be immediately evident on initial admission.

16.6.1 Recommendations

1. Monitor blood sugar level 8 hourly for the first 72 hours after stroke in all patients—both diabetic and non-diabetic, to determine the presence of transient hyperglycaemia.
2. Treat with insulin if the blood sugar rises above 10 mmol/l, aiming for a blood glucose within the range 5–8 mmol/l. This is most effectively done by insulin sliding scale—generally using normal saline where possible. The sliding scale may need to be adjusted to avoid the use of dextrose where practical. Dextrose is generally not recommended for use in acute stroke.

3. For established diabetics, where possible continue with established hypoglycaemic treatment. Where the patient is 'nil by mouth' and it is impossible to administer oral hypoglycaemics give insulin, via sliding scale.

16.7 Protocol for the Management of Oxygenation and Positioning After Acute Stroke

16.7.1 Recommendations

1. Patients with acute stroke should have an initial specialist assessment for positioning as soon as possible and within 4 h of arrival at hospital.
2. Healthcare professionals responsible for the initial assessment of patients with acute stroke should be trained in how to position patients appropriately, taking into account the degree of their physical impairment after stroke.
3. When lying or sitting, patients with acute stroke should be positioned to minimise the risk of aspiration and other respiratory complications, shoulder pain and subluxation, contractures, and skin pressure ulceration.
4. Patients with acute stroke should be helped to sit up in bed, and as soon as possible positioned correctly in a chair.
5. Patients with acute stroke should only receive supplemental oxygen if their oxygen saturation is below 95% and there is no contraindication.
6. Where oxygen saturations are low look for an underlying cause, e.g., previous chronic pulmonary disease, pulmonary embolism, pneumonia,

16.8 Protocol for the Management of Deep Venous Thrombosis (DVT) Prophylaxis after Acute Stroke

Deep vein thrombosis (DVT) and pulmonary embolism (PE) are common complications of hemiplegic stroke with up to 50% of patients having thrombus in either the calf or thigh of the paretic limb. The risk of symptomatic intracerebral haemorrhage outweighs the benefit from the prevention of venous thromboembolism (VTE) with routine anticoagulation with low dose heparin (including low molecular weight heparin) following acute ischaemic stroke. It is also not possible to predict which patients with acute stroke may be at sufficiently high risk of VTE compared to haemorrhagic complications to inform the targeted use of heparin treatment in selected patients. The CLOTS 1 and 2 trials showed that graduated compression stockings were ineffective in preventing VTE or improving functional outcome in stroke. The landmark randomised controlled CLOTS 3 trial showed that intermittent pneumatic compression (IPC) in immobile patients in the first 30 days after stroke is an effective treatment for reducing proximal DVT and improves survival but not functional outcomes. Healthcare professionals should explain to the patient or their family members or carers that IPC reduces the risk of DVT and may provide an increase in survival, but it will not help them recover from their stroke, and there may be an associated increased risk of surviving with severe disability.

If proximal DVT does occur in a patient with ischaemic stroke, the risk of PE is high and such patients should receive treatment-dose anticoagulation. If DVT occurs in a patient with ICH there are no randomised trial data to support any particular treatment, but single-centre case series have reported that in such cases a vena caval filter is probably safe and effective for the prevention of PE. There is no evidence to guide the management of patients with ICH and PE, and the decision to use or to avoid the use of anticoagulant treatment can only be made on the physician's individualised assessment of the balance of risk and benefit.

16.8.1 Recommendations

1. Patients with immobility after acute stroke should be given intermittent pneumatic compression within 3 days of admission to hospital for the prevention of deep vein thrombosis. Treatment should be continuous for 30 days or until the patient is mobile or discharged, whichever is sooner.
2. Patients with immobility after acute stroke should not be routinely given low molecular weight heparin or graduated compression stockings (either full length or below knee) for the prevention of deep vein thrombosis.
3. Patients with ischaemic stroke and symptomatic deep vein thrombosis or pulmonary embolism should be given anticoagulation treatment provided there are no contraindications.
4. Patients with intracerebral haemorrhage and symptomatic deep vein thrombosis or pulmonary embolism should be given treatment with a vena caval filter.

16.9 Protocol for the Management of Thrombolysis

Patients should receive thrombolysis within 4.5 h of confirmed stroke onset unless after this time advanced imaging shows that there is salvageable brain tissue. All patients should have had a CT brain scan prior to treatment to confirm an ischaemic stroke and should have an examination and NIHSS score prior to treatment. Speed of treatment is essential for a good outcome after thrombolysis therefore hospital processes should allow rapid assessment and treatment of patients with thrombolysis.

16.9.1 Recommendations

1. All healthcare staff involved in thrombolysis should be trained in the hospital thrombolysis protocol, patient monitoring, and management of post-thrombolysis complications.
2. Patients having received thrombolysis should have the following treatment:

(a) No antiplatelets or anticoagulants for at least 24 h or until the repeat CT confirms there is no haemorrhagic changes.
(b) No arterial puncture for at least 24 h (unless essential).
(c) No urinary catheterisation unless for urinary retention.
(d) Blood pressure should be actively managed to below 180 mmHg systolic and 110 mmHg diastolic.
(e) Neurological observations:
    Every 15 min for 2 h, every 30 min for 6 h then hourly until 24 h
(f) Close nursing observations for complications of thrombolysis including angioedema, anaphylaxis, intra- and extracranial haemorrhage.
(g) Treatment for an anaphylactoid reaction including chlorphenamine, adrenaline, and hydrocortisone should be easily available near to the patient.
(h) Where extracranial haemorrhage is suspected, a full medical examination should take place. Any peripheral areas may require pressure support or bandaging. A suspected internal bleed may require further imaging or discussion with surgeons. Where the haemorrhage is suspected to be severe or life threatening the provision of fresh frozen plasma or cryoprecipitate may be necessary and haematology should be involved.
(i) For a suspected intracerebral haemorrhage, a repeat CT scan should take place within an hour and a management plan agreed.
(j) If the patient develops post-thrombolysis complications, the infusion should be stopped if still in progress.

3. Data should be collected on all thrombolysed patients including onset to treatment time, door to needle time, NIHSS on admission and at 24 h, pre-morbid and discharge Modified Rankin score.
4. Regular governance meetings should take place for stroke clinicians to discuss thrombolysis cases, present patients, and review service improvements required to improve the speed of treatment. This meeting should also review any thrombolysis related side effects such as symptomatic intracerebral haemorrhage.

16.10 Protocol for the Management of Swallowing After Stroke

The correct management of dysphagia after stroke can significantly improve patient's morbidity and mortality. The prevention of aspiration is a core component of stroke care.

16.10.1 Recommendations

1. All stroke patients should have a swallow screen performed by specially trained healthcare staff within 4 h of admission.
2. Patients should not receive any food, fluids or medication by mouth until the swallow screen has been completed.
3. Where the patient has failed the swallow screen, an alternative management plan to ensure adequate nutrition should be initiated within 24 h of hospital admission.
4. A nasogastric tube should be inserted if the patient is unable to maintain their oral nutrition intake.
5. Alternative hydration should be commenced within 4 h of admission if the patient is unable to maintain oral hydration—see hydration protocol.
6. If the patient can tolerate modified consistency diet and liquids, this should be initiated with regular reviews to ensure the swallow remains safe. If there are any signs of coughing, increased respiratory rate, wet voice or aspiration, the modified diet and liquids should be reviewed, and the patient considered to be placed nil by mouth.
7. Patients on modified diet and liquids should have a chest examination by doctors at least daily to ensure there are no clinical signs of aspiration.
8. Regular blood results should be performed to ensure there are no biochemical signs of aspiration or infection.

16.11 Protocol for the Management of Hyperlipidaemia After Acute Stroke

16.11.1 Recommendations

1. Patients with acute ischaemic stroke should receive high intensity statin treatment with atorvastatin 20–80 mg daily as soon as they can swallow medication safely. Treatment should target a > 40% reduction in non-HDL cholesterol and if not achieved within 3 months:
   (a) discuss adherence and timing of dose.
   (b) optimise adherence to dietary and lifestyle measures.
   (c) consider increasing to a high intensity dose if not prescribed from the outset.
2. All patients who have had an ischaemic stroke or TIA should receive advice on lifestyle factors that may modify lipid levels, including diet, physical activity, weight, alcohol, and smoking.
3. Patients with primary intracerebral haemorrhage should only be started on statin treatment based on their cardiovascular disease risk and not for secondary prevention of intracerebral haemorrhage.

4. Do not offer fibrates, bile acid sequestrants, nicotinic acid or omega-3 fatty acid compounds to individuals who have had TIA or stroke.

16.12 Protocol for the Management of Positioning and Early Mobilisation after Stroke

Therapeutic positioning aims to optimise recovery after stroke by reducing the likelihood of post-stroke complications. These include pressure damage, oedema, shoulder injury, pain and discomfort, and contractures. Good positioning can improve respiratory function, promote hydration and nutrition, and social interaction.

There are a number of detrimental effects of prolonged bed rest and immobility in hospitalised patients including muscle weakness, reduced respiratory function, postural hypotension, and increased risk of deep vein thrombosis. Early mobilisation after stroke aims to reduce the risks of immobility and minimise post-stroke complications thereby optimising recovery post-stroke.

16.12.1 Recommendations

1. Healthcare professionals responsible for the initial assessment of patients with acute stroke should be trained in how to position patients appropriately, taking into account the degree of their physical impairment after stroke (RCP 2016).
2. Patients with acute stroke (both ischaemia and haemorrhagic) should be helped and supported to sit upright as soon as they are awake and medically stable. This will help to reduce the risk of respiratory complications such as aspiration and lung collapse, prevent skin damage, and promote hydration and nutrition.
3. A supine position in bed is the least recommended position for stroke patients due to the increased likelihood of aspiration.
4. Sitting upright (above 45 degrees) will provide benefits for improved lung expansion and oxygenation, reduced aspiration risk, improved safety for eating and drinking, and improved social interaction (Tyson and Nightingale, 2004, McGlinchey et al., 2015).
5. Patients with acute stroke should be sat out of bed and supported to stand and walk as soon as possible, unless medically unstable. This should include frequent, short daily mobilisations with appropriate staffing, and equipment.
6. Safe seating of stroke patients should be considered as an essential component of care. Patients should be sat out of bed in a position that is erect, symmetrical, and aligned.

16.13 Protocol for the Management of Incontinence and Constipation After Stroke

A structured nurse-led protocol for the management of continence is recommended and can improve the quality of care for patients.

16.13.1 Recommendations

1. Urinary catheters should be avoided—unless essential for urinary retention or critical fluid balance monitoring.
2. Urinary catheters should be removed at the earliest opportunity when they are no longer required.
3. An assessment of urinary and faecal incontinence should be completed within 2 weeks of hospital admission to incorporate:
   (a) Pre-morbid history of bladder and bowel disturbance.
   (b) Continence monitoring to determine pattern of incontinence.
   (c) Rectal examination.
   (d) Post-void residual bladder volume ultrasound (for urinary incontinence).
   (e) Urinalysis to exclude urinary tract infection (for urinary incontinence).

   The results of the assessment should indicate the likely causes of incontinence, e.g., urge, stress, neurogenic, functional incontinence. The cause of incontinence will influence the treatment plan for each patient.
4. A plan for managing incontinence should be completed within 2 weeks of hospital admission based upon the continence assessment and likely causes of incontinence. The continence plans may include prompted toileting, timed toileting, bladder retraining, use of suitable supportive equipment. Medication should also be considered if appropriate to support bladder tone or detrusor muscle instability. The decision to use incontinence pads without toileting should be made only after opportunities to promote continence over several weeks have failed.
5. Patients should have daily monitoring of their bowel habits after stroke to include the frequency of bowel actions and the type of stool. A stool type chart such as the Bristol stool chart [3] (Fig. 16.3) should be used. This will allow early identification of constipation.
6. Laxatives should be prescribed to ensure regular bowel actions with an aim of avoiding constipation. The choice of laxatives will vary for each patient but should consider any pre-morbid laxatives used and the stool chart results. The choice of laxatives should consider whether the stool requires a softener, an emollient or a bulk forming laxative.
7. If constipation develops, the patient should receive either suppositories or an enema as soon as this is identified. Oral laxatives should be reviewed and increased to prevent further episodes of constipation. Hydration should also be reviewed.

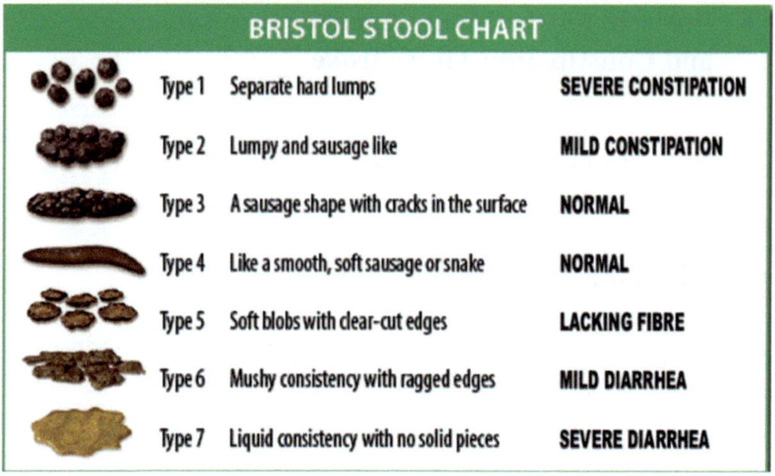

Fig. 16.3 By Cabot Health, Bristol Stool Chart - http://cdn.intechopen.com/pdfs-wm/46082.pdf, CC BY-SA 3.0, https://commons.wikimedia.org/w/index.php?curid=41761316

16.14 Protocol for the Insertion of Urinary Catheters

Urinary catheters should be avoided unless indicated as they are associated with increased morbidity and mortality after stroke. They increase the likelihood of a urinary tract infection and are likely to lead to bladder incompetence and increase problems with urinary incontinence. Urinary catheters should not be used to manage urinary incontinence.

16.14.1 Recommendations

1. Urinary catheters should only be inserted for the following indications:
   (a) Urinary retention—confirmed clinically and with post-void residual bladder scan.
   (b) Critical fluid balance such as associated with an acute kidney injury or acute renal failure.
   (c) Extensive pressure sore of grade 3 or 4 in the sacral area which would deteriorate further with urinary incontinence.
2. Where required urinary catheters should be inserted using aseptic technique by appropriately trained staff. The date of the insertion should be clearly documented.
3. Catheter care should be provided daily to observe for any signs of infection and catheter bags should be emptied regularly. Catheter bags should be leg bags and attached securely to the patient's leg.

4. Urinary catheters should be removed as soon as they are no longer required. There is no indication for flip-flop valves or catheter occlusions such as using a spigot to improve bladder tone prior to catheter removal.
5. Following urinary catheter removal a continence management plan should be initiated to manage continence—see continence protocol.

16.15 Protocol for Use of Anti-Thrombotic and Anticoagulant Medication in Acute Stroke

16.15.1 Recommendations

1. For patients with ischaemic stroke or TIA and without paroxysmal or permanent AF:

   (a) clopidogrel should be the standard anti-thrombotic treatment at a dose of 75 mg daily,
   (b) offer aspirin 75 mg daily in combination with modified release dipyridamole 200 mg twice daily for those who are unable to tolerate clopidogrel,
   (c) offer aspirin 75 mg daily, if both clopidogrel and modified release dipyridamole are contraindicated or not tolerated,
   (d) offer modified release dipyridamole 200 mg twice daily, if both clopidogrel and aspirin are contraindicated or not tolerated,
   (e) the combination of aspirin and clopidogrel is not recommended unless there is another indication such as acute coronary syndrome or recent coronary stent procedure.

2. Antiplatelet therapy can be started or continued in patients with haemorrhagic infarction unless the clinician feels that the risk outweighs the benefits. Haemorrhage within an ischaemic infarct does not in itself constitute a contraindication to commencing or continuing antiplatelet therapy.
3. For patients with ischaemic stroke or TIA in paroxysmal, persistent or permanent atrial fibrillation (valvular or nonvalvular) or atrial flutter, anticoagulation should be the standard treatment. Anticoagulation:

   (a) should not be given after stroke or TIA until brain imaging has excluded haemorrhage.
   (b) should not be commenced in patients with uncontrolled hypertension,
   (c) of patients with disabling ischaemic stroke should be deferred until at least 14 days have passed from the onset; aspirin 300 mg daily should be used until this time.
   (d) of patients with non-disabling ischaemic stroke should be deferred for an interval at the discretion of the prescriber, but no later than 14 days from the onset.

(e) should be commenced immediately following a TIA once brain imaging has ruled out haemorrhage, using an agent with a rapid onset such as low molecular weight heparin or an oral direct thrombin or factor Xa inhibitor (the latter confined to patients with nonvalvular AF).

4. Anticoagulation should not be used for patients with stroke or TIA in sinus rhythm unless there is another indication such as a major cardiac source of embolism, cerebral venous thrombosis or arterial dissection.
5. Anticoagulation therapy for patients with TIA or stroke should be with:

   (a) adjusted-dose warfarin, target INR 2.5 (range 2.0–3.0), with a target time in the therapeutic range (TTR) of >72% or,
   (b) an oral direct thrombin inhibitor or factor Xa inhibitor (nonvalvular AF only).

6. For patients with cardioembolic stroke for whom treatment with anticoagulation is considered inappropriate:

   (a) antiplatelet treatment should not be used as an alternative for patients with absolute contraindications to anticoagulation (e.g., undiagnosed bleeding),
   (b) measures should be taken to reduce bleeding risk, using a tool such as HAS-BLED [4] (Fig. 16.4) to identify modifiable risk factors for patients with relative contraindications to anticoagulation. If after intervention for relevant risk factors, the bleeding risk is considered too high for anticoagulation, antiplatelet treatment should not be used as an alternative.

7. Anti-thrombotic treatment for patients with recurrent TIA or stroke should be the same as for those who have had a single event. More intensive antiplatelet therapy or anticoagulation treatment should only be given as part of a clinical trial or in exceptional clinical circumstances.

The HAS-BLED score is designed to assess the 1-year risk of major bleeding in patients with atrial fibrillation and therapeutic anticoagulation. Major bleeding is characterized as follows: intracranial hemorrhage, need for hospitalization, relevant hemoglobin drop, need for transfusion.
For risk stratification of ischemic stroke and thromboembolism in patients with atrial fibrillation, the **CHA_2DS_2-VASc score** can be used.

Hypertension	No	Yes (+1)
Abnormal renal function Dialysis, kidney transplantation, creatinine ≥ 200 µmol/l (≥ 2.26 mg/dl)	No	Yes (+1)
Abnormal liver function Liver disease, bilirubin > 2× ULN with ASAT/ALAT/AP > 3× ULN	No	Yes (+1)
Stroke history	No	Yes (+1)
Previous major Bleeding or predisposition to bleeding	No	Yes (+1)
Labile INR	No	Yes (+1)
Age > 65 years	No	Yes (+1)
Medications predisposing to bleeding Antiplatelet agents, NSAID	No	Yes (+1)
Alcohol ≥ 8 units/week	No	Yes (+1)

ULN = upper limit of normal, ASAT = aspartate transaminase, ALAT = alanine transaminase, AP = alkaline phosphatase, INR = international normalized ratio, NSAID = non-steroidal anti-inflammatory drugs

Fig. 16.4 HAS-BLED Score [3]

Interpretation

Points	Bleedings per 100 patient-years [1]	Risk for major bleeding [3]	Recommendation
0	1.13	0.9 %	Low risk for major bleeding Anticoagulation should be considered
1	1.02	3.4 %	Moderate risk for major bleeding Anticoagulation may be considered
2	1.88	4.1 %	
3	3.74	5.8 %	High risk of major bleeding Caution with anticoagulation. Alternatives should be considered.
4	8.7	8.9 %	
5	12.5	9.1 %	
> 5	-	-	Very high risk of major bleeding

Fig. 16.4 (continued)

16.16 Managing the Hemiplegic Shoulder and Post-Stroke Shoulder Pain

In stroke, the lack of muscle activation can result in weakness, muscle atrophy, and lack of use which can result in joint stiffness and oedema. Due to the hanging weight of the arm and lack of muscle activation, the shoulder joint structures can stretch and develop a partial dislocation or subluxation. Subluxation is associated with poor upper limb functional recovery and therefore it is important to carefully handle the upper limb after stroke to prevent damage to the soft tissue structures. Around one quarter of stroke patients develop hemiplegic shoulder pain which is often preventable with careful handling and positioning

16.16.1 Recommendations

1. Any patient with functional loss in their upper limb should have the risk of developing shoulder pain reduced by ensuring that everyone handles the weak upper limb correctly, avoiding pulling, and excessive movement.
2. Hemiplegic upper limbs should be positioned consistently to ensure adequate support at all joints of the upper limb, e.g., on a pillow or table.

3. Healthcare staff should be trained on the management and positioning of the affected upper limb both in bed, in the chair and during mobilisation.
4. Supportive slings may provide support during transfers and mobilising but should be balanced with the risk of developing increased muscle tightness and joint stiffness. Where not required the sling should be removed after mobilising to allow good positioning of the arm and avoiding shortening of the muscles in a flexed position.
5. Shoulder examination should be completed by appropriately trained staff to identify any signs of shoulder subluxation and to alter the management plan accordingly.
6. Patients should be routinely assessed by appropriately trained staff to determine if they have any post-stroke shoulder pain. The assessment should include a determination of the triggers, severity, and type of pain. Visual assessment tools will be required for patients with dysphasia. If pain is suspected or confirmed, a pain monitoring plan should monitor the frequency and severity of pain.
7. Oral analgesics should be commenced to coincide with the triggers for pain for example before mobilising or therapy sessions. The choice of analgesic will vary according to the type of pain present.
   (a) Simple analgesics such as paracetamol should be considered in the first instance.
   (b) Neuroleptic agents may be beneficial for neuropathic pain but should be balanced with the side effects particularly drowsiness.
   (c) Opiates should be considered carefully with the increased risk of constipation and delirium.
   (d) Analgesic patches such as lidocaine or buprenorphine patches for the affected area may be a helpful option.

16.17 Protocol for the Prevention of Pressure Sores

Stroke patients are at high risk of skin breakdown due to the effects of pressure, shearing, and friction. The prevention of pressure sores should be a core component of stroke unit care and should commence on hospital admission.

16.17.1 Recommendations

1. All stroke patients should have an assessment of their pressure sore risk within 12 h of admission. This should be with a standardised, validated tool such as the Waterlow score [5]. https://www.cgakit.com/_files/ugd/2a1cfa_e542f9127895455682b2e3191b34a6ba.pdf

2. A thorough skin inspection should also be performed within 12 h to identify any pre-existing areas of skin breakdown or wounds. Any wounds present should have a management plan initiated to prevent their further deterioration.
3. Patients identified at high risk of pressure area breakdown following the assessment should have a management plan in place which addresses the following areas:
   (a) Regular repositioning in bed and in the chair—likely to require 1–2 hourly position changes.
   (b) Provision of a foam bed mattress, at least 6inches thick.
   (c) Daily skin inspection to identify redness, discolouration or signs of skin breakdown.
   (d) Management of any incontinence to ensure skin moisture is reduced. Regular management of incontinence may help to prevent this.
   (e) Barrier creams which may reduce the effects of moisture.
   (f) Massage should not be used in the affected areas as this will increase the tissue damage.
4. Where skin breakdown occurs, the management plan should increase the interventions such as increased frequency of repositioning. A wound assessment should take place to document the size, depth, grade and condition of the wound. An appropriate dressing should be applied to aim for wound healing. The dressing used will depend upon the nature of the wound and may require a dressing to encourage desloughing or granulation.
5. Family members should receive training from healthcare staff on the identification of the signs of skin breakdown and the specific preventative plan for their relative. Visual information on leaflets can help to support understanding.

16.18 Protocol for the Management of Privacy and Dignity

Patients should be provided with privacy and dignity during their hospital stay.

16.18.1 Recommendations

1. Patients should be offered privacy during treatment including curtain/screen privacy from other patients during clinical examinations, personal care such as washing and dressing, management of incontinence.
2. There should be sufficient curtains or screens to ensure patients always have access to privacy. No patient should receive personal care or clinical examinations without privacy.
3. All family members should be advised on the protocol for maintaining privacy and should be encouraged to adhere to the use of curtains and screens.

4. Patients should be cared for in single sex areas. Male and female patients should not share a bedroom area. An exception may be required for the hyper-acute stroke area for the first 24 h but male and female segregation within the area may still be possible.
5. All patients will be treated equally regardless of their ethnicity, culture, gender, sexuality or religion.
6. Healthcare staff should introduce themselves to each patient at the start of each shift or ward round. The introduction should include their name and role within the stroke service e.g. doctor, nurse, therapist.
7. Patients and family members should be encouraged to ask questions of the healthcare team to ensure they understand their condition and their treatment plan.
8. Regular updates on the patient's clinical condition should be provided to the patient and their family.
9. Clinical information about patients should remain confidential within the healthcare team and only shared with others with patient consent.

16.19 Copies of Scores Used in Protocols

16.20 Bristol Stool Chart [3]

References

1. Teasdale G, Jennett B. Assessment of coma and impaired consciousness, A practical scale. Lancet. 1974;2(7872):81–4.
2. Brott T, Adams HP Jr, Olinger CP, Marler JR, Barsan WG, Biller J, et al. Measurements of acute cerebral infarction: a clinical examination scale. Stroke. 1989;20:864–70.
3. Cabot Health, Bristol Stool Chart—http://cdn.intechopen.com/pdfs-wm/46082.pdf. CC BY-SA 3.0. https://commons.wikimedia.org/w/index.php?curid=41761316.
4. Lip GY. Implications of the CHA(2)DS(2)-VASc and HAS-BLED scores for thromboprophylaxis in atrial fibrillation. Am J Med. 2011;124(2):111–4.
5. Waterlow J. Pressure sores: a risk assessment card. Nurs Times. 1985;81:49–55.

Chapter 17
Longer Term Impact of Stroke

An Quang Nguyen, Thuan Duc Nguyen, Ton Duy Mai, and Ngoc Huy Nguyen

17.1 Introduction

Very few patients who have a stroke have no long-term sequalae even if they make a full neurological recovery. Everyone will realise that they have had an illness that could have killed them or left them with long-term disability. Every stroke survivor will have concerns about whether and when they will have a further event. Having a stroke even with ‘full recovery’ has consequences for employment, buying life insurance and for many it has an impact on relationships. This chapter covers the epidemiology and management of the long-term consequences of stroke and highlights areas where we need further research.

A. Q. Nguyen (✉)
Phutho Medical College, Phutho, Vietnam
e-mail: longdangtrang@gmail.com

T. D. Nguyen
Neurology Department, Military Hospital 103, Vietnam Military Medical University, Hanoi, Vietnam

T. D. Mai
Stroke Center, Bach Mai Hospital, Hanoi, Vietnam

VNU University of Medicine and Pharmacy, Hanoi, Vietnam

Hanoi Medical University, Hanoi, Vietnam

N. H. Nguyen
VNU University of Medicine and Pharmacy, Hanoi, Vietnam

Phutho Department of Health, Phutho, Vietnam
e-mail: ngochuynguyen8888@gmail.com

A. Rudd et al. (eds.), *Stroke Management in Vietnam*,
https://doi.org/10.1007/978-981-96-0221-6_17

17.2 Long-Term Effects of Stroke

17.2.1 Self-Reported Outcomes

A population-based survey in south London UK [1] reported that one-third of survivors were severely or moderately disabled and two-fifths of survivors were more disabled than they had been at 3 months after their stroke. The range of problems identified by the patients is summarized in Fig. 17.1.

The survey using two population based registries in the UK (SLSR) and the Oxford Vascular Registry (OXVASC) and a national cohort recruited through a random selection of patients from the Medical Research Council General Practice Research Framework by McKevitt et al. [1] found that 51% reported having no unmet needs between 3 months and 2 years after stroke. Of those reporting unmet needs, the number ranged from 1 to 13, with a median of 3 (Table 17.1) 52% of those surveyed, who were still in employment at the time of the stroke, were unable to return to work or had reduced their hours and 67% reported reduced participation in leisure activities. Thirty-one percent reported increased expenses. Forty-two percent reported a negative change in relationship with their partner, and 26% reported negative changes in family relationships. Patients living in deprived areas of the UK were significantly more likely to report long-term problems compared to those in affluent areas. Comparable data have not been found for patients in Vietnam.

17.2.2 Long-term Survival After Stroke

Crichton's paper 2016 [2] reports survival up to 15 years after first stroke for 2625 patients from the South London Stroke Register which is a population-based register with very high case ascertainment. It includes data for patients with all strokes including all ischaemic types, primary intracerebral haemorrhage, and subarachnoid haemorrhage. Slightly less than a quarter of patients are still alive 15 years after their initial stroke but for an illness where the average age of onset in this group was 73 years, it is not surprising that the survival rates were relatively low up to 15 years. Unfortunately, data for an age matched healthy cohort is not provided in the paper to show the extent to which the stroke contributed to the mortality rate.

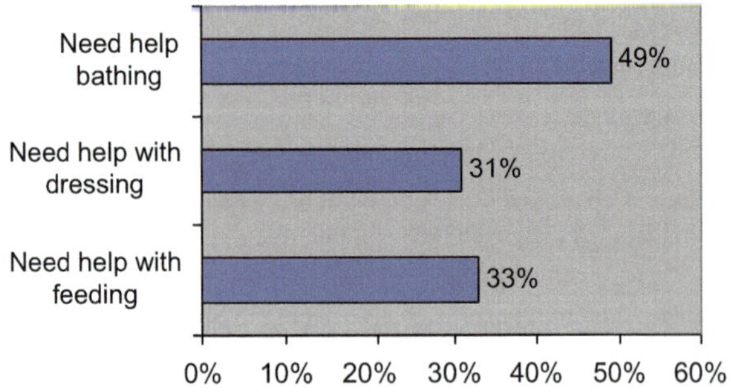

Fig. 17.1 Problems with activities of daily living reported by patients from the South London Stroke Register (SLSR) at 6 months after stroke

Table 17.1 Range of unmet needs 6 months after stroke from UK

	N reporting problem (weighted %)	Need unmet (%)	Need met to some extent (%)
Mobility	321 (58.4)	25	43
Falls	265 (43.9)	21	47
Incontinence	217 (37.2)	21	40
Pain	249 (39.5)	15	51
Emotional	244 (38.4)	39	34
Speech	194 (34.3)	28	33
Sight	212 (37.2)	26	39
Fatigue	301 (51.7)	43	36
Concentration	260 (44.7)	43	41
Memory	260 (42.8)	59	25
Reading	148 (23.2)	34	43

Another more recent population based cohort from Australia and New Zealand [3] provided data on survival by age, sex, and stroke subtype up to 10 years after first stroke for 313,162 patients (Fig. 17.2). Overall, 36.4% survived to 10 years so fairly comparable to the UK data.

17.2.3 Long-term Disability and Quality of Life

Again, no data were found on the prevalence of disability after stroke for Vietnamese populations. While the data from high income countries may differ, it does provide useful information for the future, particularly for a very rapidly developing economy such as Vietnam. The Crichton paper from South London [2] reports data on the prevalence of disability, activity, depression, and anxiety for the cohort divided into two groups, the entire period of 0–15 years and then separately for those patients who survived to 10 years looking at the pattern of disability between 10 and 15 years. Of 2625 people having first-ever stroke, 262 21% survived to 15 years. By 15 years, 61% (95% CI 55% to 67%) of the survivors were male, with a median age of stroke onset of 58 years (IQR 48–66). 87% of the 15-year survivors were living at home and 33.8% (26.2–42.4%) had mild disability, 14.3% (9.2–21.4%) moderate disability and 15.0% (9.9–22.3%) severe disability. The prevalence of disability increased with time but 1 in 10 of the 15-year survivors had lived with moderate-severe disability since their stroke. At 15 years, the prevalence of cognitive impairment was 30.0% (19.5–43.1%), depression 39.1% (30.9–47.9%), and anxiety 34.9% (27.0–43.8%), and survivors reported greater loss of physical than mental quality of life.

A separate paper, but using the same population register by Wolfe et al. [4] reported more granular data on the range of disabilities experienced by the patients (Fig. 17.3).

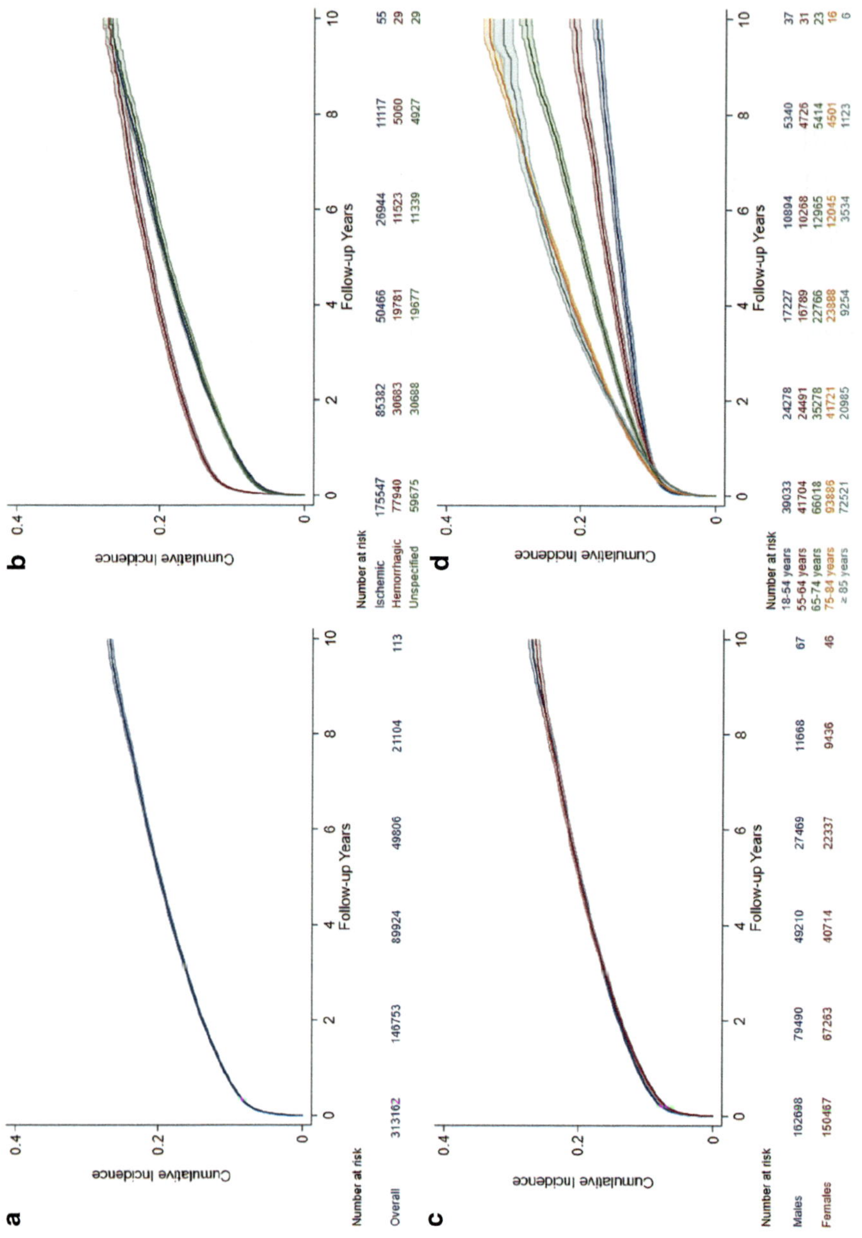

Fig. 17.2 Survival probability after a stroke hospitalisation. (**a**) All patients; (**b**) by stroke subtypes; (**c**) by sex; (**d**) by age [3]

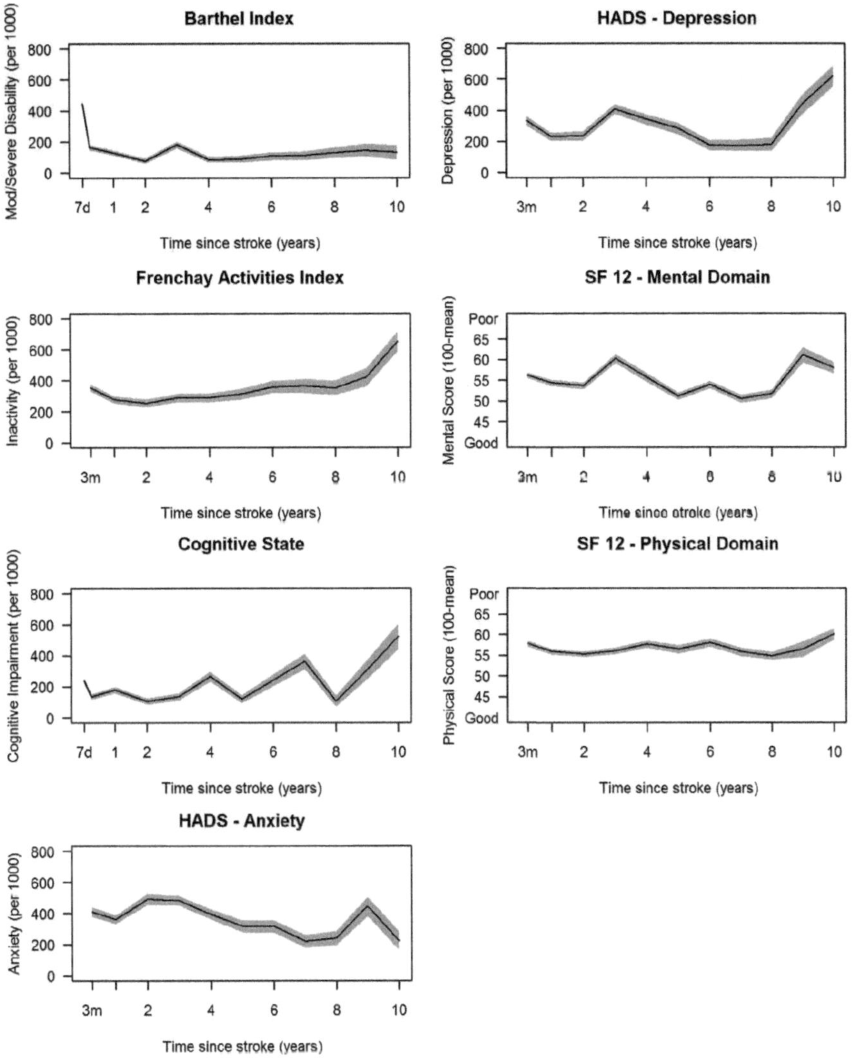

Fig. 17.3 Data on 10-year outcomes. HADS is the Hospital Anxiety and Depression score, Frenchay Activities Index scores performance on activities of daily living, SF12 is a score measuring Health Related Quality of Life [4]

17.3 Patterns of Recovery After Stroke

Recovery of impairments after stroke can continue for many months after the acute event. Language, sensory, and higher cognitive deficits are often slower to recover than motor deficits but there is huge individual variation that is affected by the type and severity of the stroke, age, prior disability and functional level, personality, access to and participation with treatment, and the development of complications. Models have been developed to try and predict recovery [5, 6] but while they may be useful for understanding populations of stroke patients, they are less useful for individual patients where labelling someone as 'untreatable' or 'likely to end up needing permanent care' may become self-fulfilling prophesies that result in poorer recovery than would be possible if rehabilitation was approached with an optimistic mind.

17.4 Stroke Complications

17.4.1 Central Post-Stroke Pain [6–8]

Central post-stroke pain (CPSP) is considered as a form of central pain, which follows a vascular event affecting the ascending pathways and/or their brainstem or cortical relays. It is usually associated with abnormal sensibility to temperature and to noxious stimulation. The term 'thalamic pain' used to be used, but it is a misleading term as it can arise from lesions in a variety of anatomical sites in the brain. Most imaging studies have shown CPSP is associated with lesions which include the ventero-posterior thalamic region Lesions involving cortical and brainstem regions may also give rise to CPSP. CPSP is also associated with medullary lesions as well as pontine and midbrain stroke, particularly infarction in the territory of the posterior inferior cerebellar artery. All forms of cerebrovascular disease have been reported to cause CPSP. However, the commonest causes include infarction in the territory of the thalamostriate artery, which involves the ventroposterior part of the thalamus, and the posterior inferior cerebellar artery (PICA) which supplies the lower brainstem.

The incidence of CPSP is extremely difficult to elucidate. There are many causes of pain following stroke and the onset of the pain may be delayed. In a prospective study of 191 patients, 8.4% developed central pain but 18% of those with somatosensory symptoms developed CPSP [9]. In a retrospective study, MacGowan [10] described CPSP in 25% of patients with brain stem stroke.

CPSP is highly variable in character, severity, and distribution. The history may be vague and 'non-anatomical' leading to a diagnosis of psychogenic pain. It is necessary to exclude underlying causes of post-stroke pain related to immobility, including shoulder and skin pain. The onset of CPSP may be highly variable with approximately 50% developing pain within a few days or during the first month, but in the remainder, the onset of pain may be delayed by up 3 years. The classical description of severe, intolerable, burning pain is common a significant number of patients experience a stinging or aching pain of less severity even with thalamic lesions. The pain is often extensive and diffuse. Others describe the pain as tearing, pricking, or lancinating. Although the pain may not be excruciating, it is frequently irritating and constant. Hyperaesthetic sensation is commonly associated with

CPSP. There may be increased sensation to a painful stimulus or allodynia if pain results from a stimulus that does not normally evoke pain.

CPSP can be extremely difficult to treat and responds poorly to a variety of physical, pharmacological, and interventional procedures. All treatments carry potential side effects some of which may be severe. They must be advised that treatment is often aimed at symptomatic relief rather than curing the pain. The first line of management is the treatment of any nociceptive component such as infection, skin changes, and abnormal posture as these enhance CPSP.

Tricyclic antidepressants are the most valuable drugs available for the treatments of CPSP and between 50 and 90% of patients derive benefit, the non-selective drugs seem to be most helpful. In a single controlled trail, 66% of patients responded to amitriptyline regardless of whether the CPSP had a thalamic or non-thalamic aetiology, but other studies of tricyclics have failed to support these results. The benefits of amitriptyline are probably independent of any depression in most patients but are dose dependent.

Antiepileptic drugs are frequently used to treat CPSP. Carbamazepine is the best studied—there is a small but significant effect in reducing central pain in a small group of patients with CPSP. Gabapentin, phenytoin, and valproate can be tried if carbamazepine is ineffective or not tolerated.

Local anaesthetics and anticonvulsants. There are occasional reports of systemic lignocaine and oral mexilitine being effective in treating CPSP.

Analgesics may be beneficial to a minority of patients and opiods are used in some with varying benefit.

Neurosurgical ablative and stimulation procedures: Many different lesioning procedures have been undertaken but no reliable technique has been found. The results are not favourable because of unacceptably high complication rates or return to postoperative pain levels after some time. While enthusiasm for ablative procedures has waned, there has been increasing use of stimulation procedures. TENS Transcutaneous electrical nerve stimulation (TENS) is simple and easy to administer, however, it can only be effective if the dorsal column—medial lemniscal pathways are still functionally intact and the patient has not lost touch and vibration sensation to the painful. Deep Brain Stimulation has not been subjected to adequate trials.

The recommendations in the UK National Stroke Guidelines [11] are:

- People with central post-stroke pain should be initially treated with amitriptyline, gabapentin or pregabalin:
  - amitriptyline starting at 10 mg/day, with gradual titration as tolerated, but no higher than 75 mg per;
  - gabapentin starting at 300 mg twice daily with titration as tolerated to a maximum of 3.6 g/day;
  - pregabalin starting at 150 mg/day with titration as tolerated but no higher than 600 mg/day in two divided doses.

- People with central post-stroke pain should be regularly reviewed including physical and psychological well-being, adverse effects, the impact on lifestyle, sleep, activities and participation, and the continued need for pharmacological treatment. If there is sufficient improvement, treatment should be continued and gradual reductions in the dose over time should be considered if improvement is sustained.

17.5 Spasticity and Contractures [12, 13]

Up to 40% of people who have significant weakness after a stroke will have some degree of spasticity. It is estimated that 15% of people will have severe disabling spasticity. The frequency depends on the size and location of the stroke and can be affected by the nursing and medical care that patients receive. Again, depending on the circumstances it can result in pain, limited motor recovery and contractures. Contractures can impede activities such as washing, dressing, walking, self-feeding, and even sitting comfortably and may be associated with pain.

The evidence for spasticity management includes a clinical guideline [14] and several RCTs of botulinum toxin some of which are summarised in systematic reviews [15, 16]. There is a Cochrane review of splinting and stretching [17] and two systematic reviews with meta-analyses of electrical stimulation [18, 19]. These show that electrical stimulation does not affect spasticity after stroke and should not be used alone for the purpose of reducing spasticity. The evidence base for splinting remains limited and therapists must be circumspect in identifying who and when to splint and when not to splint. A best practice guideline on splinting has also been produced by the UK College of Occupational Therapists & Association of Chartered Physiotherapists in Neurology [20].

Splints should only be assessed, fitted, and reviewed by appropriately skilled staff. Botulinum toxin administration improves spasticity, range of movement, and ease of care (i.e., passive function) but not active function. It is an expensive treatment, needing to be given usually every 3 months by experts in its administration. For it to be effective, it also needs to be followed by an active stretching and exercise programme, best delivered by physiotherapists with neurology expertise.

The recommendations from the UK National Stroke Guidelines [11] include the following:

- People with motor weakness after stroke should be assessed for spasticity as a cause of pain, as a factor limiting activities or care, and as a risk factor for the development of contractures.
- People with spasticity after stroke should be monitored to determine the extent of the problem and the effect of simple measures to reduce spasticity, e.g., positioning, passive movement, active movement (with monitoring of the range of movement and alteration in function), and/or pain control.

- People with persistent or progressive focal spasticity after stroke affecting one or two areas for whom a therapeutic goal can be identified (e.g., ease of care, pain) should be offered intramuscular botulinum toxin. This should be within a specialist multidisciplinary team and be accompanied by rehabilitation therapy and/or splinting or casting for up to 12 weeks after the injections. Goal attainment should be assessed 3–4 months after the injections and further treatment planned according to response.
- People with generalised or diffuse spasticity after stroke should be offered treatment with skeletal muscle relaxants (e.g., baclofen, tizanidine) and monitored for adverse effects, in particular, sedation and increased weakness. Combinations of anti-spasticity medication should only be initiated by healthcare professionals with specific expertise in managing spasticity.
- People with stroke with increased tone that is reducing passive or active movement around a joint should have the range of passive joint movement assessed. They should only be offered splinting or casting following individualised assessment and with monitoring by appropriately skilled staff.
- H People with stroke should not be routinely offered splinting for the arm and hand.
- I People with spasticity in the upper or lower limbs after stroke should not be treated with electrical stimulation to reduce spasticity.

17.6 Shoulder Subluxation and Pain

Hemiplegic shoulder pain affects 30–65% of people with stroke and is often associated with upper limb weakness, gleno-humeral subluxation, and a restricted range of shoulder movement [21]. It is associated with reduced function and recovery of the arm and may make physiotherapy more difficult and painful [22, 23]. While it is associated with subluxation of the shoulder joint, the two are not always present together. Subluxation can occur without pain and pain can occur without subluxation. Prevention is essential, particularly where the patient initially has reduced muscle tone. Mishandling of the patient by pulling on a paralysed flaccid arm can do major damage. So, all staff and relatives who might be moving and handling patients should be taught the correct techniques so that this does not happen.

Supporting the arm on elbow rests while the patient is sitting is good practice but there is no evidence that strapping the shoulder is of any use.

The literature on hemiplegic shoulder pain and shoulder subluxation in stroke consists of small trials and systematic reviews that evaluate interventions such as electrical stimulation of the long head of biceps [24]. A high quality systematic review and meta-analysis of 11 trials including 432 participants provided moderate to good evidence that neuromuscular stimulation can reduce shoulder subluxation for people when used in the acute or subacute stages of stroke (i.e., up to 6 months) [25]. The meta-analysis was underpowered to test the effects for people with chronic stroke and the impact on pain and function. Further research is needed to establish the optimal stimulation parameters and dose of stimulation.

Subacromial injections of corticosteroid [26] or local injections of botulinum toxin [27]. Have also been tested. Botulinum toxin injections showed some positive benefits in reducing pain and improving shoulder function and range of motion but low statistical power means that this intervention cannot be confidently recommended and larger high quality RCTs are required. There is little evidence to support shoulder strapping as a way of preventing or treating shoulder subluxation.

The UK guidelines recommend [11]:

- People with functional loss in their arm after stroke should have the risk of shoulder pain reduced by:
  - Careful positioning of the arm, with the weight of the limb supported, including the use of wheelchair arm rests.
  - Ensuring that healthcare staff and family/carers handle the affected arm correctly, avoiding mechanical stress, and excessive range of movement.
  - Avoiding the use of overhead arm slings/shoulder supports and pulleys.
- People who develop shoulder pain after stroke should:
  - Be assessed for causes and these should be managed accordingly, including musculoskeletal issues, subluxation, and spasticity.
- People with shoulder pain after stroke should only be offered intra-articular steroid injections if they also have inflammatory arthritis.
- People with inferior shoulder subluxation within 6 months of hemiplegic stroke should be considered for neuromuscular electrical stimulation, unless contraindicated.

17.7 Post-Stroke Seizures [28]

Seizures after stroke are divided into those that occur early after the stroke (usually defined as within the first 7–14 days) and better referred to as acute symptomatic seizures (ASS) and those that occur late or better termed unprovoked seizures (US). Following stroke, acute symptomatic seizures (manifestation within 7 days) and epilepsy, i.e., occurrence of at least one unprovoked seizure (manifestation after more than 7 days), are reported in 3–6% and up to 12% of patients, respectively. Incidence of acute symptomatic seizures is higher in intracranial haemorrhage (10–16%) than in ischaemic stroke (2–4%). The rates quoted above are those for symptomatic events. If asymptomatic seizures, only detected by doing EEG recording, are included rates are significantly higher. ASS are not sufficient to make a diagnosis of epilepsy as they are usually provoked by the acute ischaemic or haemorrhagic event and once the early structural and metabolic changes have resolved the seizures stop and often do not recur. Acute symptomatic seizures and unprovoked seizure may be associated with unfavourable functional outcome and increased mortality. The European Stroke Organisation has issued evidence-based guidelines on the management of post-stroke seizures and epilepsy [29]. No adequately powered randomised controlled trials were identified and so the evidence for all their recommendations is very low. In most instances, they suggest not giving antiepileptic drugs for ASS. Due to high incidence of seizure recurrence after one post-stroke unprovoked seizure, secondary antiepileptic drugs prophylaxis should be considered using conventional anticonvulsant drugs. Adequately powered randomised controlled trials are required to assess interventions for post-stroke seizure management [29].

17.8 Urinary and Faecal Incontinence

Patients after stroke often experience variable degrees of urinary frequency, urgency, or incontinence due to a number of causes. Neurogenic bladder can lead to incomplete bladder emptying. Patients often become constipated which can impair bladder emptying and patients with clouding of consciousness may lose bladder control. Immobility, particularly if there are insufficient staff around to help may lead to incontinence, as may significant communication problems. 25% of stroke patients have urinary incontinence at discharge and 15% are still incontinent at 1 year [30]. Urinary incontinence 30 days after a stroke is associated with almost four times the 1-year mortality of continent stroke survivors. Incontinence of urine greatly increases the risk of skin breakdown and pressure ulceration and is associated with high levels of depression and anxiety both for the patient and their carers. Incontinence of faeces is associated with more severe stroke and is more difficult to manage [31]. Constipation is common, occurring in 55% of people within the first month of stroke and can compound urinary and faecal incontinence.

The first stage in the management of both urinary and faecal incontinence is to try and establish the cause. With regard to faecal incontinence, has the patient become constipated and developed faecal impaction with overflow? If they are constipated, is it because of the immobility. Is it because they are being asked to defaecate on a bed pan while lying in bed (nearly impossible!)? Is the patient frightened to open their bowels because there is insufficient privacy and they are embarrassed to do it in public? Has the patient lost perineal sensation or awareness? For those patients with urinary incontinence, are they emptying their bladder adequately and if not is there significant urinary retention? If so, is the cause a neurogenic bladder or could there be another cause such as outflow obstruction from an enlarged prostate. Is there a urinary tract infection irritating the bladder, causing urgency and premature voiding? One certain way of the patient remaining incontinent is if a urinary catheter is inserted. While it may be necessary for patients with acute retention, although intermittent catheterisation is preferred, there are few other circumstances where an indwelling catheter is justified for the treatment of post-stroke incontinence.

A 2013 review of bowel management strategies [32] identified three small studies of varying quality, and concluded that the evidence was limited but a structured nurse-led approach may be effective. In a review of therapeutic education for people with stroke, Daviet et al. [33] concluded from small non-randomised studies that a nurse-targeted education programme may improve longer term continence. A small study by Guo et al. [34] examined the use of transcutaneous electrical nerve stimulation for the treatment of urinary incontinence over 6 months and found an improvement in nocturia, urgency, and frequency. The evidence-based recommendations in the UK National Clinical Guidelines [11] are as follows:

- Stroke unit staff should be trained in the use of standardised assessment and management protocols for urinary and faecal incontinence and constipation in people with stroke.
- People with stroke should not have an indwelling (urethral) catheter inserted unless indicated to relieve urinary retention or when fluid balance is critical.
- People with stroke who have continued loss of bladder and/or bowel control 2 weeks after onset should be reassessed to identify the cause of incontinence, and be involved in deriving a treatment plan (with their family/carers if appropriate). The treatment plan should include:
  - treatment of any identified cause of incontinence;
  - training for the person with stroke and/or their family/carers in the management of incontinence;
  - referral for specialist treatments and behavioural adaptations if the person is able to participate;
  - adequate arrangements for the continued supply of continence aids and services.
- People with stroke with continued loss of urinary continence should be offered behavioural interventions and adaptations prior to considering pharmaceutical and long-term catheter options, such as:
  - timed toileting;
  - prompted voiding;
  - review of caffeine intake;
  - bladder retraining;
  - pelvic floor exercises;
- People with stroke with constipation should be offered:
  - Advice on diet, fluid intake, and exercise
  - Regulated routine of toileting
  - medication review to minimise use of constipating medication;
  - oral laxatives
  - a structured bowel management programme which includes nurse-led bowel care interventions;
  - education and information for the person with stroke and their family/carers.

17.9 Venous Thromboembolism

The rates of deep venous thrombosis (DVT) and pulmonary embolism (PE) after stroke cited in the literature vary hugely depending on the patient population, especially stroke severity, and how hard clinicians look for thrombosis. In one study [35] where MRI direct thrombus imaging was used and which is very sensitive at identifying both DVT and PE reported that 50% of patient with hemiplegia had a DVT in the paretic leg, although many of these were below knee. Furthermore, it was reported that even though very few of these had been detected by the patients' physicians when the researcher examined each patient carefully including measurement of calf and thigh circumference many of them did demonstrate classical signs of DVT.

The risk of symptomatic intracerebral haemorrhage outweighs the benefit from the prevention of venous thromboembolism (VTE) with routine anticoagulation with low-dose heparin (including low molecular weight heparin) following acute ischaemic stroke [36]. It is also not possible to predict which patients with acute stroke may be at sufficiently high risk of VTE compared to haemorrhagic complications to inform the targeted use of heparin treatment in selected patients [37]. This assessment of the evidence differs from the American and European guidelines but our view is that the UK guidelines are the correct ones. The CLOTS 1 and 2 trials showed that graduated compression stocKing's were ineffective in preventing VTE or improving functional outcome in stroke [38]. The CLOTS 3 trial [39] showed that intermittent pneumatic compression (IPC) using sequential compression with venous refill technology in immobile patients in the first 30 days after stroke is an effective treatment for reducing proximal DVT and improves survival but not functional outcomes. The recommendations from the UK guidelines [11] for the prevention and management of venous thromboembolism are:

- Patients with immobility after acute stroke should be offered intermittent pneumatic compression within 3 days of admission to hospital for the prevention of deep vein thrombosis. Treatment should be continuous for 30 days or until the patient is mobile or discharged, whichever is sooner.
- Patients with immobility after acute stroke should not be routinely given low molecular weight heparin or graduated compression stocKing's (either full length or below knee) for the prevention of deep vein thrombosis.
- Patients with ischaemic stroke and symptomatic deep vein thrombosis or pulmonary embolism should receive anticoagulant treatment provided there are no contraindications.
- Patients with intracerebral haemorrhage and symptomatic deep vein thrombosis or pulmonary embolism should receive treatment with a vena caval filter.

17.10 Pressure Sores

Pressure sores should be seen as a failure in the quality of care (Fig. 17.4). The only circumstance where they are unavoidable is where a patient has had very delayed admission to hospital because they were unable to call for help after the acute stroke. The risk factors for developing pressure sores include immobility, age especially with thin fragile skin, incontinence of urine and faeces, poor manual handling of immobile patients, sensory and cognitive impairment, fever and infections, malnutrition, dehydration, obesity, and low body weight. Prevention of pressure sores is essential because once they have developed they are often very difficult to treat. All

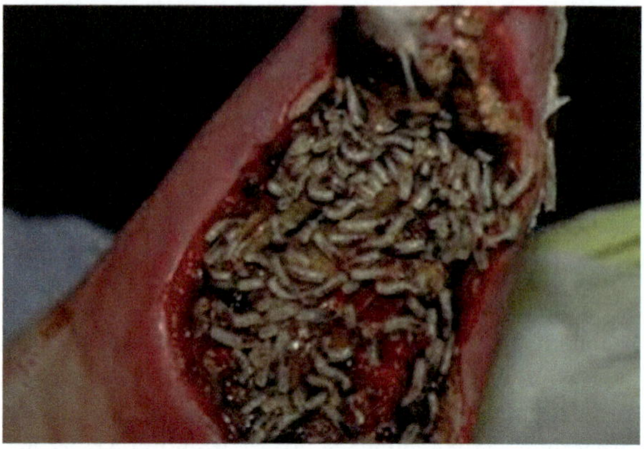

Fig. 17.4 Large heel pressure sore infected with maggots

patients should be screened using a validated score to assess their risk such as the Waterlow score [40] and identify those who require higher dependency nursing and specialised equipment. This assessment should be done on admission and repeated regularly until the patient is no longer at significant risk. Hospitals should keep an adequate supply of high quality pressure relieving mattresses. Nurses should be trained to manage pressure sore prevention and to recognise the early signs.

Once a sore has become established, there is no magic treatment. It almost does not matter what is put on to the sore, so long as it is not the patient. Pressure relief is the most important along with good skin hygiene, effective management of incontinence preferably without the use of an indwelling catheter and maintaining adequate nutrition.

Occurrence of pressure sores should be an important marker of quality of care and should be regularly audited.

17.11 Fatigue and Apathy

Post-stroke fatigue is characterised by a disproportionate sense of tiredness, a lack of energy, and a need to rest that is greater than usual. Clearly, there are similarities with post covid fatigue and other post viral fatigue syndromes although no common mechanisms have been found. There is no consensus on how to define post-stroke fatigue, but it does need to be differentiated from post-stroke apathy which is a reduction in goal-directed activity in behavioural, cognitive or social dimensions of a person's life in comparison to their previous level of functioning. Apathy occurs in about one third of people with stroke and has a negative impact on functional outcomes and is under-recognised and poorly understood [41].

Post-stroke fatigue can profoundly impact the lives of people with stroke, particularly their return to work, activities of daily living mood, cognitive function as well as the lives of the people who live with them. Post-stroke fatigue is common and may be the sole residual problem in people who have made an otherwise good recovery. Between 35% and 92% of people with stroke are estimated to have post-stroke fatigue [42]. Post-stroke fatigue may present early or later after stroke, while early-onset fatigue persists in a proportion of cases [43].

Post-stroke fatigue appears to be multifactorial and may fluctuate over the course of the day and vary in severity. It is commonly associated with pre-stroke fatigue, age, female gender, pain, and sleep disorder. There is no consensus or any strong evidence to indicate how it is best treated but having health professionals who believe in its existence is important. Patients should be asked about whether it is present and some attempt to measure its severity should be attempted. Associated problems such as sleep disorder and depression both of which may be treatable should be addressed. The evidence for treatment is summarised in the Cochrane review [44] and a more recent meta-analysis [45]. There is clear evidence that fluoxetine and therefore probably other antidepressants should not be used as it is not effective, and increases the likelihood of falls, fractures and epileptic seizures. There is some suggestion that acupuncture may help but the evidence is not sufficiently strong to recommend its routine use.

Apathy, as with fatigue often fails to be recognised by clinicians. Again, it is probably multifactorial and may be associated with depression, anxiety and cognitive impairment. There are no evidence-based interventions that have been shown to work so more research is badly needed. It is important that the approaches to treatment are considered by the whole multidisciplinary team and of course take into consideration the views of the patient and their carers.

17.12 Cognitive Impairment [46]

Stroke can have an impact on many facets of cognition including memory, attention, and concentration, perception, and executive function. Memory loss is a characteristic feature of dementia, which affects about 20% of people after stroke often in those patients with pre-existing diffuse cerebrovascular disease. Careful assessment of the whole range of cognitive abilities is important as it is important, for example, to differentiate memory loss secondary to dementia from memory loss associated with poor sleep fatigue and impaired concentration. About 10% of patients develop cognitive impairment after the initial stroke and about 30% at the end of 1 year. Risk factors for developing dementia include advanced age, previous stroke, lacunar infarction, diabetes mellitus, and left hemisphere stroke.

17.13 Headache

This is a topic that is relatively poorly addressed by the research literature. One recent paper [47] studied 529 patients with first-ever ischaemic stroke to establish the frequency of headache lasting at least 3 months. At 3 months, 61 patients (11.5%) had a headache. Of these 6 were suffering headaches that had existed pre-stroke so the overall incidence was 10.4%. Many of the patients ended up taking excessive amounts of medication. The factors associated with headaches were lack of sleep, 29.1% and cerebellar infarction (18.2%).

17.14 Depression and Anxiety

Mood disturbance is very common after stroke. It may present as low mood, depression, anxiety, or emotionalism. Many people with stroke have psychological distress that does not meet diagnostic criteria for depression and anxiety but which nevertheless disrupts their lives. Healthcare professionals should be aware that mood disturbance after stroke can arise because of psychosocial factors (e.g., disability, loss, trauma), or because of neurochemical changes in the brain, or both.

Depression affects about one-third of people with stroke and frequently persists long-term [48]. Anxiety affects about 25% of people after stroke but may only become evident after several months [49]. A survey of long-term needs found that nearly three-quarters of people with emotional difficulties felt their needs had not been fully met [1]. There are three important high quality Cochrane reviews. One on the treatment of anxiety [50] and two on preventing and treating depression [51, 52]. For anxiety, the Cochrane review of three studies indicated that psychological interventions and medication treatments appear useful, but the studies were of low quality. SSRIs reduce anxiety but no single SSRI is superior to any other.

The Cochrane review of depression prevention in 19 RCTs with 1771 patients found that there was low quality evidence that selective serotonin reuptake inhibitors (SSRIs) can prevent depression in some people at risk of depression after stroke but there remains uncertainty over the balance of benefits and risk of adverse events. There have been three large scale RCTs of fluoxetine in the first days following stroke [53–55]. The trials were designed to assess functional recovery but collected information on the incidence of depression. Two of the studies suggested that medication therapy could reduce depression, but at the cost of more serious adverse events, principally seizures, and hip fracture.

A Cochrane review of depression treatment [52] of 49 trials and over 3000 patients synthesised low quality (high risk of bias) evidence that non-invasive brain stimulation and psychological interventions may be of benefit in the treatment of depression, in addition to pharmacological treatment with SSRIs. Psychological interventions were evaluated as a standalone treatment and were found to be as effective as combined therapy (SSRI and psychological therapy). The recommendation in the UK National Stroke Guidelines [11] derived from this evidence include:

- A Healthcare professionals should be aware of the psychological needs of people with stroke and their family/carers, and routinely provide education, advice, and emotional support for them. Multidisciplinary teams should embed measures that promote physical and mental well-being including increased social interaction, activities to support rebuilding of self-confidence and self-esteem, increased exercise, and mind-body interventions such as relaxation, mindfulness, Tai Chi, and yoga.

- People with stroke should be routinely screened for anxiety and depression using standardised tools, the results of which should be used alongside other sources of information to inform clinical formulation of treatment and support needs.
- People with stroke should be offered one-to-one motivational interviewing or problem-solving therapy, adapted as necessary for people with aphasia or cognitive impairment, as part of a multidisciplinary rehabilitation approach to prevent depression.
- People with stroke should not be routinely offered SSRIs for the prevention of depression, but SSRIs may be considered when other preventative approaches are not appropriate (e.g., in people with severe cognitive or language impairment) or when the risk of depression is high (e.g., in people with a previous history of depression).
- People with depression after stroke should be offered psychological interventions (motivational interviewing, cognitive behavioural therapy or problem-solving therapy)

17.15 Emotionalism

Around 20% of people with stroke are affected in the 6 months and although frequency decreases by 12 months, more than 10% remain affected [56]. It is often very distressing for both the patient and their family. While it typically occurs in association with bilateral anterior frontal cortical lesions or subcortical disease leading to white matter tract disruption and bilateral frontal cortical disconnection, it has been associated with lesions almost anywhere in the brain. There has been very little research into it and no randomised studies since the Cochrane review in 2010 [56]. There is not strong evidence to support the use of antidepressants but most clinicians think that judicious use is justified. People with severe or persistent emotionalism after stroke should be given antidepressant medication, monitoring effectiveness by the frequency of crying. They should be monitored for adverse effects and treated for at least 4 months beyond initial recovery. If the patients' emotionalism has not improved after 2–4 weeks check whether they are taking the drug and either increase the dose or change to an alternative antidepressant. There is no evidence to suggest that any particular antidepressant is any better than any other.

17.16 Sleep [57]

Sleep apnoea is a risk factor for stroke and if present before the stroke is likely to continue after it. Insomnia is common in stroke patients and affects 20–56% of them. About 18% of the people reported new-onset insomnia after their stroke. Insomnia typically occurs in the setting of the acute phase of the stroke. There is a higher prevalence after right hemispheric strokes as well as those within the thalamus or brainstem. But probably more frequently sleep problems arise from anxiety following a major life event, being in hospital where sleep is always disturbed, difficulty getting comfortable because of impaired movement and sensory abnormalities including pain. There may also be disturbed circadian rhythms. The loss of the normal routine of daytime activity followed by night time somnolence is also a major issue.

In addition to insomnia hypersomnolence can also be an issue, particularly after thalamic stroke especially bilateral thalamic lesions.

17.17 Sex and Relationships [11]

The physical and psychological impact of stroke can affect personal identity and relationships with sexual partners. Sexual dysfunction is common after stroke, affecting both the person with stroke and their partner. It is typically multifactorial including other vascular disease, altered sensation, limited mobility, the effects of medication, mood changes, and fear of precipitating further strokes. Sex and sexual dysfunction after stroke is often not discussed because of reluctance on the part of both the patient, their partner and the health professional. It is important to overcome the barriers to addressing the issues as there are often solutions. The first and most important is to reassure patients and partners that sexual activity is safe and is extremely unlikely to precipitate a further stroke or heart attack. For patients with impaired mobility advice about alternative sexual positions can be helpful. Although it is probably sensible to avoid the use of a phosphodiesterase type 5 inhibitor such as sildenafil for the first 3 months after the acute stroke, after that time, so long as major risk factors such as hypertension are controlled there is no reason to withhold it.

17.18 Visual Problems

Visual problems after stroke are common. In a multicentre prospective cohort study, 58% of people with stroke were found to have visual problems and about half of them, regardless of the visual impairment type, were visually asymptomatic [58, 59]. Visual problems include altered acuity, field loss such as hemianopia and disruption of eye movements causing diplopia, nystagmus, blurred vision, and loss of depth perception. Perceptual disorders such as visual agnosia should be distinguished from visual impairments. Visual disturbance has a significant impact on confidence, safety and independence and should therefore remain a focus for all members of the multidisciplinary team to support with identification, adjustment and adaptation. People with visual changes following stroke who were previously driving should be advised to seek specialist advice about whether it is safe to drive and whether their condition means that they do not comply with Vietnamese laws about driving.

For people with visual field loss after stroke, interventions are focussed on compensating for the visual field defect by changing their behaviour or activity, substituting for the defect by using devices such as prisms to shift the field of view from the affected side, or restoring the visual field through repetitive stimulation of the affected field of vision. Compensatory training includes both visual scanning training, which involves repetitive symmetrical movements to each (right/left) side and visual search training, which involves repeatedly looking for (searching) for objects on each side. A Cochrane review found that there is limited, low quality evidence that compensatory training, and in particular visual scanning and search training, may be more beneficial than placebo [60].

17.19 Dysphagia

Dysphagia is common after acute stroke with an incidence between 40 and 78%. There is an association between dysphagia and poor outcomes including a higher risk of longer hospital stay, chest infection, disability and death Evidence from national audit in the UK shows that delays in the screening and assessment of dysphagia are associated with an increased risk of stroke-associated pneumonia [61]. Prompt detection of dysphagia in patients with acute stroke is therefore essential.

The majority of people with dysphagia after stroke will recover, in part due to bilateral cortical representation of neurological pathways) but a proportion will have persistent abnormal swallow and continued aspiration at 6 months [62] and a small proportion, particularly those with brainstem lesions, will have chronic and severe swallowing difficulty. People with persistent swallowing problems may avoid eating in social settings and thus lose the physical and social pleasures connected with food and drink. This section is not addressing the acute management of dysphagia. For those people whose dysphagia persists longer term, the UK National Stroke Guidelines [11] make the following recommendations:

- People with swallowing difficulty after stroke should be considered for swallowing rehabilitation by a specialist in dysphagia management. This should be based on a thorough assessment of dysphagia, such as by a speech and language therapist, to decide on the most appropriate behavioural intervention, and may include a variety of muscle strengthening and/or skill training exercises.
- People with dysphagia after stroke may be considered for neuromuscular electrical stimulation as an adjunct to behavioural rehabilitation where the device is available and it can be delivered by a trained healthcare professional.
- People with difficulties feeding themselves after stroke should be assessed and provided with the appropriate equipment and assistance (including physical help and verbal encouragement) to promote independent and safe feeding.
- People with stroke should be considered for gastrostomy feeding if they:

  - need, but are unable to tolerate, nasogastric tube feeding, even after a trial with a nasal bridle if appropriate and other measures such as taping the tube or increased supervision;
  - are unable to swallow adequate food and fluids orally by 4 weeks from the onset of stroke and gastrostomy feeding is considered to be required long-term;

- People with stroke receiving end-of-life (palliative) care should not have burdensome restrictions on oral food or fluids if those restrictions would exacerbate suffering. In particular, following assessment this may involve a decision, taken together with the person with stroke, their family/carers and the multidisciplinary team, to allow oral food or fluids despite risks including aspiration and choking.

17.20 Needs of Families and Carers [63]

Carers' needs are frequently unrecognised and both physical and psychological morbidities are high. Failure to identify and manage these problems can result in the home situation for the patient becoming untenable. Carers need information, skills training, emotional support, regular respite, advice about support, and easy access to aids and equipment. There may also be the need to try and identify some financial support. The first stage is to ensure that carers are not forgotten when the stroke patient is followed up.

17.21 Summary

The effects of stroke are for many patients long lasting and disabling. They include things which are clearly visible but also things which are less evident, especially psychological and cognitive issues. These are easily missed if the patient is not followed up long term by clinicians who have a detailed knowledge of the long-term effects of stroke. Many of the long-term effects are treatable but they need to be recognised in order to treat them. The specialty of stroke is not just about learning how to thrombolyse and perform thrombectomy. It is also about managing the patient's long-term problems.

References

1. McKevitt C, Fudge N, et al. Self-reported long-term needs after stroke. Stroke. 2011;42(5):1398–403.
2. Crichton SL, Bray BD, et al. Patient outcomes up to 15 years after stroke: survival, disability, quality of life, cognition and mental health. J Neurol Neurosurg Psychiatry. 2016;87(10):1091–8.

3. Peng Y, Ngo L, et al. Long-term survival, stroke recurrence, and life expectancy after an acute stroke in Australia and New Zealand from 2008-2017: a population-wide cohort study. Stroke. 2022;53(8):2538–48.
4. Wolfe CD, Crichton SL, et al. Estimates of outcomes up to ten years after stroke: analysis from the prospective South London Stroke Register. PLoS Med. 2011;8(5):e1001033.
5. Tilling K, Sterne JA, et al. A new method for predicting recovery after stroke. Stroke. 2001;32(12):2867–73.
6. Klit H, Finnerup NB, Jensen TS. Central post-stroke pain: clinical characteristics, pathophysiology, and management. Lancet Neurol. 2009;8(9):857–68.
7. Mulla SM, Wang L, et al. Management of central poststroke pain: systematic review of randomized controlled trials. Stroke. 2015;46(10):2853–60.
8. Liampas A, Velidakis N, et al. Prevalence and management challenges in central post-stroke neuropathic pain: a systematic review and meta-analysis. Adv Ther. 2020;37:3278–91.
9. Andersen G, Vestergaard K, et al. Incidence of central post-stroke pain. Pain. 1995;61:187–93.
10. MacGowan DJL, Janal MN, et al. Central post-stroke pain and Wallenberg's lateral medullary infarction: frequency, character, and determinants in 63 patients. Neurology. 1997;49:120–5.
11. UK National Clinical Guidelines for Stroke. 2023. https://www.strokeguideline.org/.
12. Glaess-Leistner S, Ri SJ, et al. Early clinical predictors of post stroke spasticity. Top Stroke Rehabil. 2021;28(7):508–18.
13. Zeng H, Chen J, Guo Y, Tan S. Prevalence and risk factors for spasticity after stroke: a systematic review and meta-analysis. Front Neurol. 2021;11:616097.
14. Royal College of Physicians, Chartered Society of Physiotherapy, British Society of Rehabilitation Medicine, & Association of Chartered Physiotherapists Interested in Neurology. Spasticity in adults: management using botulinum toxin. National Guidelines. Royal College of Physicians. 2018. https://www.rcplondon.ac.uk/guidelines-policy/spasticity-adults-management-using-botulinum-toxin.
15. Elia AE, Filippini G, et al. Botulinum neurotoxins for post-stroke spasticity in adults: a systematic review. Mov Disord. 2009;4(6):801–12.
16. Rosales RL, Kong KH, et al. Botulinum toxin injection for hypertonicity of the upper extremity within 12 weeks after stroke: a randomized controlled trial. Neurorehabil Neural Repair. 2012;26(7):812–21.
17. Katalinic OM, Harvey LA, Herbert RD. Effectiveness of stretch for the treatment and prevention of contractures in people with neurological conditions: a systematic review. Phys Ther. 2011;91(1):11–24.
18. Johnston TE, Keller S, et al. A clinical practice guideline for the use of ankle-foot orthoses and functional electrical stimulation post-stroke. J Neurol Phys Ther. 2021;45(2):112–96.
19. Tang Y, Wang L, et al. Optimal method of electrical stimulation for the treatment of upper limb dysfunction after stroke: a systematic review and Bayesian network meta-analysis of randomized controlled trials. Neuropsychiatr Dis Treat. 2012;17:2937–54.
20. College of Occupational Therapists, & Association of Chartered Physiotherapists in Neurology. Splinting for the prevention and correction of contractures in adults with neurological dysfunction. 2015. https://www.acpin.net/pdfs/Splinting_Guidelines.pdf.
21. Kumar R, Metter EJ, et al. Shoulder pain in hemiplegia: the role of exercise. Am J Phys Exercise Rehabil. 1990;69:205–8.
22. Adey-Wakeling Z, Liu E, et al. Hemiplegic shoulder pain reduces quality of life after acute stroke: a prospective population-based study. Am J Phys Med Rehabil. 2016;95(10):758–63.
23. Paolucci S, Iosa M, et al. Prevalence and time course of post-stroke pain: a multicenter prospective hospital-based study. Pain Med. 2016;17(5):924–30.
24. Manigandan JB, Ganesh GS, et al. Effect of electrical stimulation to long head of biceps in reducing gleno humeral subluxation after stroke. NeuroRehabilitation. 2014;34(2):245–52.
25. Lee JH, Baker L, et al. Effectiveness of neuromuscular electrical stimulation for management of shoulder subluxation post-stroke: a systematic review with meta-analysis. Clin Rehabil. 2017;31(11):1431–44.

26. Rah UW, Yoon SH, et al. Subacromial corticosteroid injection on poststroke hemiplegic shoulder pain: a randomized, triple-blind, placebo-controlled trial. Arch Phys Med Rehabil. 2012;93(6):949–56.
27. Singh JA, Fitzgerald PM. Botulinum toxin for shoulder pain. Cochrane Database Syst Rev. 2010;9:CD008271.
28. Holtkamp M, Beghi E, et al. Current advances on mechanisms and treatment of post-stroke seizures. Acta Epileptol. 2021;3:4. https://doi.org/10.1186/s42494-021-00047-z.
29. European Stroke Organisation. European Stroke Organisation guidelines for the management of post-stroke seizures and epilepsy. Eur Stroke J. 2017;2(2):103–15.
30. Patel M, Coshall C, et al. Natural history and effects on 2-year outcomes of urinary incontinence after stroke. Stroke. 2001;32:122–7.
31. Harari D, Coshall C, et al. New-onset fecal incontinence after stroke: prevalence, natural history, risk factors, and impact. Stroke. 2003;34:144–50.
32. Lim SF, Childs C. A systematic review of the effectiveness of bowel management strategies for constipation in adults with stroke. Int J Nurs Stud. 2013;50(7):1004–10.
33. Daviet JC, Bonan I, et al. Therapeutic patient education for stroke survivors: non-pharmacological management. A literature review. Ann Phys Rehabil Med. 2012;55(9-10):641–56.
34. Guo ZF, Liu Y, et al. Transcutaneous electrical nerve stimulation in the treatment of patients with poststroke urinary incontinence. Clin Interv Aging. 2014;9:851–6.
35. Kelly J, Rudd A, et al. Venous thromboembolism after acute ischaemic stroke. A prospective study using magnetic resonance direct thrombus imaging. Stroke. 2004;35:2320–6.
36. Geeganage CM, Sprigg N, et al. Balance of symptomatic pulmonary embolism and symptomatic intracerebral hemorrhage with low-dose anticoagulation in recent ischemic stroke: a systematic review and meta-analysis of randomized controlled trials. J Stroke Cerebrovasc Dis. 2013;22(7):1018–27.
37. Whiteley WN, Adams HP, et al. Targeted use of heparin, heparinoids, or low-molecular-weight heparin to improve outcome after acute ischaemic stroke: an individual patient data meta-analysis of randomised controlled trials. Lancet Neurol. 2013;12(6):539–45.
38. CLOTS Trials Collaboration. The effect of graduated compression stocKing's on long-term outcomes after stroke: the CLOTS trials 1 and 2. Stroke. 2013;44(4):1075–9.
39. CLOTS Trials Collaboration. Effect of intermittent pneumatic compression on disability, living circumstances, quality of life, and hospital costs after stroke: secondary analyses from CLOTS 3, a randomised trial. Lancet Neurol. 2014;13(12):1186–92.
40. Papanikolaou P, Lyne P, Anthony D. Risk assessment scales for pressure ulcers: a methodological review. Int J Nurs Stud. 2007;44(2):285–96.
41. Tay J, Morris RG, Markus HS. Apathy after stroke: diagnosis, mechanisms, consequences, and treatment. Int J Stroke. 2021;16(5):510–8.
42. Duncan F, Wu S, Mead GE. Frequency and natural history of fatigue after stroke: a systematic review of longitudinal studies. J Psychosom Res. 2012;73(1):18–27.
43. Wu S, Mead G, et al. Model of understanding fatigue after stroke. Stroke. 2015;46(3):893–8.
44. Legg LA, Tilney R, et al. Selective serotonin reuptake inhibitors (SSRIs) for stroke recovery. Cochrane Database Syst Rev. 2019;11:CD009286.
45. Chen K, Marsh EB. Chronic post-stroke fatigue: it may no longer be about the stroke itself. Clin Neurol Neurosurg. 2018;174:192–7.
46. El Husseini N, Katzan IL, et al. Cognitive impairment after ischemic and hemorrhagic stroke: a scientific statement from the American Heart Association/American Stroke Association. Stroke. 2023;54(6):e272–91.
47. Lebedeva ER, Ushenin AV, Gurary NM, Gilev DV, Olesen J. Diagnostic criteria for acute headache attributed to ischemic stroke and for sentinel headache before ischemic stroke. J Headache Pain. 2022;23(1):11.
48. Ayerbe L, Ayis S, et al. The long-term outcomes of depression up to 10 years after stroke; the South London Stroke Register. J Neurol Neurosurg Psychiatry. 2014;85(5):514–21.

49. Knapp P, Campbell Burton CA, et al. Interventions for treating anxiety after stroke. Cochrane Database Syst Rev. 2017;5(5):CD008860.
50. Campbell Burton CA, et al. Interventions for treating anxiety after stroke. Cochrane Database Syst Rev. 2011;12:CD008860.
51. Allida S, Cox KL, et al. Pharmacological, psychological and non-invasive brain stimulation interventions for preventing depression after stroke. Cochrane Database Syst Rev. 2020;5(5):Cd003689.
52. Allida S, Cox KL, et al. Pharmacological, psychological, and non-invasive brain stimulation interventions for treating depression after stroke. Cochrane Database Syst Rev. 2020;1:CD003437.
53. Dennis M, Forbes J, et al. Fluoxetine to improve functional outcomes in patients after acute stroke: The FOCUS RCT. Health Technol Assess. 2020;24(22):1–94.
54. Lundström E, Isaksson E, et al. Safety and efficacy of fluoxetine on functional recovery after acute stroke (EFFECTS): a randomised, double-blind, placebo-controlled trial. Lancet Neurol. 2020;19(8):661–9.
55. Almeida OP, Hankey GJ, et al. Depression outcomes among patients treated with fluoxetine for stroke recovery: the affinity randomized clinical trial. JAMA Neurol. 2021;78(9):1072–9.
56. Hackett ML, Yang M, et al. Pharmaceutical interventions for emotionalism after stroke. Cochrane Database Syst Rev. 2010;2:CD003690.
57. Hepburn M, Bollu PC, et al. Sleep medicine: stroke and sleep. Mo Med. 2018;115(6):527–32. PMID: 30643347; PMCID: PMC6312177.
58. Rowe FJ, Hepworth LR, et al. High incidence and prevalence of visual problems after acute stroke: an epidemiology study with implications for service delivery. PLoS One. 2021;14(3):e0213035.
59. Rowe F, Hepworth L, et al. Impact of visual impairment following stroke (IVIS study): a prospective clinical profile of central and peripheral visual deficits, eye movement abnormalities and visual perceptual deficits. Disabil Rehabil. 2020;44:1–15.
60. Pollock A, Hazelton C, et al. Interventions for visual field defects in people with stroke. Cochrane Database Syst Rev. 2019;5:CD008388.
61. Bray BD, Smith CJ, et al. The association between delays in screening for and assessing dysphagia after acute stroke, and the risk of stroke-associated pneumonia. J Neurol Neurosurg Psychiatry. 2017;88(1):25–30.
62. Mann G, Hankey GJ, Cameron D. Swallowing function after stroke: prognosis and prognostic factors at 6 months. Stroke. 2019;30(4):744–8.
63. Legg LA, Quinn TJ, et al. Non-pharmacological interventions for caregivers of stroke survivors. Cochrane Database Syst Rev. 2011;10:CD008179.

Chapter 18
Pharmacology and Stroke

Anthony Rudd, Thong Van Nguyen, Ton Duy Mai, and Ha Thu Vu Phan

18.1 Introduction

The number of drugs which a physician needs to be familiar with when managing stroke is fairly small. In Vietnam, there are several drugs in common use that are not used much in Europe and the USA. The evidence for some of the commonly used drugs will be reviewed in this chapter. Much of the information will overlap with information elsewhere in this book. We are not reviewing drugs used to treat complications after stroke, such as drugs for spasticity or seizures and we are not covering drugs for diabetes or some other risk factors. A good summary can be found in the review by Bansal et al. 2013 [1].

Whenever available use generic drugs that are no longer subject to patent as these are likely to be significantly cheaper and will be just as effective. When drug patents are about to expire pharmaceutical companies often produce a non-significant variant on the original drug and will try and persuade physicians that it is important that this new version is much better than anything else available. Always review the

A. Rudd (✉)
King's College, London, UK
e-mail: anthony.rudd@kcl.ac.uk

T. Van Nguyen
Stroke Center, Phutho General Hospital, Phutho, Vietnam

Vietnam Stroke Association, Hanoi, Vietnam

T. D. Mai
Stroke Center, Bach Mai hospital, Hanoi, Vietnam

VNU University of Medicine and Pharmacy, Hanoi, Vietnam

Hanoi Medical University, Hanoi, Vietnam

H. T. V. Phan
Phutho Department of Health, Phutho, Vietnam

A. Rudd et al. (eds.), *Stroke Management in Vietnam*,
https://doi.org/10.1007/978-981-96-0221-6_18

primary evidence yourself and do not be persuaded by carefully prepared glossy graphs and tables produced by industry. Ask the question is this drug really better than the cheaper alternatives? Just because something is new it does not mean that it is better. The drugs before they are released will have had to undergo testing to ensure that they are safe, but the regulatory agencies will not usually have assessed whether the drug is offering something significant that is not already available. Health expenditure is always constrained. If it is the patient paying for the drug, they are more likely to take it if they can afford it. If the state or insurance companies are paying, then again their funds are limited and if they spend all their money on expensive new drugs that offer little additional benefit then there will be less to spend on effective treatments.

18.2 Drugs Used for Stroke Prevention

18.2.1 Antiplatelet Drugs: Aspirin, Clopidogrel, Dipyridamole, Cilostazol, Ticagrelor, Ticlopidine

18.2.1.1 Primary Prevention

Aspirin is the drug that has been used most frequently and for the longest time for stroke prevention. There seems to be little benefit for the use of low-dose aspirin for primary prevention of stroke [2]. In the Aspirin in Reducing Events in the Elderly (ASPREE) which was a randomized, double-blind, placebo-controlled trial of daily low-dose aspirin used in over 19 thousand people free of symptomatic cardiovascular disease aspirin did not produce a statistically significant reduction in the incidence of ischemic stroke (hazard ratio [HR], 0.89; 95% CI, 0.71–1.11). It did, however, produce a statistically significant increase in intracranial bleeding among the individuals given aspirin (108 individuals [1.1%]) compared with those receiving placebo (79 individuals [0.8%]; HR, 1.38; 95% CI, 1.03–1.84). This lack of benefit was confirmed in a meta-analysis of 11 trials which included patients of all ages [3] (Judge et al. 2020).

18.2.1.2 Secondary Prevention

Antiplatelet treatment has been proven beyond doubt in multiple trials for secondary prevention of both transient ischaemic attack (TIA) and stroke, both acutely and for the longer term.

Acute Stroke

The Cochrane review of antiplatelet drug use acutely after stroke showed definite benefit especially when started within 48 h of onset of symptoms [4]. A total of 11 studies were included in the review with a total of 42,226 participants. Aspirin, at a dose of 160–300 mg daily, started within 48 hours of the onset of stroke symptoms, saved lives, and reduced the risk of further stroke, occurring in the first 2 weeks, without increasing the risk of haemorrhagic complications. For every 1000 people treated with aspirin, 13 people would avoid death or dependency [number needed to treat (NNT) for an additional beneficial outcome 79]. Almost all the trials were ones that used aspirin rather than any other antiplatelet agent. But a review by Paciaroni et al. 2019 [5] suggested that clopidogrel was associated with fewer side effects especially longer term when used as a single agent compared to aspirin alone.

Long-Term Antiplatelet Treatment

A meta-analysis of 57 RCTs [6] (Del Giovani et al) with 165,533 participants showed that compared to placebo or no treatment, cilostazol, clopidogrel, dipyridamole + aspirin, ticagrelor, ticlopidine, and aspirin ≤ 150 mg/day significantly reduced the risk of all strokes (odds ratios, ORs, and absolute risk difference, ARD): cilostazol 0.51 (95% confidence interval, CI, 0.37 to 0.71; 3.6% fewer), clopidogrel 0.63 (95% CI, 0.49 to 0.79; 2.7% fewer), dipyridamole + aspirin 0.65 (95% CI, 0.55 to 0.78; 2.5% fewer), ticagrelor 0.68 (95% CI, 0.50 to 0.93; 2.3% fewer), ticlopidine 0.74 (95% CI 0.59 to 0.93; 1.9% fewer), aspirin ≤ 150 mg/day 0.79 (95% CI, 0.66 to 0.95; 1.5% fewer). Aspirin > 150 mg/day and the combinations clopidogrel/aspirin, ticagrelor/aspirin, also decrease all strokes but increase the risk of haemorrhagic events. Only aspirin > 150 mg/day significantly reduced all-cause mortality (OR 0.86, 95% CI 0.76 to 0.97; ARD 0.9%, 95%CI 1.5–0.2% fewer, moderate confidence). Compared to aspirin ≤ 150 mg/day, clopidogrel significantly reduced the risk of all strokes, cardiovascular events, and intracranial haemorrhage outcomes. Cilostazol also appeared to provide advantages, but data are limited to the Asian population. Dipyridamole is most effective when given with aspirin with the main trial showing benefit using the modified release form of the dipyridamole. However, it is a drug that often causes side effects, particularly headache and is overall less well tolerated than aspirin or clopidogrel.

Considering the benefits and harms ratio, cilostazol, clopidogrel, dipyridamole + aspirin, ticagrelor, ticlopidine, and aspirin ≤ 150 mg/day appear to be the best choices as antiplatelet drugs for secondary prevention of patients with ischemic stroke or TIA. It is difficult to recommend one regime over any other based on outcome data alone so it seems sensible to use the regime that is cheapest. Aspirin should be available at minimal cost and clopidogrel, now that it is available in generic form is also relatively inexpensive.

Multiple Antiplatelet Drug Therapy Vs. Single Drug for Acute Stroke

The Cochrane review included 15 RCTs with a total of 17,091 participants [7]. Most of the studies compared aspirin combined with dipyridamole or clopidogrel with aspirin or clopidogrel alone. Compared with fewer antiplatelet agents, multiple antiplatelet agents were associated with a significantly lower risk of stroke recurrence (5.78% versus 7.84%, risk ratio (RR) 0.73, 95% confidence interval (CI) 0.66 to 0.82; $P < 0.001$); with no significant difference in vascular death. There was a higher risk of intracranial haemorrhage (0.42% versus 0.21%, RR 1.92, 95% CI 1.05 to 3.50; $P = 0.03$;) and extracranial haemorrhage (6.38% versus 2.81%, RR 2.25, 95% CI 1.88 to 2.70; $P < 0.001$; high-certainty evidence) with multiple antiplatelet agents. The authors conclusions were that multiple antiplatelet agents are more effective in reducing stroke recurrence but increase the risk of haemorrhage compared to one antiplatelet agent. The benefit in reduction of stroke recurrence seems to outweigh the harm for dual antiplatelet agents initiated in the acute setting and continued for 1 month.

For patients with non-valvular atrial fibrillation, there is a modest benefit of about a 25% reduction in risk of stroke but this is much less than the benefits obtained through the use of anticoagulants [8].

18.2.1.3 Anticoagulants: Warfarin, Dabigatran, Rivaroxaban, Apixaban, and Endoxaban

There is strong evidence to suggest that unless strongly contraindicated patients with non-valvular atrial fibrillation should be treated with an oral anticoagulant using either warfarin or one of the direct oral anticoagulants (rivaroxaban, dabigatran, apixaban, endoxaban). Overall anticoagulants reduce the risk of stroke by about two-thirds [9]. There are advantages and disadvantages for all of these choices. Warfarin has been in use for many years, there is wide experience in its use, and it is relatively easy to reverse using fairly easily available treatments at relatively low cost. It is also easy to measure whether the patient has been taking the treatment. It is also a low cost drug although the costs increase when consideration is given to the costs of supervision and monitoring efficacy.

The Direct Oral Anticoagulants (DOAC) are more expensive, are less easy to reverse and it is more difficult to assess whether the drug has been taken. However, they are much easier for the patient to take, there is no need for individual dose monitoring and their absorption and metabolism are not affected by foods, other medications or comorbidities apart from renal failure. A systematic review of 49 trials [10] (Khouja et al. 2022) evaluated efficacy, safety, and cost effectiveness. Generally, the direct OACs, particularly apixaban (5 mg twice daily), were more effective and safer than warfarin in preventing AF-related stroke. The evidence suggested that some direct OACs may reduce the risk of bleeding, compared with warfarin. Patients were more adherent to direct OACs than warfarin. The authors conclusion was that for stroke prevention in AF, DOACs seemed to be more effective and safer than warfarin and that apixaban (5 mg twice daily) had the best profile. This was confirmed in a review by Lopez-Lopez et al. 2017 [11].

Heparin

Heparin is rarely needed for stroke prevention. If anticoagulation is needed and the patient cannot take drugs orally, then warfarin or a DOAC can be given via a naso-gastric tube or gastrostomy tube. If these options are not possible, then treatment dose low molecular weight heparin (LMWH) can be used. Heparin is, however, often prescribed after acute stroke to prevent venous thromboembolism. However, the evidence for this is weak as although it does prevent deep venous thrombosis and pulmonary embolism it increases the risk of intracranial haemorrhage. The evidence-based alternative of using intermittent pneumatic compression on the legs is more effective and safer [12].

Heparin is also used for venous stroke where it is usually highly effective. It is usually given by infusion of unfractionated heparin. Heparin (usually LMWH) is also recommended for patients with stroke related to antiphospholipid syndrome [12].

18.3 Antihypertensives

Over 50% of patients admitted with stroke will have hypertension either previously known or diagnosed at the time of the stroke. There is a long list of antihypertensive drugs available for use after stroke. The most important thing is to lower the blood pressure without causing any major side effects to the patient. And given that the type of blood pressure tablet is relatively unimportant then cost should be considered as one of the major deciding factors in the choice of medication [12]. African or Caribbean patients are often unresponsive to beta blockers and ACE inhibitors and so for them these drugs should not be used first line. The UK National Stroke Guidelines make the following recommendations [13]:

- For people with stroke or TIA aged 55 or over, or of African or Caribbean origin at any age, antihypertensive treatment should be initiated with a long-acting dihydropyridine calcium-channel blocker or a thiazide-like diuretic. If target blood pressure is not achieved, an angiotensin converting enzyme inhibitor or angiotensin II receptor blocker should be added.
- For people with stroke or TIA not of African or Caribbean origin and younger than 55 years, antihypertensive treatment should be initiated with an angiotensin converting enzyme inhibitor or an angiotensin II receptor blocker.

18.4 Lipid Lowering: Rosuvastatin, Atorvastatin, Simvastatin, Fluvastatin, Rosuvastatin, Pravastatin, Pitavastatin, Lovastatin, Ezetimibe

Most patients after ischaemic stroke will benefit from lipid lowering agents. High intensity statins such as atorvastatin are the usual drugs of choice. Most patients tolerate statins well but although the evidence of an association is weak some patients do complain of myalgia after taking them. There is little difference between the statins, so the choice again should include a consideration of cost. An alternative to statins is ezetimibe which can also be added to a statin if the statin alone at high dose is ineffective. If the combination of a statin and ezetimibe still fail to reduce lipids to satisfactory levels, then adding a proprotein convertase subtilisin/kexin type 9 (PCSK9) inhibitor such as evolocumab is justified. If there are persistently raised triglyceride levels, then adding icosapent ethyl might also reduce cardiovascular morbidity [14].

18.5 Polypill

There is increasing evidence for the use of a polypill for both primary and secondary stroke prevention particularly in low-and middle-income countries (LMIC). The polypill concept proposed by Wald and Law in 2003 [15] had a central theme of modifying cardiovascular risk at a population level by treating everyone ≥55 years without consideration of measured blood pressure or lipids as well as those with established cardiovascular disease with a single, daily administered pill. The cardiovascular polypill for prevention of atherosclerotic cardiovascular disease typically comprises of a statin, antihypertensive agents, aspirin, and folic acid. The projections based on clinical trial and meta-analytic data were that a polypill containing three classes of antihypertensive medications, a statin, aspirin, and folic acid could reduce the occurrence of stroke by 80% and ischemic heart disease by 88% [16]. Large multicentre trials in LMIC and high-income country (HIC) settings have now clearly demonstrated the beneficial effects of the cardiovascular polypill versus placebo (or usual care) in reducing primary stroke risk by 50%. For survivors of a recent myocardial infarction residing in HICs, the polypill reduced risk of major cardiovascular events by 25% due to improved treatment adherence. But data on the clinical efficacy of the polypill for secondary stroke prevention are scanty both in HICs and LMICs.

18.6 Acute Treatment

18.6.1 Thrombolytics: Alteplase, Tenecteplase, Streptokinase, Urokinase

There is very strong evidence to support the use of alteplase (recombinant tissue plasminogen activator) and tenecteplase after acute stroke subject to some strict criteria described in the chapter on the management of acute stroke [17]. When used by clinicians without the correct knowledge and skills they are potentially dangerous drugs that could kill the patient. When used correctly they can transform a patient living a life with long-term disability to someone who is independent.

Streptokinase should not be used as a thrombolytic after acute stroke. Trials done in the too high but until and unless further studies are done it cannot be recommended. There is very limited evidence to support the use of urokinase and so again it cannot be recommended even though it is significantly cheaper than alteplase and tenecteplase.

18.7 Anti-Oedema Drugs: Mannitol, Dexamethasone, Hypertonic Saline (Natri Chloride 3%

The evidence to support the use of any of these drugs to either prevent or treat strokerelated oedema is very weak. Dexamethasone does not help cytotoxic oedema which is the cause of oedema after stroke. Vasogenic oedema from malignancy can be exquisitely sensitive to dexamethasone but after stroke it is only likely to make the patient worse by interfering with glucose metabolism. There is more logic to using mannitol, but the Cochrane review concluded that with only three small trials involving 226 participants, there was not enough evidence to decide if mannitol improves survival or prevents disability after stroke [18]. The treatment can cause several adverse effects and therefore should not be used outside of clinical trial settings. This view was further reinforced by the research by Papagianni et al. 2018 [19] who found that administration of mannitol to patients with ischemic stroke-related cerebral oedema did not appear to affect the functional outcome and might increase mortality, independently of stroke severity.

There is no evidence to support the use of hypertonic saline either. If there is oedema severe enough to cause major deterioration over and above that caused by the infarct itself, then the only evidence-based treatment is surgical decompression by hemicraniectomy.

18.8 Prothrombotic Drugs: Tranexamic Acid, Etamsylate

Tranexamic acid has been tested in a randomized controlled trial after primary intracerebral haemorrhage. The TICH-2 trial [20] tested whether tranexamic acid as a haemostatic agent could reduce the risk of rebleeding after ICH. This trial involving 2325 patients was negative for the primary outcome measure of functional status at 90 days although it did reduce 7 day mortality but not 90 day. Its use cannot be recommended at the moment. We have been unable to find any clinical trials to support the use of Etamsylate.

18.9 'Nutrition for the Brain'

18.9.1 Cerebrolysin

Cerebrolysin is widely used in Vietnam and China for patients with acute ischaemic stroke. Cerebrolysin, and the cerebrolysin-like agent Cortexin, are mixtures of proteins, peptides, and amino acids purified from animal brains. Some of the proteins in Cerebrolysin or Cortexin are found naturally in the human brain and for this reason it is thought that they may help to protect and repair brain cells after ischemic stroke. The Cochrane review published in 2023 [21] found seven studies in 1773 people who had an acute ischaemic stroke. The studies looked at the effect of giving Cerebrolysin in addition to standard therapy during the first 48 h after a stroke. The studies compared this treatment with standard therapy alone or standard therapy plus placebo.

Meta-analysis of the trials found no evidence that the drug was in any way beneficial in terms of reducing mortality, morbidity, or improving quality of life. There was some suggestion that patients receiving cerebrolysin had more significant side effects than patients who received standard therapy either with or without placebo.

18.9.2 Luotai

Luotai is the brand name of Panax notoginseng. A meta-analysis of 206 studies involving, 21,759 elderly ischaemic stroke patients, all done in China suggested a marginal benefit in terms of reducing long-term disability for patients receiving the drug [22]. The studies were generally of low quality both in terms of size of cohort and in terms of the conduct of the trials. There was also significant heterogeneity in the studies. Despite the large number of reported studies, the case for using the drug is not yet proven and in our view the drug should only be given as part of a well conducted trial.

A case controlled study was registered in 2019 being conducted in several hospitals in Vietnam but no results have yet been published.

18.9.3 *Citicoline*

A Cochrane review published in 2021 [23] identified ten RCTs including 4281 participants. They included trials of the drug being given orally, intravenously or both compared to placebo or standard care. Citicoline doses ranged between 500 mg and 2000 mg per day. All the trials were assessed as having a high level of potential bias. A pooled analysis of eight trials indicated that there was little or no difference in all-cause mortality comparing citicoline with placebo (17.3% versus 18.5%; RR 0.94, 95% CI 0.83 to 1.07); Four trials showed that citicoline may not increase the proportion of patients with a moderate or lower degree of disability or dependence compared with placebo. Four trials suggested that citicoline resulted in no difference in functional recovery, according to the Barthel Index, compared with placebo (32.78% versus 30.70%; RR 1.03, 95% CI 0.94 to 1.13. The authors conclusions were that there may be little to no difference between citicoline and its controls regarding all-cause mortality, disability or dependence in daily activities, functional recovery, neurological function, and severe adverse events, based on low-certainty evidence. None of the included trials assessed quality of life and the safety profile of citicoline remains.

Our conclusion based on this evidence that again this drug should not be used outside well designed clinical trials.

18.9.4 *Choline Alfoscerate*

A systematic review identified five clinical trials that included 2544 patients with acute stroke treated with choline alphoscerate for between 1 and 6 months [24]. Outcomes were measures of cognition and functional recovery. Three of the trials did not use any control group. There was a trend towards improved outcomes in the treated group, but the design and quality of the studies was such that it would be unwise to recommend routine treatment with the drug until further studies are performed using appropriate control groups.

18.9.5 *Neuroai*

Traditional Chinese medicine (TCM) MLC601 has shown promising results on functional recovery of patients after stroke but mainly in animal studies. A systematic review by González-Fraile et al. 2016 [25] identified five randomised controlled

Table 18.1 Summary of evidence base for drugs used in stroke patients. Note this does not include medication for comorbidities such as diabetes or for longer term complications such as spasticity or epilepsy

Drugs with a good evidence base	Drugs that should not be used or only as part of a trial
Antiplatelet drugs: Aspirin, dipyridamole, clopidogrel, cilostazol, ticagrelor, ticlopidine	Anti-oedema drugs: Mannitol, hypertonic saline, dexamethasone
Anticoagulants: Warfarin, rivaroxaban, apixaban, dabigatran, endoxaban, heparin	Prothrombotic drugs: Tranexamic acid, Etamsylate
Antihypertensives	Cerebrolysin
Lipid lowering drugs: Rosuvastatin, atorvastatin, simvastatin, fluvastatin, rosuvastatin, pravastatin, pitavastatin, lovastatin	Citicoline
	Choline alfoscerate
	Neuroaid

trials but only three comparing the drug with placebo with a total 1370 patients. The quality of the studies was moderate but there was considerable heterogeneity. The conclusion was that the current evidence suggests MLC601 does not outperform placebo on functional recovery after stroke particularly when the placebo-controlled trials are considered.

18.10 Conclusions

There is good evidence for the use of antiplatelet drugs, anticoagulant drugs, antihypertensives, and lipid lowering drugs for some patients for secondary prevention of stroke. Intravenous thrombolysis with either alteplase or tenecteplase has proven benefit. But there is insufficient evidence or in some cases clear evidence of lack of benefit for anti-oedema drugs, neuroprotective type drugs or brain 'nutrients (Table 18.1)'. In many cases, there is justification to conduct further trials and clinicians are encouraged to participate in these so long as they are of high quality and likely to properly address the question being asked.

References

1. Bansal S, Sangha KS, Khatri P. Drug treatment of acute ischemic stroke. Am J Cardiovasc Drugs. 2013;13(1):57–69.
2. Cloud GC, Williamson JD, Thao LTP, et al. Low-dose aspirin and the risk of stroke and intracerebral bleeding in healthy older people: secondary analysis of a randomized clinical trial. JAMA Netw Open. 2023;6(7):e2325803.
3. Judge C, Ruttledge S, Murphy R, et al. Aspirin for primary prevention of stroke in individuals without cardiovascular disease-a meta-analysis. Int J Stroke. 2020;15(1):9–17.

4. Minhas JS, Chithiramohan T, Wang X, et al. Oral antiplatelet therapy for acute ischaemic stroke. Cochrane Database Syst Rev. 2022;1:CD000029. https://doi.org/10.1002/14651858.CD000029.pub4.
5. Paciaroni M, Ince B, Hu B, et al. Benefits and risks of Clopidogrel vs. aspirin monotherapy after recent ischemic stroke: a systematic review and meta-analysis. Cardiovasc Ther. 2019;2019:1607181.
6. Del Giovane C, Boncoraglio GB, Bertù L, et al. Antiplatelet drugs for secondary prevention in patients with ischemic stroke or transient ischemic attack: a systematic review and network meta-analysis. BMC Neurol. 2021;21(1):319.
7. Naqvi IA, Kamal AK, Rehman H. Multiple versus fewer antiplatelet agents for preventing early recurrence after ischaemic stroke or transient ischaemic attack. Cochrane Database Syst Rev. 2020;8(8):CD009716. https://doi.org/10.1002/14651858.CD009716.pub2. PMID: 32813275; PMCID: PMC7437397.
8. Aguilar MI, Hart R. Antiplatelet therapy for preventing stroke in patients with non-valvular atrial fibrillation and no previous history of stroke or transient ischemic attacks. Cochrane Database Syst Rev. 2005;4:CD001925. https://doi.org/10.1002/14651858.CD001925.pub2.
9. Piccini JP, Fonarow GC. Preventing stroke in patients with atrial fibrillation—a steep climb away from achieving peak performance. JAMA Cardiol. 2016;1(1):63–4.
10. Khouja C, Brunton G, Richardson M, et al. Oral anticoagulants: a systematic overview of reviews on efficacy and safety, genotyping, self-monitoring, and stakeholder experiences. Syst Rev. 2022;11:23.
11. López-López JA, Sterne JAC, Thom HHZ, et al. Oral anticoagulants for prevention of stroke in atrial fibrillation: systematic review, network meta-analysis, and cost effectiveness analysis. BMJ. 2017;359:j5058.
12. Boncoraglio GB, Del Giovane C, Tramacere I. Antihypertensive drugs for secondary prevention after ischemic stroke or transient ischemic attack: a systematic review and meta-analysis. Stroke. 2021;52(6):1974–82.
13. UK National Clinical Guidelines for Stroke. 2023. https://www.strokeguideline.org/.
14. Tsankof A, Tziomalos K. The role of lipid-lowering treatment in the secondary prevention of ischemic stroke. Diseases. 2021;10(1):3.
15. Wald NJ, Law MR. A strategy to reduce cardiovascular disease by more than 80%. BMJ. 2003;326:1419.
16. Sarfo FS, Nichols M, Opare-Addo PA, Ovbiagele B. Polypill programs to prevent stroke and cut costs in low income countries: moving from clinical efficacy to pragmatic implementation. Stroke. 2023;54(2):407–14.
17. Wardlaw JM, Murray V, Berge E, del Zoppo GJ. Thrombolysis for acute ischaemic stroke. Cochrane Database Syst Rev. 2014;2014(7):CD000213.
18. Bereczki D, Liu M, Fernandes do Prado G, Fekete I. Mannitol for acute stroke. Cochrane Database Syst Rev. 2007;3:CD001153. https://doi.org/10.1002/14651858.CD001153.pub2.
19. Papagianni M, Tziomalos K, Kostaki S, et al. Treatment with mannitol is associated with increased risk for in-hospital mortality in patients with acute ischemic stroke and cerebral edema. Am J Cardiovasc Drugs. 2018;18(5):397–403.
20. Sprigg N, Flaherty K, Appleton JP, et al. Tranexamic acid for hyperacute primary intra cerebral Haemorrhage (TICH-2): an international randomised, placebo-controlled, phase 3 superiority trial. Lancet. 2018;391:2107–15.
21. Ziganshina LE, Abakumova T, Nurkhametova D, Ivanchenko K. Cerebrolysin for acute ischaemic stroke. Cochrane Database Syst Rev. 2023;10:CD007026. https://doi.org/10.1002/14651858.CD007026.pub7.
22. Guan P, Gui D, Xu Y. Evaluation on the efficacy and safety of Panax Notoginseng Saponins in the treatment of stroke among elderly people: a systematic review and meta-analysis of 206 randomized controlled trials. Evid Based Complement Alternat Med. 2023;2023:4312489.
23. Martí-Carvajal AJ, Valli C, Martí-Amarista CE, et al. Citicoline for treating people with acute ischemic stroke. Cochrane Database Syst Rev. 2020;8(8):CD013066.

24. Sagaro GG, Amenta F. Choline-containing phospholipids in stroke treatment: a systematic review and meta-analysis. J Clin Med. 2023;12(8):2875.
25. González-Fraile E, Martín-Carrasco M, Ballesteros J. Efficacy of MLC601 on functional recovery after stroke: a systematic review and meta-analysis of randomized controlled trials. Brain Inj. 2016;30(3):267–70.